# Mutagenicity, Carcinogenicity, and Teratogenicity of Industrial Pollutants

# Mutagenicity, Carcinogenicity, and Teratogenicity of Industrial Pollutants

Edited by
**Micheline Kirsch-Volders**
*Free University of Brussels*
*Brussels, Belgium*

**Plenum Press • New York and London**
**Published in Conjunction with the Belgian Environmental Mutagen Society**

Library of Congress Cataloging in Publication Data

Main entry under title:

Mutagenicity, carcinogenicity, and teratogenicity of industrial pollutants.

"Published in conjunction with the Belgian Environmental Mutagen Society."
Includes bibliographical references and index.
1. Industrial toxicology. 2. Pollution—Toxicology. 3. Chemical mutagenesis. 4. Car-
cinogens. 5. Teratogenic agents. I. Kirsch-Volders, Micheline. II. Belgian Environ-
mental Mutagen Society. [DNLM: 1. Carcinogens, Environmental—Adverse effects. 2.
Chromosome aberrations. 3. Environmental pollutants—Adverse effects. 4.
Mutagens—Adverse effects. 5. Teratogens—Adverse effects. QZ 202 M992]
RA1229.M87 1983                    615.9′02                    83-11126
ISBN 0-306-41148-2

© 1984 Plenum Press, New York
A Division of Plenum Publishing Corporation
233 Spring Street, New York, N.Y. 10013

Printed in the United States of America

# Contributors

**N. Degraeve** • University of Liège, Genetics Department, Liège, Belgium.

**M. Duverger-van Bogaert** • Laboratory of Toxicology, Tour Erlich, Brussels, Belgium.

**G. B. Gerber** • Department of Radiobiology, CEN-SCK, Mol, Belgium.

**J. de Gerlache** • Laboratoire de Biochemie Toxicologique et Cancerologique, U.C.L., Brussels, Belgium.

**P. Jacquet** • Department of Radiobiology, CEN-SCK, Mol, Belgium.

**P. Jeggo** • Département de Biologie Moléculaire, U.L.B., and M.R.C. National Institutes of Medical Research, Department of Genetics, Mill Hill, London, England.

**M. Kirsch-Volders** • Laboratorium voor Antropogenetika, V.U.B., Brussels, Belgium.

**A. Lafontaine** • Institute for Hygiene and Epidemiology, Brussels, Belgium.

**M. Lambotte-Vandepaer** • Laboratory of Toxicology, Tour Erlich, Brussels, Belgium.

**M. Lans** • Laboratoire de Biochemie Toxicologique et Cancerologique, U.C.L. Brussels, Belgium.

**R. R. Lauwerys** • Medical and Industrial Toxicology Unit, University of Louvain, Brussels, Belgium.

**A. Léonard** • Department of Radiobiology, CEN-SCK, Mol, Belgium.

**C. de Meester** • Laboratory of Toxicology, Tour Erlich, Brussels, Belgium.

**M. Mercier** • International Program for Chemical Safety, Management Unit, W.H.O. Geneva, Switzerland.

**J. Moutschen-Dahmen** • University of Liège, Genetics Department, Liège, Belgium.

**M. Moutschen-Dahmen** • University of Liège, Genetics Department, Liège, Belgium.

**F. Poncelet** • Laboratory of Toxicology, Tour Erlich, Brussels, Belgium.

**M. Radman** • Département de Biologie, U.L.B., and Laboratoire de Génétique, Université Paris Sud, Faculté des Sciences, Orsey, France.

**Charles Susanne** • Free University Brussels, Laboratory of Human Genetics Brussels, Belgium.

**L. Verschaeve** • Laboratorium voor Antropogenetika, V.U.B., Brussels, Belgium.

This book is dedicated to our colleague and friend,

**Prof. Dr. Fernand Poncelet,**

President of the Belgian Environmental Mutagen Society,
who died in an accident in October 1982

# Preface

This book is intended for anyone who cares about the health of people exposed to industrial pollutants. Attention is given to those pollutants which present a possible risk to the genetic material of exposed workers. Chapters are devoted to heavy metals such as arsenic, beryllium, cadmium, chromium, lead, mercury, nickel, etc.; insecticides (chlorinated, organophosphorus, and carbonate insecticides); monomers such as vinyl-chloride, acrylonitrile, styrene, vinylidene chloride, butadiene, chlorobutadiene, hexachlorobutadiene, etc.; and halogenated hydrocarbon solvents such as chloroform, carbon tetrachloride, trichloroethylene, 1,2-dichloroethane, tetrachloroethylene, dichloromethane, and 1,1,1-trichloroethane.

The main aim of this work is to provide the physician, the biologist, the pharmacologist, or anyone involved in genetic toxicology with a useful compendium of up-to-date information and references.

Efforts are made to open the field to nonspecialists. An introductory chapter deals with the mechanisms whereby a given compound, reaching genetic material, either directly or indirectly, may increase the risk of a cancer developing in the exposed individual and of abnormalities being passed on to his or her progeny.

Efforts are also made to allow easy and efficient reading for those who are not interested in detailed results. Comparative tables provide the following data on the compounds studied: chemical properties, production, occurrence, accepted standards in the industry, and positive or negative results with different test systems.

Finally, senior research workers might find good descriptions in this book of the most recent results from mutagenesis and carcinogenesis testing in plant, nonmammalian, and mammalian systems.

I hope that this book will contribute to a better link between university research workers and industrial teams who have to reconcile the necessity of production with the health of workers. This is not only our wish, but also the well-defined proposal of the International Environmental Mutagen Society and our local section, the Belgian Environmental Mutagen Society.

M. Kirsch-Volders
*Brussels*

# Contents

## PART III: CHROMOSOMAL ALTERATIONS AND CARCINOGENESIS

*Chapter 2*

**Mutagenicity, Carcinogenicity, and Teratogenicity of Industrially Used Metals**

A. Léonard, G. B. Gerber, P. Jacquet, and R. R. Lauwerys

## Chapter 3
## Mutagenicity, Carcinogenicity, and Teratogenicity of Insecticides
J. Moutschen-Dahmen, M. Moutschen-Dahmen, and
   N. Degraeve

## Chapter 4
## Mutagenicity, Carcinogenicity, and Teratogenicity of Industrially Important Monomers

F. Poncelet, M. Duverger-van Bogaert, M. Lambotte-Vandepaer, and C. de Meester

## Chapter 5
## Mutagenicity, Carcinogenicity, and Teratogenicity of Halogenated Hydrocarbon Solvents
M. Mercier, M. Lans, and J. de Gerlache

# Introduction

## Mutagenesis as a Health Problem

### C. Susanne

Man has been able to make tools for at least 5 million years, to make fire for at least a half-million years, and practice farming and agriculture for at least 10,000 years. In a sense, it is a long time ago that man developed control over ecological factors. Even pollution is not a new problem, since agriculture itself cannot avoid altering the naturally balanced ecosystems. Pollution is certainly not limited to advanced civilization (Brothwell, 1972). Since the neolithicum, forests have been permanently destroyed by fire and the ground has been degraded (North Africa, the Middle East). Irrigation of fields has been known for 5000 years in Egypt and Mesopotamia, and resulted in an increase of schistosomiasis. Growth of populations resulted in new urban environments and air pollution. Since chimneys were absent in primitive houses, evidence of anthracosis has been found in some Egyptian mummies. Lead poisoning was already known during the Roman period.

However, the problems created by pollution are surely more serious in our industrial societies, where energy and efforts are needed to control its effects. One aspect of pollution is difficult to study because the effects are not observed directly, but sometimes appear years later in terms of cancer or congenital diseases. Mutagens are introduced in our environment and could potentially increase the frequency of mutations. These mutations are modifications of the DNA at gene level (point-mutations: classical recessive, dominant, sex-linked mutations), at chromosome level (modification of structure such as deletions, translocations, dicentrics, ringchromosomes), or at genome level (modification of the number of chromosomes). These different types of mutations occur in somatic cells and might, for example, lead to cancer or alterations in germinal cells which, in turn, may give rise to congenital diseases. Moreover, they have a definitive and additive character.

---

**C. Susanne** • Free University Brussels, Laboratory of Human Genetics, Brussels, Belgium.

The potential increase in the frequency of mutations is today an important problem, not only in relation to the amount of potential mutagens, but also because better protection against infectious diseases has led to the relative increase of congenital diseases.

Mutagenesis is a health problem also, due to the fact that some similar mechanisms are involved in carcinogenesis and teratogenesis. Many authors correlate somatic mutations with the mechanisms for carcinogenesis (Cairns, 1975; Magnee, 1977). Since the work of Boveri (1914), we know that chromosomal aberrations are frequent in tumors.

The promotor–inductor hypothesis for carcinogenesis illustrates this idea. Moreover, the breakage syndromes (Bloom, Fanconi, etc.) are shown to present higher risk for cancer. Also, most carcinogens are mutagens (Ames et al., 1973). Finally, one cannot exclude the possibility that interactions with RNA or proteins might result in epigenetic mechanisms of aberrant differentiation (Weinstein et al., 1975).

Teratogenic agents may be exogenous factors inducing abnormal embryogenesis, but may also be endogenous, such as point mutations or chromosomal aberrations. Radiation, some chemicals, and certain viral infections are teratogenic, but are also carcinogenic and mutagenic as well. However, for many agents, the mechanisms of teratogenesis are not related to those of mutagenesis or of carcinogenesis (Kalter, 1975; Poswillo, 1976).

Mutagenic mechanisms involve anything that damages DNA or interferes with the structure of the DNA, or with cell-division. They involve not only the replication of DNA but also transcription and repair. Mutagenic conditions include, for instance, modifications of nucleotides resulting in mispairing and base pair substitutions, local misalignments in base pairing (Frameshift mutations), modifications of bases leading to aborted DNA synthesis, and different factors influencing DNA metabolism (for instance, deprivation of some bases, analogues of amino acids, alkylation of enzymes of DNA metabolism).

Cells are, however, able *to protect themselves against* defective replications and DNA damage by DNA repair processes. In human cells, the two processes of excision repair and post-replication repair are considered important. Other processes perhaps also occur such as photoreactivation and SOS repair. In excision repair, which is an error-free repair system, a damaged single-strand region is replaced by a new strand of bases (Lindhal, 1976). It involves various enzymatic mechanisms needed for recognition of damaged sites, for nuclease action, and also for dissociation of DNA from the histones of nucleosomes (Cleaver, 1977). The molecular mechanisms of the post-replication repair are less well understood. Perturbations of DNA replication are observed in damaged cells, and *de novo* replication fills the gaps produced by the abnormal replication. Post-replication repair might be partially error-free, but is sometimes error-prone (SOS repair). These repair systems are generally error-free, but when confronted with excessive doses of mutagenic factors they may saturate, resulting in mutations.

In spite of the existence of repair systems, ionizing radiation has been shown to be mutagenic. It induces single or double breaks in the phospho-diester strands. The mutagenic nature of ionizing radiation is not discussed by geneticists or biologists, at least at the qualitative level. The interpretation of the quantitative effects of radiation is, however, far more difficult, and estimations of these genetic effects have been published by international commissions (Unscear, 1972).

Our knowledge of the effects of irradiation is certainly not complete, but it is much more comprehensive than our knowledge of chemical mutagens. International associations have been formed to coordinate the studies of these factors (Environmental Mutagen Society, European Environmental Mutagen Society), but intensive work is still needed.

Mutagenic chemicals can themselves be intrinsically mutagenic, or can become mutagenic after activation by enzymatic reactions of the tissues or of the intestinal flora of the host. Thus, when methods are used to detect mutagenic effects, the use of microorganisms which lack the requisite enzymes for activation will give misleading results, and, in this cell, the use of an activation system is desirable.

Many tests have been developed to give rather rapid and *accurate results*. Chromosomal aberrations can be studied in animals exposed *in vivo*. This type of experiment allows comparison of genetic risks in somatic (bone-marrow), and germinal cells (spermatocytes). Other tests on animals for dominant lethals or numerical sex chromosome anomalies are useful too. As far as extrapolation to man is concerned, the use of experimental animals phylogenetically closer to man must be recommended. Of course, man himself can be used when accidentally exposed.

*In vitro* tests can be performed on bacteria or mammalian cells. The Ames test, for instance, uses a histidine mutation in *Salmonella typhimurium*. Different mammalian cell lines, such as Chinese hamster CHO or V79, human lymphocytes, or HELA cells are also routinely used. However, as already discussed, the addition of an activation system is necessary.

The choice of a test system is important, but no less important is the choice between the different cytological techniques recently developed to reveal the genetic changes.

One of these techniques reveals genetic exchange between sister double-stranded DNA molecules at the chromosomal level (sister chromatid exchange) (Perry *et al.*, 1974). These changes occur spontaneously, but higher frequencies are induced by numerous chemical mutagens, even when the cells are exposed to low concentrations. Sister chromatid exchanges develop as a consequence of DNA lesions, but only a minority of exchanges will result in the development of aberrations.

These different techniques help lead to a better knowledge of mutagenicity and to a better definition of norms. But many problems are not yet solved. These include the problems of extrapolation from *in vitro* results to *in vivo* situations, from results on experimental animals to human beings, and from somatic to germinal mutations. It is also clear that, until now, most energy has been directed towards solving the problems of acute or subacute exposure. In the future, much effort will be needed to study the effects of chronic exposure, which has a direct bearing on national health. Moreover, most studies are designed to analyze the effect of only one factor or agent, and not the global influence of two (or more) different mutagenic agents. The global influence of two chemicals is not necessarily equal to the sum of the two independent influences; a former or simultaneous exposure may inhibit, modify, or stimulate the influence of the other chemical.

Society must realize that this health problem is important. Yearly, about 250,000 new chemical agents are produced and, of these, about 300 are biologically active, and are introduced into our environment without a precise knowledge of their mutagenic (or carcinogenic) effects. It is no longer possible to hide behind our ignorance.

## REFERENCES

Ames, B. N., Durston, W. E., Yamasaki, E., and Lee, F. D., 1973, Carcinogens are mutagens: A simple test system combining liver homogenates for activation and bacteria for detection, *Proc. Nat. Acad. Sci. US.* **70**:2281–2285.

Boveri, T, 1914, *Zur Frage der Entstehung maligner Tumoren*, Gustav Fisher, Jena, pp. 64.

Brothwell, D., 1972, The question of pollution in earlier and less developed societies, in *Population and Pollution* (edited by P. R. Cox and J. Peel). Academic Press, New York, pp. 15–27.

Cairns, J., 1975, Mutation, selection and natural history of cancer, *Nature* **225**:197–200.

Cleaver, J. E., 1977, DNA repair processes and their impairment in some human diseases, in *Progress in Genetic Toxicology*, (edited by D. Scott, B. A. Bridges, and F. H. Sobels), Elsevier, New York, pp. 29–42.

Kalter, H., 1975, Some relations between teratogenesis and mutagenesis, *Mutation Res.* **33**:29–36.

Lindhal, T., 1976, A new class of enzymes acting on damaged DNA, *Nature* **259**:64–66.

Magee, M., 1977, The relationship between mutagenesis, carcinogenesis and teratogenesis, in *Progress in Genetic Toxicology* (edited by D. Scott, B. A. Bridges, and F. H. Sobels), Elsevier, New York, pp. 15–27.

Perry, P., and Evans, H. J., 1974, New Giemsa method for the differential staining of sister chromatids, *Nature* **251**:156–158.

Poswillo, G., 1976, Mechanisms and pathogenesis of malformations, *Brit. Med. Bull.* **32**:59–64.

Unscear, 1972, United Nations scientific committee on the effects of atomic radiation ionizing radiation: Levels and effects, *Report to the General Assembly with Annexes*, United Nations, New York.

Weinstein, I. B., Yamaguchi, N., Gebert, R., and Kaighn, M. E., 1975, Use of epithelial cultures for studies on the mechanism of transformation by chemical carcinogens, *In vitro* **2**:130–141.

Chapter 1

# Molecular Mechanisms of Mutagenesis and Carcinogenesis

M. Kirsch-Volders, M. Radman, P. Jeggo, and L. Verschaeve

## PART I: CELLULAR FACTORS WHICH MODIFY THE EXPRESSION OF MUTAGENIC ACTION INTO GENETIC LESIONS

A given mutagen interacting with the cell may induce different types of genetic lesions, ranging from a single-base modification, which might completely be restored in its initial form, to a chromatid break or to the loss of a chromosome.

The interactions which are genetically important are those which result in a hereditary modification of the DNA sequences. The estimation of genetic risks inherent in exposure to environmental mutagens is therefore based on measurements of submicroscopic modification of DNA sequences (point mutations) by cloning of revertants and on the identification of structural (chromosome mutation) and numerical (genome mutation) chromosome aberrations with a light microscope.

Whether the interactions of environmental mutagens with the cell machinery are transformed or not into point, chromosome, or genome

M. Kirsch-Volders • Laboratorium voor Antropogenetika, V.U.B., Pleinlaan 2, 1050 Brussels, Belgium.    M. Radman • Département de Biologie, U.L.B. and Laboratoire de Génétique, Université Paris Sud, Faculté des Sciences, Bt. 400, Orsey, France.    P. Jeggo • Département de Biologie Moléculaire, U.L.B. and M.R.C., National Institutes of Medical Research, Department of Genetics, Mill Hill, London, England.    L. Verschaeve • Laboratorium voor Antropogenetika, V.U.B., Pleinlaan 2, 1050 Brussels, Belgium. This work was supported by a grant from Euratom and a contract with IAEA, Vienna.

mutations is dependent on different cellular factors which will be discussed in this chapter.

## 1. THE NATURE OF THE TARGET

In the study of mutagenesis, emphasis has undoubtedly been given to agents which *directly* affect *DNA*. The current classification divides these mutational mechanisms into four main categories: DNA breakage; nucleotide modifications leading to direct mispairing, and thus generating base pair substitutions; local base pairing misalignments which generate either frame shift mutations or amino acid insertions and deletions; and nucleoside modifications leading to such poor base pairing that DNA synthesis is aborted, whereupon mutagenic repair systems may intervene.

*Indirect* mutagenesis by agents which interfere either with repair enzymes, with the enzymes of DNA synthesis, or with the spindle has been studied less.

### 1.1. Direct Mutagenesis with DNA as Target

It is important to realize that, even in *the simplest model* of chromosome structure, a chromatid consists of a single long DNA molecule, and that a discontinuity in such a structure must be a DNA double-strand event. Therefore, a chromosome aberration must be generated either by a double-strand break (DSB) at once, or as a result of defective-gap filling; a mechanism must produce a discontinuity at a similar locus into the nascent strand.

The *secondary structure of the chromosome* consists of 140 base pair (bp) sequences of DNA each associated with one octameric histone complex (nucleosome), and separated from its neighbors by spacer DNA (15 to 100 bp). The chromatin is further coiled in association with histone $H_1$ and nonhistones as high mobility groups (HMG) of proteins to generate higher levels of organization (for review, see Kornberg, 1977; Felsenberg, 1978; Lilley and Pardon, 1979; Bak *et al.*, 1979). The final compaction of DNA in metaphase chromosomes might be maintained by residual nonhistone proteins as suggested in the recently described "scaffold" structures observed in histone depleted metaphase chromosomes (Paulson and Laemmli, 1977; Hadlaczky *et al.*, 1981): The metaphase chromosome appears as numerous and extensive loops of DNA radiating from a coarsely fibrous structure bearing a shape resembling that of a typical chromosome and containing a characteristic sct of proteins.

Experiments performed by Comings (1980) suggest, however, that the "chromosome scaffold" might be an artifact of aggregation of nonhistone proteins following the rapid release of histone and DNA.

Some attempts were made to analyze *the impact of chromosome structure on the sensitivity of DNA and chromosome regions*;

(i) *At nucleosomal level*, it might be interesting to know whether a mutagen interacts preferentially with nucleosomal or spacer DNA. Cech and Pardue (1977) showed, for instance, that the DNA between nucleosomes is the major reaction site of me$_3$-psoralen, a drug which reacts randomly with pyrimidines in DNA. Also, Bodell (1977), with methyl methanesulfonate, found more DNA damage in the internucleosomal DNA.

(ii) *Random or nonrandom induction of chromosome lesions was extensively studied on chromosomes banded* either by fluorescent staining as quinacrine mustard (Q-banding), or by Giemsa staining after different treatments to obtain either G-banding of R-banding. Q-banding and G-banding give quite similar banding patterns with an exception for some special loci; R-banding on the other hand shows dark bands on the places which are lightly stained with Q or G-banding and vice versa (for review, see Comings, 1978; Schwarzacher, 1979). The localization of chromosome breaks on chromosomes banded by two complementary techniques can indicate whether breaks are induced specifically on some chromosome regions. It is, however, necessary to recall that a chromosome band contains an average number of $8.15 \times 10^6$ bp, and that for this reason, it is difficult to estimate which genetic lesion corresponds to a chromosome break.

The numerous results obtained for the distribution of spontaneous, congenital, radio-induced, and chemically induced chromosome breaks and sister chromatid exchanges (SCE) in human cells are collected in Table I. It is quite clear that the chromosome lesions (SCEs and breaks) *do not occur at random along the chromosomes*: Most authors report that they occur preferentially on the clear bands regardless of the banding used. The latter, therefore, might well be a bias of observation. In general, the hypothesis can be accepted that the transition zone between the dark G-band and the dark R-band might be the most sensitive point in the chromatid. Since this zone probably corresponds to the junction between euchromatin (R positive band) and heterochromatin (G positive band), it was suggested that more rapid repair occurs in the euchromatin, resulting in fewer aberrations; the very slow blocked repair in heterochromatin leads to incomplete aberrations, whereas the delayed repair in junctions allows the formation of SCEs and of complete aberrations (Brøgger, 1977).

Comparison of the *distribution of chromosome damage on the different chromosomes* raises the question of agent specificity, which was already discussed by Brøgger (1977). The chromosome damage is indeed different for the different agents considered. Mitomycin C is the only chemical which

## Table I
## Localization of Spontaneous, Congenital, Radio-Induced, Chemically Induced Chromosome Aberrations and Sister Chromatic Exchanges

| Chromosome region excess — Number of works | telomeres | centromeres | telom. and centrom. | Chromosome band excess — Number of works | $G^+$, or $R^-$ or $Q^+$ | band junction | $G^+ = G^-$ | $G^-$ or $R^+$ or $Q^-$ | Number of works | 1 | 2 | 3 | 4 | 5 | 6 | 7 | 8 | 9 | 10 | 11 | 12 | 13 | 14 | 15 | 16 | 17 | 18 | 19 | 20 | 21 | 22 | X | Y |
|---|---|---|---|---|---|---|---|---|---|---|---|---|---|---|---|---|---|---|---|---|---|---|---|---|---|---|---|---|---|---|---|---|---|
| **Chromosome aberrations** | | | | | | | | | | | | | | | | (a) Spontaneous | | | | | | | | | | | | | | | | | |
| 1 | | | | 3 | 1 | — | 1 | 1 | 6 | 2 | 5 | 1 | 2 | 3 | 1 | 1 | 1 | | | | | 3 | | | 6 | 1 | | | | | | | 3 |
| | | | | | | | | | | | | | | | | (b) Congenital | | | | | | | | | | | | | | | | | |
| *Reciprocal translocations* | | | | | | | | | | | | | | | | | | | | | | | | | | | | | | | | | |
| 6 | 1 | 1 | 2 | 5 | — | 1 | — | 4 | 7 | | 2 | | | | | 2 | 1 | 1 | | | 2 | | | | | 1 | | | 1 | 1 | | | |
| *Bloom's syndrome* | | | | | | | | | | | | | | | | | | | | | | | | | | | | | | | | | |
| 1 | — | 1 | — | 1 | | | | | 1 | 1 | | | | | | | | | | | | | | | | | | | | | | | |
| *1 Late replicating areas* | | | | | | | | | | | | | | | | | | | | | | | | | | | | | | | | | |
| *Fanconi's anemia* | | | | | | | | | | | | | | | | | | | | | | | | | | | | | | | | | |
| 2 | 1 | | | 2 | 1 | 1 | | | 2 | 2 | 1 | 1 | | 2 | | 1 | | 1 | | | 2 | | | | | | | | | | | | |
| | | | | | | | | | | | | | | | | (c) Radio-induced | | | | | | | | | | | | | | | | | |
| 3 | 3 | 2 | | 5 | 2 | | | 3 | 6 | 3 | 2 | 1 | | | | 1 | 1 | 1 | | 1 | 1 | 1 | 2 | 1 | | 2 | 1 | 1 | | 1 | | | 1 |
| | | | | | | | | | | | | | | | | (d) Chemically-induced | | | | | | | | | | | | | | | | | |
| *Mitomycin-C* | | | | | | | | | | | | | | | | | | | | | | | | | | | | | | | | | |
| 3 | | | 3 | 5 | | | | | 5 | 5 | | | | | | 1 | 5 | | | | | 1 | 1 | 1 | 5 | 1 | | 1 | 1 | 1 | 1 | | |
| *Thio-Tepa, Tepa* | | | | | | | | | | | | | | | | | | | | | | | | | | | | | | | | | |
| 1 | 1 | | | 2 | | | | | 2 | 1 | 1 | 2 | 1 | 1 | | | | | | 1 | 1 | | | 1 | 1 | 1 | | 1 | | | | | |
| *Clorambucil* | | | | | | | | | | | | | | | | | | | | | | | | | | | | | | | | | |
| | | | | 1 | | | | | 1 | | | | | | | | | 1 | | | | | | | | | | | | | | | |
| *Cyclophosphamide* | | | | | | | | | | | | | | | | | | | | | | | | | | | | | | | | | |
| | | | | 1 | | | | | 1 | | | | | | | | | | | | | | 1 | | | | | | | | | | |
| *Caffeine* | | | | | | | | | | | | | | | | | | | | | | | | | | | | | | | | | |
| | | | | 1 | | | | | | 1 | | | | | | | | | | | | | 1 | | | | | | | | | | |
| *Quinacrine mustard* | | | | | | | | | | | | | | | | | | | | | | | | | | | | | | | | | |
| | | | | 1 | 1 | | | | | | | | | | | | | | | | | | | | | | | | | | | | |
| **Sister chromatid exchanges** | | | | | | | | | | | | | | | | | | | | | | | | | | | | | | | | | |
| *Spontaneous* | | | | | | | | | | | | | | | | | | | | | | | | | | | | | | | | | |
| 9 | 6 | | | 7 | 1 | 4 | — | 1 | 3 | 3 | 1 | 1 | 1 | 2 | | 1 | | 1 | | | | | | | 1 | 1 | | | | | | | |

*Bloom, Fanconi's anemia, ataxia telangectasia*
As in spontaneous: length dependent on large chromosomes: fewer than expected on the small chromosomes.

[a] Aula and Von Koskull, 1976; Ayme et al., 1976; Giraud et al., 1976; Lubs and Samuelson, 1967; Mattei et al., 1979; Obe and Luers, 1972.

[b] Aurias et al., 1978; Evans et al., 1978; Friedrich and Nielsen, 1973; Jacobs et al., 1974; Nagakome et al., 1976; Nielsen and Rasmussen, 1976; Stoll, 1980.

[c] Lindgren, 1981; Shiraishi and Sandberg, 1977.

[d] Dutrillaux et al., 1977; Von Koskull et al., 1973.

[e] Buckton, 1976; Caspersson et al., 1972; Cooke et al., 1975; Dubos et al., 1978; Holmberg and Jonasson, 1973; Kucerova and Poliukova, 1976; San Roman and Bobrow, 1973; Seabright, 1973.

[f] Bourgeois, 1974; Funes–Craviato, 1974; Morad et al., 1973; Schaap et al., 1980; Vogel and Schroeder, 1974.

| | | | | | | | | | | | | | | | | | | | | | | | | |
|---|---|---|---|---|---|---|---|---|---|---|---|---|---|---|---|---|---|---|---|---|---|---|---|---|
| Chromosome number | | | | | | | | | | | | | | | | | | | | | | | | |
| Deficit | | | | | | | | | | | | | | | | | | | | | | | | |
| 1 | 2 | 3 | 4 | 5 | 6 | 7 | 8 | 9 | 10 | 11 | 12 | 13 | 14 | 15 | 16 | 17 | 18 | 19 | 20 | 21 | 22 | X | Y | References |
| (a) Spontaneous | | | | | | | | | | | | | | | | | | | | | | | | |
| | 1 | | 1 | 1 | | 1 | | | | | 1 | 1 | | | 1 | 2 | 2 | 3 | 2 | 2 | 1 | 3 | | [a] |
| (b) Congenital | | | | | | | | | | | | | | | | | | | | | | | | |
| 2 | 1 | 3 | | 2 | | 1 | | | | | 1 | | | | 1 | 1 | | | | 2 | 2 | | | [h] |
| | | | | | | | | | | | | | | | | | | | | | | | | [c] |
| | | | | | | | | | | | | | | | | | | | | | | | | [d] |
| (c) Radio induced | | | | | | | | | | | | | | | | | | | | | | | | |
| | | | | | | | | | | | | | | 1 | | | | | 1 | 2 | | | | [e] |
| (d) Chemically-induced | | | | | | | | | | | | | | | | | | | | | | | | |
| | | 1 | | | | | | | | | 1 | 1 | 1 | | | | | 1 | 1 | 1 | 1 | | | [f] |
| 1 | | | | | 1 | | | | | | 1 | 1 | 1 | | | | | | 1 | 1 | | | | [g] |
| | | | | | | | | | | | | | | | | | | | | | | | | [h] |
| | | | | | | | | | | | | | | | | | | | | | | | | [i] |
| | | | | | | | | | | | | | | | | | | | | | | | | [j] |
| | | | | | | | | | | | | | | | | | | | | | | | | [k] |
| | | | | | | | | | | | 1 | 1 | 1 | 1 | 1 | 1 | 1 | | | | | | | [l] |
| | | | | | | | | | | | | | | | | | | | | | | | | [m] |

[g] Funes-Craviato et al., 1974; Kucerova et al., 1976.

[h] Revees and Margoles, 1973.

[i] Morad and El Zawahri, 1977.

[j] Weinstein et al., 1973.

[k] Savage et al., 1974.

[l] Crossen et al., 1977; Dutrillaux et al., 1977; Galloway and Evans, 1975; Herreros and Gianelli, 1967; Kim, 1974; Latt, 1974; Morgan and Crossen, 1977; Pathak et al., 1975; Schnedl et al., 1976; Smyth and Evans, 1976; Sperling et al., 1975; Tice et al., 1975.

[m] Haglund and Zech, 1979; Shiraishi and Sandberg, 1977.

affects centromeres and, preferentially, the secondary constrictions of chromosomes 1,9, and 16 (*c*-heterochromatin rich chromosomes). *X ray*-induced lesions differ from experiment to experiment, probably as a result of different irradiation times through the cell cycle; x rays affect both centromeres and telomeres. As far as *spontaneous* aberrations and congenital aberrations are concerned, it is noticeable that the same weak points for structural rearrangement are mentioned several times and, moreover, correspond to the most frequent radiation and chemically-induced lesions. Finally, *Fanconi's anemia* also presents specific hot spots with some excess on telomeres.

Correspondence between SCE and chromosome breaks is difficult to affirm, but they both are preferentially located at the G–R interface; moreover, in Fanconi's anemia (Dutrillaux *et al.*, 1977) and in Bloom's syndrome (Shiraishy and Sandberg, 1977) evidence is presented that some of the break points are common. However, conflicting with these data are the observations (for review, see Schubert and Rieger, 1981) that (i) heterochromatin-containing regions are less preferred sites for SCEs than for chromatid aberrations, and (ii) that chromatid aberrations obtained after treatment with the same mutagens are much more preferentially distributed than SCEs.

(iii) As far as chromosome organization must be analyzed for its influence on mutagenic events, it is necessary to recall the *possible protective role of C-heterochromatin versus euchromatin regions.* C-heterochromatin, the part of the genome which intensively stains by C-banding procedures, consists of condensed late-replicating, highly-repetitive DNA sequences which are highly polymorphic, contain few, if any, structural genes, and which probably never transcribe. One of the possible roles of these C-heterochromatins is that of a bodyguard (Hsu, 1975); C-heterochromatin would form a layer of dispensable shield on the outer surface of the nucleolus. Mutagens, clastogens, or even viruses attacking the nucleus must first interact with the constitutive heterochromatin which in this way would protect the underlaying euchromatic genes by absorbing damage, particularly from chemical clastogens. The peripheral position of C-heterochromatic-rich regions in human metaphases, and the excess of chromosome damage after treatment with some chemicals (but not with others) in those areas which contain repetitive DNA sequences support this hypothesis.

## 1.2. Indirect Mutagenesis through Non-DNA Targets

### 1.2.1. Spindle Inhibitors

**1.2.1a. Problems Associated with the Study of Spindle Inhibitors.** Mitotic poisons, which do not act upon the hereditary material itself cannot, for that reason, be considered true mutagens. They indeed will act on the spindle apparatus, centrioles, and other nuclear organelles. Since no good assay systems for their detection exist, due to the lack of a spindle apparatus in bacterial systems, for example, their study has been neglected until recently. It is now recognized, however, that mitotic poisons could contribute as much to mutagenesis as true mutagens (Sawada and Ishidate, 1978; de Serres, 1979).

Since an influence on mitotic processes may be achieved in several different ways, and since an enormous number of mitotic poisons exist with unknown or insufficiently known characteristics, a clear classification is actually not possible to make. Attempts to define mitotic poisons have been undertaken by various authors. *Turbagenic compounds* are defined by Brøgger (1979) as compounds disturbing mitotic processes, whether the mechanism of action is the inhibition of spindle apparatus formation and function, the disordering of chromosome segregations, etc. One important class of surviving cells from such errors are aneuploid cells. Deysson (1968, 1976) talks about *antimitotic compounds*, indicating that every compound that lowers the number of mitoses in a cell population could be so classified, again regardless of the mechanism of this reduction. *Mitoclasic effects* are exerted when the spindle mechanism is partly or completely inhibited. Mitoses where the spindle apparatus are completely inhibited are designated as *stathmokinesis* or *C-mitosis* (colchicine effect). A classification of the major groups of turbagenic compounds will be given later on.

Before discussing observable effects provoked by turbagens, it should be mentioned that mutagenic chemicals may not only be classified into clastogens on the one hand and turbagens on the other hand, but that different compounds may be both clastogenic and turbagenic. Among the substances which seem to be only turbagenic, are colchicine, vincristine, mercapto-ethanol, and inhalation anaesthetics such as halothane, enflurane, and methoxyflurane. Agents that are clastogenic as well as turbagenic are, for example, ethidium bromide, actinomycin D, propidium dioxide, and possibly all the DNA intercalating substances. Reference to the above mentioned compounds is given in Brøgger (1979). We will now, however, only pay attention to turbagenesis.

### 1.2.1b. Morphological Features Observed After Exposure to Turbagens.
The following different morphological features may account for a turbagenic effect:

*C-mitosis (colchicine effect, stathmokinesis, or scattered metaphase chromosomes).* Due to the inhibition of tubuline polymerization, the cell cycle will be arrested in metaphase. Overcontracted chromosomes are seen dispersed over the cell. C-mitosis is obtained after exposure to various chemical and physical factors (e.g., colchicine, colcemid, vincristine, rota-none, etc.), and is frequently observed in malignant tissues (Oksala and

Therman, 1974). Since the cell may enter the following interphase without anaphase movement, polyploidy may result. This is especially seen in plants (Sawada and Ishidate, 1978). After removal of the C-mitotic drug, the spindle apparatus may regenerate. Multipolarity may, however, be seen due to the migration of mature daughter centrioles, each organizing the spindle apparatus.

*Endoreduplication.* This originates from at least two chromosome replications without the occurrence of mitosis. Chromosome reproduction may then be regarded as the only relic of the normal cell cycle. In many plant cells endoreduplication is perfectly viable. In animal cells it is less commonly observed, although it is frequent in animal tumors. Mercaptopyruvate, 6-mercaptopurine, colchicine, and ethidiumbromide are some examples of endoreplication-inducing substances.

*Abnormal spindle formation.* Multipolarity is obtained after treatment of the cells with, for example, low doses of colchicine, high doses of X rays, and probably all anesthetics or other compounds that act upon the centrioles. Normal centriole migration during prophase is hampered, and procentrioles may mature and organize the spindle apparatus. A partial disturbing of the spindle apparatus or of the spindle–chromosome interaction may, furthermore, account for nondisjunction, for example heavy metals may be mentioned in this respect.

*Chromosome decondensation and stickiness.* The failure of proper condensation of specific chromosome regions may induce chromosome banding after cell exposure to different environmental agents. A well known example is given by actinomycin D which induces G-band patterns on chromosomes (Shafer, 1973) and which is also known to induce a severe degree of decondensation of metaphase chromosome (Arrighi and Hsu, 1975). Other compounds may induce chromosome banding. Mercury chloride, for example, was shown to induce a "G-band-like" banding pattern in human lymphocytes exposed to the drug for 3 hr during the $G_1$–S stage of the cell cycle (Verschaeve and Susanne, 1978).

Chromatin threads of sticky chromosomes were shown to be intermingled, preventing normal anaphase movement. Although the spindle apparatus is present, a situation may eventually be obtained similar to that of the colchicine effect.

*Premature chromosome condensation.* According to Brøgger (1979), premature chromosome condensation may be regarded as a new parameter of chromosome damage which may be classified as a manifestation of turbagenicity.

### 1.2.2. Action on Enzymatic Processes

Besides spindle inhibitors, a number of mutagens may also act quite indirectly upon the genetic material by acting on enzymes of, for example,

DNA synthesis. Since this mutagenicity may be highly variable with respect to the test organism, and since the enzymes of DNA synthesis are likely to be more varied in nature than DNA itself, their study and/or detection is much more difficult than that of other mutagens. However, some examples may be given of substances acting on enzyme systems. Certain metal cations, beryllium and manganese, for example, may, besides a direct interaction with DNA itself, exert their mutagenicity by interaction with enzymatic error-avoidance mechanisms. Some amino acid analogues produce defective enzymes of DNA metabolism, and may be mutagenic for that reason. Deoxyribonucleoside triphosphate inbalances during DNA synthesis would be expected to be mutagenic. Thymine deprivation appears to promote mutagenesis in *E. coli* or in phage T4. Interactions with repair mechanisms influencing or inducing direct error-prone repair may partly be reponsible for this action (Drake, 1977).

## 1.3. Role of the Cell Cycle

A classification of chromosome aberrations was provided by Evans (1962, 1974) and by Savage (1976), distinguishing between the different chromatid-type (one chromatid is damaged at a given location) and the chromosome-type aberrations (both sister chromatids are damaged at the same location).

Since replication duplicates the genetic information of the $G_1$ single chromatid into the $G_2$ sister chromatid in S phase, one must expect—as observed in irradiation experiments—that chromosomes of cells irradiated in $G_1$ show chromosome-type aberrations, while the chromosomes of cells irradiated in $G_2$ show chromatid-type aberrations; irradiation in S phase produces a mixture of both types of aberrations.

The situation with aberrations induced by chemicals is not so simple. Besides a few chemicals which produce a similar pattern of aberrations to that of irradiation, most chemicals, including the so called "radiomimetic alkylating agents," at first are effective in producing aberrations only in $G_1$ and S, not in $G_2$ phase, and later produce, even in $G_1$, only chromatid-type aberrations. This might signify that most chemicals interact preferentially with S phase-related processes.

Exposure to mutagens at different stages of the cell cycle will thus modify the types of aberrations produced, not only *as a function of the DNA duplication* effect, but also *as a function of the different types of repair systems active either in the $G_1$ and/or S phase*.

## 1.4. Interspecies Differences

The ideal animal species for studies on mutagenicity, carcinogenicity, and teratogenicity, would be the one whose biological response to the test substance is identical to that of humans. In practice, however, rats, mice, and Syrian hamsters are extensively used, not because of their biochemical, physiological, or anatomical similarities with man, but rather for such practical features as small size, low cost, short life span, and easy reproduction. Nevertheless, our extensive biological knowledge of these species, including genetic characteristics, spontaneous tumor incidences, and susceptibilities to tumor induction makes them quite adequate study material. Of course primates and dogs are also used, but their routine use is difficult (For details, see Feron *et al.*, 1980).

Extrapolation of data collected on the mutagen sensitivity of animals to that of human risk, however, remains difficult. The different available studies (Röhrborn and Hansmann, 1971; Goetz *et al.*, 1975; Hansmann *et al.*, 1975; Scott *et al.*, 1975) clearly demonstrate that both subtle and large differences in sensitivity to chromosome aberration production exist not only between species, but also between different strains of the same species and between cell lines derived from a common tumor. The reasons for these different sensitivities are not well understood. As far as chemicals are concerned, genetic differences, differences in metabolism, detoxification, and repair capacities may vary among the species (Sasaki, 1973; Brewen, 1976). For ionizing radiation, consistent results were obtained by Brewen *et al.* (1973) and Abrahamson *et al.* (1973). They concluded, respectively, that the sensitivity to the induction of dicentric chromosomes by ionizing radiation in blood lymphocytes of different mammalian species is related to the effective chromosome arm number, and that per locus per rad (low LET) radiation-induced forward mutation rates in organisms, whose DNA content varies by a factor of about 1,000, is proportional to genome size.

A more recent revaluation of genetic radiation hazards in man (Schalet and Sankaranarayanan, 1976) argues against easy correlation between DNA content and radio-sensibility: In some species the yield of dicentric chromosomes is directly related to the chromosome arm number, in others not (Van Buul and Natarajan, 1980).

Finally, it must be recalled that, in addition to the problem of interspecies differences, the choice of a strain may be important in a particular bio-assay. The use of outbred or inbred strains, and the high spontaneous incidences of a particular type of tumor in a particular strain must be taken into account.

In conclusion, it is recommended that one test a material in different strains and in at least two different species (Feron *et al.*, 1980).

## 2. THE NATURE OF THE MUTAGEN

### 2.1. True Mutagens

Several excellent reviews (Drake and Baltz, 1976; Evans, 1977a; Drake, 1977; Bostock and Sumner, 1978) analyze in detail the type of chromosome damage induced by the *different classical mutagens*. These data are summarized here to present a synthetic comparative insight.

*X rays.*   In intact cells, both prokaryotic and eukaryotic, it has now been fairly established that the most important lesion produced by X rays is the breakage of the DNA molecule. These breaks may be single or double strand breaks, but the former are about 10 times more frequent than the latter. It is still not certain, however, whether the initial lesion produced by X rays is already a DNA break; indeed, X irradiation can also produce apyrimidic sites which are spontaneously transformed into single-strand breaks.

In addition to DNA breakage, X rays can also cause base damage by interacting preferentially with thymine.

*UV light.*   Although in nonbiological conditions, a wide variety of changes are induced by UV, in biological conditions the most important changes are the formation of pyrimidine dimers (T–T, T–C, C–C). These may be intrastrand or interstrand dimers.

Other base damage and DNA–protein cross-links also seem to be UV induced in eukaryotes. In any case, DNA breakage is not directly induced by UV itself; the DNA break has to be made by the repair system.

*Chemicals.*   The result of the interaction of a chemical with a target is evidently dependent on the molecular structure of the chemical compound. Therefore, the effects of chemicals will be highly variable. Different attempts to classify chemicals on the basis of induced molecular damage were made (Regan and Setlow, 1974; Cleaver, 1975). Table II summarizes the most relevant data about the initial lesions and the genetic effects produced by the important classes of chemical mutagens.

If one considers, however, that chemicals are metabolized in the cells (see Section 1.4); that one chemical can have different types of effects; that a fraction or the totality of the damage can be repaired (see Section 1.3); and that the translation of DNA damage into chromosome aberrations is not understood (see Section 2), it will be evident that the proposed classification is a tentative, simplified, and incomplete one.


## 2.2. Turbagens

The action of turbagens is less well known and less documented than the biochemistry of the mutagens which interact directly with DNA. An attempt will be made here to gather knowledge about this problem. Since a very great number of chemicals are turbagenic, and since a turbagenic action may be exerted in many ways, it is not possible to discuss these compounds all together or to give a satisfactory classification. An attempt at classification will, however, be given below according to major groups of chemicals, and if possible, according to predominant effects.

*Colchicine.*   Since colchicine is the most extensively studied turbagenic

## Table II

### Relation Between Type of Mutagen with DNA as Target, Type of Induced DNA Lesions, and Type of Obtained Mutation

| | Type of DNA lesion | | | | | |
|---|---|---|---|---|---|---|
| | DNA base damage | | | Cross-link | | |
| Type of mutagen | Reduction of strength of binding | Destruction of base | Modification of base: mispairing | DNA—DNA | DNA—protein | Intercalation between two bases |
| Alkylating agents | | | | | | |
| Monoalkyl | + | | + | | | |
| Bifunctional | + | | + | + | | |
| Multifunctional | + | | + | + | | |
| Mispairing agents | | | | | | |
| Nitrous acids | | | + | + | | |
| Hydroxylamine | | | + | | | |
| 2-aminopurine | | | + | | | |
| BuDr | + | | | | | |
| Effects via formation of organic peroxides and free radicals | | | | | | |

| Type of mutation | Point mutation | Chromosome aberration | Frame-shift mutation |
|---|---|---|---|
| | | a-purinic gap ↓ SSB or DSB ↓ Chromosome aberration | |
| Formaldehyde | | + | |
| Ethoxycaffeine | | + | |
| Urethane | | + | |
| Intercalating agents | | | |
| Acridines | | | + |
| Phenanthridines (ethydium bromide) | | | + |
| Polycyclichydro-carbons (carcinogenic properties) | | | + |

compound it is worth being mentioned first, although we will not attempt to discuss its action thoroughly since this would bring us far beyond the scope of this report. In any event, one expects that the reason for the specificity of action on tubulin may be explained stereochemically. Each dimer of tubulin, building the spindle apparatus, has a single site for colchicine binding. This site is furthermore the receptor site for another microtubule (MT) poison, *podophyllotoxin*. Binding of colchicine to this site may prevent the proper organization of tubuline dimers into MT. Colchicine, furthermore, prevents the separation of centriole pairs into appropriate poles at prophase. Much evidence has been obtained recently, however, indicating that colchicine is not only capable of inhibiting MT formation, but also of destroying already formed MT; the doses of colchicine capable of performing the latter will, however, be greater than those preventing MT assembly (Dustin, 1978). *Colcemid*, which is essentially similar in structure and effects to colchicine, was shown to disrupt normal chromosome distribution patterns, probably due to inhibition or disassembly of some, but not all spindle fibers attached to chromosomes. It is likely that, with increasingly higher doses of colcemid, more extensive spindle fiber deficit would be incurred, and more chromosomes would display randomization of location and misalignment (Rodman *et al.*, 1980).

   *Sulfhydryl-binding drugs and metals.* Since it was shown that arsenical derivatives arrest mitosis by inactivation of the spindle, many other compounds were found to have the same or similar effect. One must mention other metals, such as lead (Gerber *et al.*, 1980), zinc (Herick, 1969; Sathaiah and Venkat Reddy, 1973), and mercury (Ramel, 1972). It is clear that the metals may affect MT by various pathways; either by combining with tubulin, or by poisoning cell enzymes necessary for MT metabolism. The fixation on sulfhydryl-groups of tubulin, glutathione, or other sulfhydryl-proteins is one, and maybe the major mode of action. This is particularly evident for arsenic, and probably also for mercury compounds. The nature of the compound may determine its effect. Thus, with regard to mercury compounds, it seems that phenylmercury is more readily bound to kinetochore MT and methylmercury to pole-to-pole MT. Mercuric chloride, on the other hand, does not seem to be particularly effective in destroying MT (Thrasher, 1973). In contrast to colchicine or colcemid, mercury will cause a much more gradual transition between normal- and C-mitotic cell division, because more alternatives in its action may be possible. Both colcemid and mercury compounds (especially organomercurials) disturb the chromosome distribution in metaphase (Verschaeve *et al.*, 1978; Rodman *et al.*, 1980). In contrast to mercury, however, colcemid does not impair in humans the tendency for the acrocentric chromosomes to associate. Addition of sulfhydryl-binding drugs to colchicine exposed cells will, at the most, enhance colchicine action only poorly

(Deysson, 1976). It is thus not surprising that, in our 1978 paper about the chromosome distribution analysis in phenylmercuryacetate exposed subjects, where colchicine was used on exposed subjects, a dissociation of the acrocentrics (not impaired by colchicine) was the most important observation. Other effects on the position of the metaphase chromosomes could be hidden by the presence of colchicine. Also, other heavy metals may disturb the normal chromosome distribution in metaphase, e.g., inorganic lead compounds (Verschaeve *et al.*, 1979).

*Alkaloids.* Many alkaloids have mitoclasic properties. Special attention must be paid, however, to the vinca alkaloids, *vincristine* (VCR) and vinblastine (VLB), which have well-known anticancer properties. Their mitotic poisoning effects are found to be very similar to those for colchicine, although some differences are noticed; for instance, in contrast to colchicine, no important rise in mitotic index is found because, along with the mitoclasic effect, an important diminution in prophase entry is observed. Furthermore, vinca alkaloids have a receptor site on the tubulin dimer which is different from the colchicine site.

*Podophyllotoxin.* It has long since been demonstrated that podophyllotoxin modifies cell division in the same way as colchicine does. This may be explained by the fixation on the same tubulin site. Podophyllotoxin, however, binds more rapidly, and, in contrast to colchicine, the binding is also more rapidly reversible and not temperature-dependent. Since podophyllotoxin has three methoxygroups, just like colchicine, and VLB or VCR contain two or three methoxygroups, one may expect that the action of these compounds is similar due to that chemical similarity.

*Griseofulvin.* Griseofulvin contains several methoxygroups, which may explain why it has an effect similar to the above mentioned chemicals. Evidence is obtained, however, that the antibiotic binds to microtubule-associated proteins (MAPs) rather than to tubulin itself (Wilson *et al.*, 1975; Roobol *et al.*, 1977). Although the observed effects are thus very similar to colchicine, colcemid, VLB, VCB, and podophyllotoxin, the mechanism of action must be different. Griseofulvin may be considered as the first reported compound inhibiting MT formation by an action on the MAPs.

That a difference in the binding site (and mode of action) can result in equal or similar effects may be illustrated by the proposed hypothesis explaining the resistance of CHO mutant cell lines to colchicine, colcemide, griseofulvin, and vinblastine (Cabral *et al.*, 1980). The CHO-resistant cell lines were thought to bear a mutation in the gene coding for $\beta$-tubulin, and we suggested that the four antimitotic drugs may all affect a critical interaction between $\beta$-tubulin and some other component in microtubule assembly. The altered $\beta$-tubulin in the CHO mutants may be able to complete this interaction even when the drugs are bound.

*Organoaliphatic compounds.*   They have long been known to influence mitosis by affecting the spindle although the threshold of the mitoclasic effect is usually very close to the threshold of toxicity (e.g., chloral hydrate). Anesthetics such as *ether* and *chloroform* are well studied mitoclasic compounds which also have a strong mitodepressive effect (Östergren, 1951). *Lidocaine* would combine reversibly with nonpolymerized tubulin and prevent the assembly of MT. Another example in this group of chemical compounds is $N_2O$, which produces typical colchicine metaphases. However, the MT were not destroyed; the centrioles remain normally located, and spindle microtubule assembly is not inhibited. Ultrastructural studies indicated that $N_2O$ blocked cells at a stage in mitosis more advanced than that produced by colcemid or other C-mitotic agents (Brinkley and Rao, 1973).

*Organic aryl compounds.*   Very many compounds belong to this class, of which *hexanitrodiphenylamine* may be mentioned. Characteristics are very similar to those of colchicine (Deysson, 1968).

*Heparin and anticoagulants.*   Many anticoagulants have antimitotic effects; however, their action on mitosis does not seem to be related to their anticoagulant properties.

*IPC (Isopropyl-N-phenylcarbamate).*   Like other carbamates (e.g., urethane) this compound has complex actions on dividing cells and DNA synthesis. It does not seem to destroy MT, but to disorientate them. All effects are reversible and do differ from those of colchicine. The receptor site and mode of action are, however, controversial.

*Melatonin.*   It was observed that this hormone was antagonistic to colchicine. Colchicine protects the cells against the inhibition of cilia regeneration caused by melatonin, and melatonin protects the organism against the lethal effects of colchicine. Again, a methoxy group has been proposed as a base for MT poisoning. Some workers, however, do not consider melatonin as being an MT poison or a mitotic inhibitor.

*Other MT poisons.*   Some substances destroy microtubules by nonspecific protein denaturation (e.g., *digitonin*). They do demonstrate that MT may be rapidly destroyed without damage to other cell structures, indicating their particular fragility. Many other MT poisons may be mentioned: *Steganicin*, for example, has a trimethoxybenzene ring and competes with colchicine. It is thought to have the same binding site as the latter (Wang *et al.*, 1976). Other examples include *rotenone*, which arrests metaphase in Chinese hamster cells and provokes identical ultrastructural changes, as does colchicine, and *chlorpromazine*, which inhibits MT assembly, colchicine binding, and the disassembling of already formed MT (Cann and Hinmann, 1975).

*Physical agents.*   Briefly, physical agents must also be mentioned. Cold, for example, disrupts spindle birefrigence, inhibits chromosome movement, and prevents microtubule formation (Roth, 1967). A similar antimitotic action by pressure probably also results in spindle microtubule inhibition and degradation (Marsland, 1966).

*Conclusion.* One may say that a great number of chemicals may be turbagenic mainly by destroying MT or inhibiting MT assembly. All kinds of morphological features may be observed with most of the single compounds. For that reason it is only possible to draw some very general conclusions. From most chemicals it can be concluded that they have a colchicinelike effect: that is particularly true for alkaloids, podophyllotoxin, and organic aryl compounds. Yet only a limited number of chemicals combine as colchicine does specifically with tubulin (e.g., vinca-alkaloids and benzimidazole derivatives). Nitrous oxide and other anesthetics will act in a later stage of the cell cycle than do colchicine and IPC. Unlike colchicine, IPC does not destroy MT but only disorients them. Like colchicine, metals—although another mechanism may be suggested—inhibit MT assembly and/or destroy preformed MT, but may also be turbagenic by a more indirect action on enzymes necessary for a normal cell-division procedure. Last but not least, griseofulvin is colchicinelike in its effects, but acts on microtubule associated proteins and may be considered unique among other turbagens in this respect.

## 3. AN OVERVIEW OF DNA REPAIR PROCESSES

We briefly summarize DNA repair processes with a particular emphasis on their influence in determining mutation frequencies. Comprehensive reviews of DNA repair are available (Hanawalt et al., 1979; Lindahl, 1979; Laval, 1980). It has become obvious that the frequency of mutations is reciprocally correlated with the efficiency of various enzymatic DNA repair and error-avoidance systems (Radman et al., 1979). On the other hand, good evidence exists for the hypothesis that a large part of induced mutations is generated as a result of cellular "decision to mutate," i.e., it is a controlled cellular process (Witkin, 1976; Radman et al., 1979). For example, it is easy to obtain *E. coli* mutants which are nonmutable by radiation and by many chemical mutagens, but which are still resistant to these agents (Witkin, 1976). Hence, nonrandomness of mutational changes, both in time (Defrais et al., 1976) and along the genome (Benzer, 1962; Coulondre and Miller, 1977) may teach us something about the role of mutagenesis in evolution.

The maintenance of genetic information depends upon the cellular capacity to (i) protect parental DNA strands from any incurring changes by DNA repair process, and (ii) perform high fidelity replication, the accuracy of which could be further improved by DNA repair using the parental strand as the master copy. In fact, such processes are operational in bacteria and probably also in mammalian cells, since astonishingly little difference has been found between various repair processes in *E. coli* and mammalian cells (Hanawalt *et al.*, 1979).

### 3.1. Prereplicative Error Correction

Prereplicative repair of DNA usually leads to the establishment of the original DNA nucleotide sequence, and hence suppresses the mutagenic potential of many mutagens. The disappearance of DNA lesions can be performed by two known principal mechanisms, lesion *reversal* and lesion *removal*. Reversal of the lesion is exemplified by the photoreactivation of UV-induced pyrimidine dimers (*in situ* monomerization of dimers) and by transalkylation (*in situ* dealkylation of an alkylated base). The enzymes involved are known (Wun and Sutherland, 1977; Olsson and Lindahl, 1980). Removal of the damaged residue (Laval, 1980) involves at least two mechanisms: (i) specific endonucleolytic cleavage of the damaged polynucleotide chain followed by exonucleolytic removal of the lesion and by DNA repair synthesis seems to apply to bulky DNA lesions; (ii) the removal of the abnormal base by an *N*-glycosylase activity without initially breaking the phosphodiester band, thus producing an apurinic–apyrimidinic (AP) site, which is then repaired by an endonuclease–exonuclease mechanism as in (i). The latter mechanism seems to act upon subtle DNA lesions and simple mispairs, such as uracil and some alkylated based (Lindahl, 1979).

### 3.2. Replicative Error Avoidance

A powerful combination of genetic and biochemical studies of phage T4 DNA polymerase mutants provided clear evidence that DNA polymerase is a high accuracy enzyme with at least two fidelity functions. Both base selection and "editing" or "proofreading" by the polymerase-associated 3′ to 5′ exonuclease activity have been identified as mechanisms of the high fidelity of DNA synthesis. Current theories (e.g., Galas and Branscomb, 1978) propose that DNA polymerases with associated 3′ to 5′ exonuclease replicate a polynucleotide chain by a random walk, forward (i.e., chain elongation) and backward (chain shortening by the exonucleolytic removal of the 3′ terminal nucleoside monophosphates), resulting from a race between polymerase and exonuclease activity. Since exonuclease activity acts preferentially on single stranded DNA [particularly in the presence of dNTPs (Burtlag and Kornberg, 1972)], 3′OH terminally mismatched bases are removed more readily than the well-matched bases, hence the proofreading. It is the relative ratio of exonuclease to polymerase activity that determines the fidelity of DNA synthesis: mutator polymerases have low, antimutator high exo–pol ratios

(Bessman *et al.*, 1974). Due to the high fidelity properties of DNA polymerases, noncoding DNA lesions in the template strand block DNA chain elongation and hence prevent mutagenesis. Whereas the inhibition of proofreading by exonuclease is not sufficient to allow "bypass" synthesis past noncoding lesions (such as AP sites), inhibition of nucleotide selection appears to promote *in vitro* a mutagenic "bypass" synthesis past AP sites (Doubleday *et al.*, 1980, 1981).

DNA polymerases are metaloenzymes containing $Zn^{++}$ and they all require $Mg^{++}$ for a faithful synthesis. Therefore, the replacement of $Zn^{++}$ and $Mg^{++}$ by other divalent cations (e.g., $Be^{++}$, $Mn^{++}$, $Co^{++}$, etc.) leads to a decrease in replicational fidelity, and this may well be the basis of metal-induced mutagenesis *in vivo* (Radman *et al.*, 1977; Loeb *et al.*, 1979). Other proteins belonging to DNA replication machinery are expected to contribute to the replicational fidelity. Mutations in the gene 32 phage T4, which codes for a DNA-binding protein, do influence the rates of spontaneous and induced mutations (Drake, 1973).

### 3.3. Post-Replicative Error Avoidance

This most recently discovered bacterial error correction mechanism has been well defined by genetic experiments using heteroduplex DNA to transfect *E. coli* cells (Radman *et al.*, 1979, 1980). This enzymatic system appears to recognize and repair by excision mismatched bases exclusively from the newly synthesized strand, the one bearing replicational errors. The discrimination between the old and new strands is based upon under-methylation of the newly synthesized DNA. Therefore, we call this process, which contributes to the accuracy of DNA synthesis by three orders of magnitude, *methylation-instructed mismatch correction*. Specific methylation involved in the major adenine methylation system, defined by the *E. coli dam* gene, methylates the GATC sequence (Lacks and Greenberg, 1977). Methylation of this sequence prevents the action of mismatch correction enzymes, and therefore the enzymes (not yet identified) probably bind to this (or an associated) sequence only when unmethylated and scan DNA for mismatches along that same strand.

*E. coli* mismatch correction-deficient mutants (Glickman and Radman, 1980) have been recently identified which, just like adenine methylation-deficient *E. coli dam⁻* mutants, show both strong spontaneous mutator and spontaneous hyperrecombination of phenotypes. Hence, a specific DNA methylation seems to stabilize genetic information.

### 3.4. Post-Replicative DNA Repair (PRR)

PRR is operationally defined as the capacity of the cellular machinery to elongate nascent DNA chains initially blocked by a noncoding lesion in the

DNA template. It is the capacity to tolerate unremoved DNA lesions. Two mechanisms have been proposed (i) In *E. coli*, it appears that the continuity of the nascent DNA chain is restored (gap-filling) by recombinational exchanges between the two daughter molecules (Rupp *et al.*, 1971); (ii) Mammalian cells show little if any such recombinational mechanisms, and a delayed "bypass" replication has been proposed as the mechanism of PRR in mammalian cells (Lehmann, 1972; Radman, 1980).

### 3.5. Direct and Indirect Mutagens

Direct mutagens cause subtle modification of DNA bases residing either in the template or in the precursors, which can miscode and cause specific errors in DNA synthesis. Base analogs (e.g, 2-aminopurine, 5-bromouracil), some oxygen alkylations (e.g., *O*-6-methyl-guanine), as well as the alkylations of cytosine and adenine produced by the metabolites of vinyl chloride monomer (Barbin *et al.*, 1980), are such subtle base modifications. Indirect mutagens cause noncoding DNA lesions which cannot be copied by the constitutive replication machinery. Such replication-inhibiting DNA lesions are produced by radiation and by the majority of well-known mutagens–carcinogens. Their low mutagenic specificity and high mutagenic potency is now being explained by the fact that these lesions induce a complex cellular response, called SOS induction, which among other effects, e.g., prophage induction and inhibition of cellular division, causes activation of a potent generalized cellular mutator effect, which in turn lead to mutation fixation opposite noncoding lesions (SOS repair), and to the mutagenesis of un-damaged DNA sequences due to the transitory low replicational fidelity (Radman *et al.*, 1979).

### 3.6. Why SOS Repair?

The SOS induction mechanism has been widely elucidated in *E. coli* (Gottesman, 1981) and a critical review has been written on the evidence for SOS induction in mammalian cells (Radman, 1980).

Why was an inducible cellular mutator system selected in evolution? We can think of two reasons: (i) to increase survival threatened by the nonrepaired bulky nonreplicative DNA lesions. Mutagenesis would then be the price paid for survival; and (ii) to increase the fitness of a population exposed to a sudden liability caused by an environmental change by producing a rapid increase in genetic variability inside the population, and hence increasing the chance that some individuals survive under new conditions (Radman, 1977). Indeed, an *E. coli* mutator strain shows higher fitness than does its low-mutation wild-type counterpart only under unfavorable, selective conditions, whereas the wild-type wins over the mutator strain under favorable conditions (Cox and

Gibson, 1974). Recombination may be SOS-inducible in higher organisms (Holliday, 1975; Fabre and Roman, 1977) and might contribute to the population fitness better than mutagenesis (e.g., Ayala, 1967). Therefore, our speculative working hypothesis is that SOS induction may be an adaptive evolutionary mechanism: a genetically programmed response to environmental insults, rapidly but transitorily creating genetic variability and hence increasing the survival changes of some selected individuals.

## 4. METABOLIZATION, SYNERGISM, AND PROTECTION

Foreign compounds entering the body may be metabolized by several mechanisms simultaneously giving rise to different products. The use of one or another metabolic pathway will be determined by the combined action of genetic as well as physiological and environmental factors.

Due to the metabolic processes, chemical compounds will thus be transformed. Mutagenic and/or carcinogenic (ultimate genotoxic) compounds may for that reason lose their genotoxic properties, but so-called "precursor genotoxic compounds" (which are not genotoxic *per se*) may as well be activated into ultimate products. *Precursor genotoxic agents*, which comprise a wide range of structurally unrelated chemicals, are usually lipophilic in nature. Since lipophilic compounds are efficiently excreted by mammals, they need to be converted into hydrophilic products in order to be effective. It is now clear that the primary mono-oxygenation reaction is the key event in the activation of many precursor genotoxic agents such as the polycyclic aromatic hydrocarbons and aflatoxin $B_1$. The activation of most classes of precursor genotoxic agents thus necessitates an initial oxygenation step. However, other types of primary metabolic reactions leading to the generation of proximate (i.e., intermediate) or ultimate genotoxic agents may occur; e.g., reduction of nitrocompounds.

Different enzymes may be involved in the metabolic transformation of the compounds. This transformation may, according to the presence or absence of the appropriate enzyme, be directed toward either activation or deactivation. In case of exposure to precursor agents, it is the balance between the activating and deactivating enzymes that is important. For many compounds, however, the balance seems to favor activation.

In most cases, *ultimate genotoxic agents* are electrophilic reactants. Two enzyme systems are present in mammalian tissues which are especially efficient in scavenging electrophiles: *S-glutathione transferases* and *epoxide hydratase*. Reactions between the nucleophilic sulfur atom of glutathione and electrophilic centers in genotoxic agents are believed to lead to a loss of activity and the rapid excretion of the formed products. Such reactions, however, do not seem to result always in detoxification.

Epoxide hydratases catalyze the hydrolysis of a carbon–oxygen bond of epoxide rings, which results in deactivation of genotoxic epoxides. In rare instances, however, the hydrated product may further be transformed into another ultimate genotoxic compound.

Chemical agents entering the body will in many instances then be transformed by the action of enzymes. One must for that reason be very careful in interpreting results of studies on mutagenesis performed as well *in vivo* as *in vitro*.

*In vitro* test systems (e.g., mammalian or bacterial cell cultures) will also for that reason usually fail to detect precursor or proximate genotoxic agents since they lack those enzyme systems present *in vivo* and responsible for activation.

Addition of mammalian tissue preparations (mainly from the liver) will mimic the *in vivo* situation. Generally, the post-mitochondrial supernatant (S9 fraction) from the liver of Aroclor-treated rats is used as an extracellular enzyme source. Although very good results were obtained using this and similar systems, one must again be careful since perturbations or faulty interpretations remain. For example, although the two most important deactivating enzymes, epoxide hydratase and S-glutathione transferases are present in the S9 fraction, at least the latter may be partly inoperative. Dilution and oxidation of glutathione during preparation of S9 may be one reason. Otherwise the S9 fraction is usually obtained from animals pretreated with microsomal enzyme inducers (e.g., Aroclor 1254). This may lead to overcompetence of certain enzymes as the mono-oxigenases and be responsible for excessive activation of precursor genotoxic agents.

*Synergistic effects*, or the simultaneous administration or exposure to different mutagenic compounds, must also be attentively considered. Indeed it is very clear that the addition of these compounds will not necessarily result in the effects being the sum of the individual effects, but that interaction between the compounds or an alteration in metabolic processes provoked by the simultaneous treatment may enhance the effects which may reach unpredictable high levels. Although very little presently is known in this respect, too many examples of synergistic actions are already known. We already mentioned that colchicine and sulfhydryl-binding substances will at the most be additive in effect, while griseofulvine potentiates the action of colchicine. Environmental factors, e.g., therapeutic drugs, alcohol, cigarette smoking, ionizing radiation, etc., may influence the metabolism and thus directly or indirectly activate or deactivate mutagenic and/or carcinogenic compounds. Further examples and a more thorough discussion of this kind of problem may be found in Wright (1980) and in Madle and Obe (1980).

Besides the metabolic transformation of a compound by the appropriate enzymes or the potentialization or addition of effects due to simultaneous exposure to different substances, some compounds may protect the cell against the deleterious (mutagenic) action of another compound. Dimercaprol (BAL), for example, will protect the cell against the C-mitotic action of mercurials (Ramel, 1969). Another example is selenium of which it is thought that a decrease in body content due to arsenic exposure may enhance cancer suceptibility (Leonard and Lauwerys, 1980). We have already reported the example of the antagonisitic action of melatonin versus colchicine; however, a thorough discussion of this kind of problem is beyond the scope of this paper.

# PART II: RELATION BETWEEN MUTATION, REPAIR, AND CHROMOSOME ABERRATION

## 5. ESTIMATION OF DNA DAMAGE

Estimation of genetic damage due to exposure of mutagens is the aim of many geneticists. Different methods with different biological systems are now available for mutagenicity testing. Several excellent books (IARC, 1980; Drake and Koch, 1976; Moutschen, 1979) discuss the advantages and disadvantages of the different assays, taking into account problems of extrapolation due to differences between species, between germinal and somatic cells, between *in vitro* and *in vivo* tests, problems of activation systems, etc. Our purpose is to summarize briefly and classify the methods which will be mentioned in the other chapters of this book. As shown in Table III, DNA damage can quantitatively and qualitatively be estimated at different levels:

*Level of gene mutation.*   Gene mutations correspond to local small modifications of the DNA sequences which can be measured by different types of assays.

*Level of structural and numerical chromosome aberrations.*   Most of the tests in eukaryotes are based on the analysis of structural and numerical chromosome aberrations after exposure to mutagens. These modifications of DNA sequences are on a large enough scale that they are visible directly under the microscope: as long as the morphology of one or more chromosomes, but not the number of chromosomes, is modified, it is considered to be a chromosome mutation: As soon as the number of chromosomes is changed, it is called a genome mutation.

The absence of specificity of some tests (for instance, dominant lethals which are the result of chromosome and/or genome mutations as well), does not at all signify that this test is less relevant for mutagenicity testing; on the

## Table III

## Classification of Principal Tests for Mutagenesis in Function of Used Biological System and Identified Genotoxic Signal

| Biological system | Mutation level (identified genotoxic signal) | | |
|---|---|---|---|
| | Gene mutation | Chromosome mutation = structural chromosome aberrations | Genome mutation = numerical chromosome aberrations |
| Plants | | Morphological changes as survival, sterility, and somatic mutations | |
| Bacteria<br>Bacillus subtilis<br>Escherichia coli; Salmonella typhimurium<br>DNA repair deficient strains (pol A, rec A, uvr A/rec A) | Mutation tests:<br>Rec-assay<br>Reversion assay<br>DNA repair tests<br><br>Tests using induction and mutagenesis of prophage λ | | |
| Yeast and molds<br>Saccharomyces cerevisiae<br>Saccharomyces pombe<br>Neurospora crassa<br>Aspergillus nidulans | Gene conversion<br>Forward mutations of base changes or deletions<br>Reverse mutations for base substitutions or frameshifts | Mitotic crossing-over | Induction of nondisjunction |
| Drosophila | Recessive lethal test:<br>(forward mutations and deletions) | Dominant lethals<br><br>Translocations<br>ring-X-chromosome loss | Loss of (rad) X- or Y-chromosome nondisjunction |

| | In vitro | |
| --- | --- | --- |
| Mammalian cells in culture<br>V₇₉ and CHO Chinese hamster cells<br>L₅₁₇₈ Y mouse cells | Locus mutations:<br>Resistance to 8-azaguanine, 6-thioguanine and ouabin<br>Resistance to 5-bromo-2'-deoxyuridine (Budr) | |
| Short-term peripheral blood lymphocyte cultures<br>Cultured fibroblast<br>Peripheral blood lymphocyte cultures | Scoring of chromosome aberrations | Scoring of aneuploidy |
| | *In vivo* | |
| Bone marrow | Scoring of chromosome aberrations<br>Micronucleus test (presence of micronuclei in polychromatic erythrocytes) | Scoring of aneuploidy |
| Animal tumor lines | | |
| Whole animals (mammals) | Heritable translocation test | Dominant lethals<br>Numerical sex chromosome anomaly test<br>Specific locus method nondisjunction |
| | Mouse spot test (*in vivo* somatic mutation test) | |

contrary it may give a better estimation of the genetic risk. However, since the relation between DNA damage and the formation of the chromosome aberrations is not well understood, it must be clear that cytogenetic tests will only give indicative information, but no proof of the mutagenicity of the tested compounds.

## 6. MECHANISMS INVOLVED IN STRUCTURAL CHROMOSOME ABERRATIONS

The term *chromosome aberrations* covers different types of modification of the chromosome structure. The first type to be considered is an interruption of the continuity of one or both *chromatids*, such as a *break (or gap)*, which implies a DNA double-strand event. The second morphological type of chromosome aberration consists of *chromosome exchanges*, where chromosomal material is displaced from one chromosome to another part of the same chromosome (exchange within a chromosome) or to another chromosome (exchange between two chromosomes). The question here is whether the exchange is subsequent or not to one or two chromosome breaks. Mutagenesis testing also now analyzes interchanges between the two chromatids of one chromosome: these *sister chromatid exchanges* (SCEs) could occur with or without loss of chromosomal material. In the following sections, mechanisms implied in the formation of chromosome gaps, chromosome breaks, and SCEs, will be discussed.

### 6.1. Chromosome Breaks and Exchanges

The first hypothesis on the mechanisms involved in the formation of chromosome aberrations was supported by the work of Karl Sax in the late 1930s: a chromosome exchange is the result of a rejoining between two chromosome ends which must *first be broken* by a mutagen (breakage first hypothesis). The existence of repair processes brought Revell (1963) to his exchange hypothesis: observed exchange events and deletions are sometimes directly due to the mutagen but are in large measure the result of intracellular recombinations (repair activities). Let us consider how these hypotheses fit with our actual knowledge about mutagen interaction with DNA and chromatin.

### 6.1.1. Chromosome Breaks

To generate chromosome breaks, you need (1) a *direct double-strand break* as expected from ionizing radiation. Indeed, sucrose-gradient centrifugations of DNA have shown that both single-strand breaks (SSB) and double-strand breaks (DSB) can occur immediately after irradiation. However, the SSB predominate the DSB at a ratio of 10:1 (Veatch and Okada, 1969); moreover, probably 98–99% of the DSB induced are repaired correctly (Scott, 1980); (2). *a defective filling, after formation of a single-strand break* (misrepair of the lesion later produces a discontinuity in the nascent strand at a similar locus to the lesion in the parent strand). The result at that moment may become a DSB. Chemicals inducing apurinic gaps, destruction of a base, and crosslinks, must be considered here (for examples, see Table II); or (3) as suggested in the exchange theory of Revell, *primary lesions which are not breaks, but altered sites* with the ability to interact in pairs. If such interaction is consummated, a physical chromosome exchange occurs, but if the interaction is incomplete, a physical discontinuity results which is seen as a chromatid break. This theory predicts that chromatid breaks would be infrequent. This is true in *Vicia faba* (Revell, 1959; Revell, 1966; Scott and Evans, 1967), but certainly not in mammalian cells (Chu *et al.*, 1962; Bhambhani *et al.*, 1973; Carrano, 1975). Detailed analysis performed by Geard (1980), however suggests that a substantial portion of chromatid breaks indeed result from interaction between pairs of damaged sites. A single chromatid break is then the result of two breaks involved in an incomplete exchange.

The main effect from the above comparison of mutagen induced chromatid breaks is that the interaction between DNA sequences from the same or from different chromatids modulate the definitive expression of mutagen lesions into genetic aberrations. As we have seen earlier, it is clear that repair processes involve interaction between two different DNA strands and that this repair may be error-free (excision repair and post-replication) or error-prone (post-replication and SOS repair). Since, moreover, the main bulk of chemical mutagens produce chromosome aberrations only if the cells pass through a replication phase, it is quite logical to relate the interstrand interactions after mutagen exposure to the post-replication repair processes which take place during the S-phase.

Since recombinational repair processes are easier to understand between two sister chromatids because evident sequence homologies do exist, the production of chromosome exchanges between different chromosomes through recombinational processes may be more difficult to accept.

### 6.1.2. Chromosome Exchanges

Even two nonhomologous chromosomes are not so different as might be expected from their constitutive genes. Indeed, the human genome consists approximatively of 35% repetitive DNA and 65% nonrepetitive DNA (Arrighi and Saunders, 1973). Half of the repetitive DNA is organized as highly repetitive DNA without known coding sequences; the other half is organized as middle repetitive DNA in which one may classify rDNA, tRNA, and promotor sequences, and is interspersed with nonrepetitive sequences coding for structural proteins.

The high repetitive sequences which can at least be partly isolated by CsCl centrifugations show similarities over the different chromosomes (Corneo *et al.*, 1968; Gosden *et al.*, 1975). Moreover, a considerable proportion of the DNA is present as inverse repeats, or palindromes averaging around 300–1200 bases in length (Evans, 1977b).

It becomes easier on these bases to construct a recombinational repair model that can result in exchanges between double-strand breaks on separate chromosomes or separate regions on the same chromosomes. Evans (1977a) presented such a model, which involves a minimum of double-strand breaks in one duplex and involves degradation, incision, and heteroduplex DNA formation between regions with sequence homology and ligation (Figure 1).

## 6.2. Chromosome Gaps

If a chromosome break can be defined as complete interruption in the chromosome continuity by displacement, less clear chromosome interruptions are often observed after treatment with ionizing radiation and certain chemicals. These chromosome aberrations vary from slight hypostainability of the chromatin to extrasecondary constriction, and finally to unstained regions without chromosome displacement. These lesions are gathered under the name of gaps.

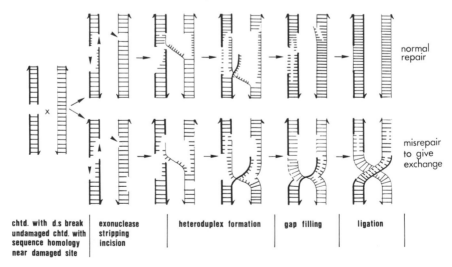

**Figure 1.** Model representation of the formation of an exchange aberration (Evans, 1977).

Under the light microscope, some gaps are crossed by chromatin fibers, but some of them look as real discontinuities; under the electron microscope, however, even these discontinuities sometimes show chromatin fibers. No clear understanding of the true nature or of the genetic importance of gaps has been obtained. Opinions on what gaps represent are quite divergent:

- Sax (1938) considered gaps as incomplete breaks maintained by chromosome matrices or other factors.
- Revell (1959) proposed that gaps correspond to the "primary events" which in exchange theory lead to breakage.
- Read (1959) considered gaps as half-chromatid or subchromatid breaks.
- Fox (1967) and Heddle and Bodycote (1970) suggested that gaps may correspond to incomplete chromatid exchanges.
- Brinkley and Shaw (1970), Brøgger (1971), and Scheid and Traut (1971) suggested that a gap is an insufficient folding of the chromosome fiber into a metaphase chromatid due either to a change in the DNA molecule (e.g., a UV-induced dimer, a combination of an alkylating agent and DNA) or a change in the packing of the proteins (nonrandom mercapto-ethanol-induced changes) (Brøgger, 1975).
- Bender et al. (1974) postulated that gaps might be SSB.

Finally, the classification of gaps into true breaks or not is very difficult and perhaps impossible with our present knowledge. Data collected about this problem are discussed clearly by Comings (1974).

## 6.3. Sister Chromatid Exchanges

The application of an easy cytogenetic technique showing the difference between sister chromatids (Latt, 1973, 1974) revealed the existence of sister chromatid exchanges and their increase after exposure to mutagens (Perry and Evans, 1974). These sister chromatid exchanges appear to involve exchange of similar sized regions of sister chromatids, but it is not yet known whether these regions are completely identical or whether the region of joining involves a butt joint or a single-strand overlap (Cleaver, 1978). In the latter case, the region of overlap would resemble single-strand recombination events. Therefore, the question rises whether SCEs are different or not from chromosome aberrations.

The main observations concerning similarities or dissimilarities between SCE and chromosome aberrations can be summarized as follows:

(1) Studies with cells from *patients with three different breakage syndromes*, Bloom's syndrome, Fanconi's anemia and, ataxia telangiectasia,

show that only Bloom's cells have an extremely high number of SCE (Chaganti *et al.*, 1974), whereas the other two are normal in this respect (Chaganti *et al.*, 1974; Galloway and Evans, 1975; Latt *et al.*, 1975).

(2) As far as *sensitivity to ionizing radiation is concerned*, it was shown that an x-ray dose which doubles the SCE frequency (about 400 rads), gives a 100-fold increase in the frequency of aberrations (Perry and Evans, 1974). Moreover, it is well-known that irradiation in $G_1$ produces chromosome-type aberrations and that irradiation in $G_2$ produces chromatid type aberrations; irradiation in S phase produces a mixture of both types of aberration. SCEs on the contrary are induced only during S phase. These data suggest that single-strand breaks (or double-strand breaks), which are the most frequent effect of ionizing radiation, are not likely candidates for being the major pathway to the production of SCEs (Wolff, 1978a).

(3) *UV-irradiation* induces long-lived lesions (mainly thymidine dimers) which, if they are not repaired, are transformed into aberrations diming the S phase (Wolff, 1978b). The lesions responsible for SCE do not seem to be thymidine dimers, since there exists no consistent relation between the amount of excision-repair ability and the sensitivity to SCE (Wolff *et al.*, 1974; De Weerd–Jasteleyn *et al.*, 1977); SCE would therefore be induced by one or more of the less common photolesions. However, studies by Kato (1974) on the photoreactivation of UV-induced damage in Potorous cells showed that the lesions, which give rise to SCE, are photoreactivable and are, therefore, probably thymidine dimers.

(4) The main results from the comparative induction of SCE and chromosome aberrations by *chemicals* arise from Latt (1974b) and Shiraishi and Sandberg (1978), who reported a distribution pattern of MMC-induced SCEs similar to the pattern of spontaneous SCEs in normal human lymphocytes and in cells of patients with Bloom's syndrome as well. However, in Xeroderma pigmentosum (XP) cells treated with alkylating agents (Sasaki, 1973; Stich and San, 1973; Wolff *et al.*, 1977), it was shown that the frequency of chromosome aberrations is directly dependent on the ability of the cells to carry out excision repair; on the contrary, the yield of SCE is high in XP cells whether or not they carry out a low or normal level of excision repair. Since the lesions responsible for SCE are long-lived, one may suggest that after excision repair has occurred normally, the lesions producing SCE are still present. Finally, in Fanconi's anemia and XP, sensitivity to SCE caused by chemical mutagens does not correlate with the sensitivity to chromatid aberration (C.A.) formation, whereas intradiplochromatid interchange formation does. These results brought Sasaki (1977) to the conclusion that there is a two-step replication-mediated repair mechanism and that SCE and CA are its cytological manifestations. In conclusion, one might summarize that SCEs are long-lived lesions which are produced during passage in S phase and which

quite probably differ from the lesions responsible for the formation of chromosome aberrations. However, a small proportion of chromatid aberrations may arise via "complete" SCEs (Schubert and Rieger, 1981). Detailed information about the nature of SCE can be found in Wolff (1978a); Evans (1978), Scott (1980), and Schubert and Rieger (1981). Models for SCE exchanges at molecular level have also been proposed. (see Figures 2(a) and 2(b)).

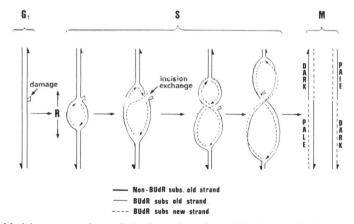

a) Replication bypass of interstrand cross link with SCE formation

(Shafer.1977) modified for clarity

| 1 | 2 | 3 | 4 | 5 | 6 |
|---|---|---|---|---|---|
| Inter-strand cross-link | Replication | Incision | Rejoining | Rejoining | Cross-link in one chromatid at SCE site |

b) Sister chromatid exchanges (SCE) may result from a variety of different DNA lesions; develop during replication (S) and involve an exchange of duplexes and not half strands.

—— Non-BUdR subs. old strand
— BUdR subs old strand.
---- BUdR subs new strand.

**Figure 2.** Model representations of the formation of an SCE: (a) Replication bypass of interstrand cross link with SCE formation, (Schaffer, 1977, and modified by Scott, 1980), (b) Sister chromatid exchanges (SCE) developing during replication (S) and involving and exchange of duplexes and not half strands (Evans, 1977).

## 7. SIGNIFICANCE OF ANEUPLOIDY

Aneuploidy may be due to different mechanisms: (i) Extensive chromosome breakage leading to chromosome loss. In this case, hyperploidy cannot be expected; (ii) Nondisjunction due to a failure of normal cell division by interaction of a turbagen with the spindle; (iii) Nondisjunction of chromosomes functionally associated in interphases (human acrocentric chromosomes) by their nucleolar organizing regions. In both cases of nondisjunction, as much hypoploidy is expected initially as hyperploidy; however, differential survival often modifies this proportion.


# PART III: CHROMOSOMAL ALTERATIONS AND CARCINOGENESIS

Epidemiological studies have demonstrated that the log–log plot of lung cancer incidence among smokers as a function of exposure time has a slope greater than one; the same may be true for the log–log plot of incidence as a function of dose (Peto, 1977). These findings and similar findings from studies of the incidence of induced tumors in mice and rats (Druckrey, 1967; Peto *et al.*, 1975) indicate that carcinogenesis is a multistep process.

It has been widely assumed that mutation represents at least one step in carcinogenesis. The evidence supporting this idea is that mutagens are carcinogens (McCann *et al.*, 1975) and, for at least some compounds, mutagenic potency is closely correlated with carcinogenic potency (Meselson and Russell, 1977). However, mutagens and certain nonmutagenic carcinogens have also been found to induce chromosomal rearrangements (Zimmermann, 1971; Ishidate and Odashima, 1977). Our aim is to examine the possibility that chromosomal rearrangement may be involved in carcinogenesis (Kinsella and Radman, 1978; Cairns, 1981).


## 8. CARCINOGENS AND CHROMOSOMAL REARRANGEMENTS

The finding that most carcinogenic agents induce base substitution and frame shift in bacterial DNA (McCann *et al.*, 1975) has led to the development of a large number of test systems designed to rapidly and inexpensively screen compounds for carcinogenic potency (Hollstein *et al.*, 1979; Montesano *et al.*, 1980). However, many of these test systems are based on genetic alterations quite distinct from base substitution and frame shift. Some test systems give positive results for some carcinogens but not for others, and some carcinogens are positive in some tests but not in others, suggesting that carcinogens may differ with respect to the types of genetic alteration they induce. Since test systems exist which detect only one or a few specific genetic alterations, the pattern of response of different systems to different carcinogens may reveal which specific types or classes of genetic alteration are involved in carcinogenesis.

Our purpose is to examine the role in carcinogenesis of those genetic alterations involving chromosomal rearrangement. For this purpose we will here define *chromosomal rearrangement* as any process of chromosomal alteration that produces either a change in nuclear DNA content or the physical exchange or reordering of pre-existing DNA sequences. Sequence alteration resulting from the insertion, deletion, or substitution of nucleotides during DNA synthesis (e.g. frame shift) is not considered to be chromosomal rearrangement. Of the mechanisms of genetic alteration involving processes capable of producing altered DNA content or sequence, only two—base substitution and frame shift—are not mechanisms of chromosomal rearrangement (Table IV). The remaining mechanisms, all mechanisms of chromosomal rearrangement, have been grouped into three classes based on specific characteristics of the processes involved. The three classes are described below. [NOTE: Because most processes of chromosomal rearrangement can involve sequence alteration, they would be classified as mutagenic by most definitions of mutation. However, homologous recombination and programmed rearrangements, such as the yeast mating-type switch (Hicks *et al.*, 1979) and the *Salmonella* flagellar antigen switch (Silverman *et al.*, 1979), are not usually thought to be mutagenic. To avoid this confusion, we have deliberately not attempted to characterize the processes of chromosomal rearrangement with respect to their ability to cause mutation].

*Homologous recombination.*   Homologous recombination involves the processes of reciprocal recombination, gene conversion, and sister chromatid exchange, which are distinct in that they can only cause the loss, amplification, or redistribution of pre-existing DNA sequences; and which are always dependent on extensive DNA homology, and capable of occurring anywhere within that homology. Processes of homologous recombination need not cause sequence alteration. (It is possible, however, that processes of homologous recombination initiating within regions of repeated DNA sequences might cause insertions or deletions).

*Nonhomologous recombination.*   Nonhomologous recombination involves processes of physical exchange or reordering of pre-existing DNA sequences that do not depend on extensive sequence homology. If any homology is involved, the process occurs at a specific site. All processes of nonhomologous recombination, including reciprocal translocation, trans-

## Table IV
### Processes of Genetic Alteration

| Process | Specific test systems[a] | Nonspecific test systems[a] |
|---|---|---|
| *Nonchromosomal rearrangement*<br>Base substitution<br>Frameshift | Ames *Salmonella*<br>*E. coli* K-12 343/113<br>Yeast haploids<br>Ouabain resistance in<br>    mammalian cells | Sperm abnormality<br>Specific locus mutation in mice<br>Drosophila recessive lethal<br>Drosophila dominant lethal<br>Dominant lethal in mice<br>Mammalian cell mutagenesis[e] |
| *Chromosomal rearrangement*<br>Homologous recombination<br>    Reciprocal recombination<br>    Gene conversion<br>    SCE | SCE<br>Yeast gene conversion<br>Yeast mitotic<br>    recombination[b]<br>Chromosome aberrations[c] | Alkaline elution<br>Unscheduled DNA synthesis<br>Transformation |
| Nonhomologous<br>    recombination<br><br>Reciprocal translocation<br>Transposition<br>Deletion<br>Insertion<br>Inversion | Micronucleus<br>Chromosome aberrations[d]<br>Heritable translocation in<br>    mice<br>Drosophila ring-<br>    X-chromosome loss<br>Drosophila translocation | |
| Ploidy change<br><br>Mitotic nondisjunction<br>Endoreduplication<br><br>Nuclear fusion | Nondisjunction in<br>    Drosophila<br>Nondisjunction in yeast<br>Drosophila sex<br>    chromosome loss<br>Sex chromosome loss<br>    in mice<br>Nondisjunction in mice | |

[a] All these systems are described in Montesano *et al.*, 1980.
[b] Only those diploid systems in which both products of an event can be recovered.
[c] Only quadriradials involving homologous sites on homologous chromosomes.
[d] Only quadriradials involving nonhomologous chromosomes or homologous chromosomes at nonhomologous sites.
[e] Except ouabain resistance.

position, deletion, insertion, and inversion, necessarily cause sequence alteration. Some transpositions, inversions, and deletions appear to be programmed in that they involve the action of specific enzyme systems on specific DNA sequences and may lead to specific changes in gene expression. Some examples of these programmed rearrangements are the yeast mating-type switch (Hicks *et al.*, 1979), the *Salmonella* flagellar antigen switch (Silverman *et al.*, 1979), G-loop inversion in bacteriophage Mu (Van de Putte *et al.*, 1980), and immunoglobin gene maturation (Davis *et al.*, 1980).

*Ploidy change.* Ploidy change involves processes such as mitotic nondisjunction, chromosome endoreduplication, and nuclear fusion, which result in the gain or loss of entire chromosomes.

The classification scheme for processes of genetic alteration presented in Table IV can also be used to classify the so-called "mutagenicity" test systems. By considering only the type of alteration to which they are sensitive, it is possible to divide the test systems into five groups (Table IV), four of which correspond to the four classes of processes of genetic alteration. Test systems in these four groups are primarily sensitive to a specific class of genetic alteration or, in some cases, to a specific type of alteration within the class. The fifth, nonspecific class consists of test systems which are sensitive to genetic alterations of more than one type and, in particular, may respond to both chromosome rearranging and nonchromosome rearranging alterations (some test systems in this class are not presented in the table).

We will use this classification of genetic alterations and mutagenicity test systems, together with the results of tests with known carcinogens, to examine the relationship between carcinogenicity and the ability to induce particular genetic alterations. The first step of this analysis is a test of the hypothesis that the ability to induce base substitution or frame shift is a general property of carcinogens. Results of the Ames *Salmonella* test, the most widely used of all the test systems, will be used as an estimate of a carcinogen's ability to induce base substitution or frame shift. McCann *et al.* (1975) have tested 174 carcinogens with Ames tests and report that 10% of them are negative. Rinkus and Legator (1979) have examined the test results of 277 carcinogens that have been tested with Ames tests and report that 23% are negative. To our knowledge, no other test system specifically sensitive to base substitution or frameshift (e.g., ouabain resistance in mammalian cells) gives positive results for carcinogens that are negative in Ames tests. Therefore, although the possibility cannot be excluded that the carcinogens which were negative in Ames tests were negative because they had not been properly activated, or because they induce specific base changes not detected by Ames strains, it appears that the ability to induce base substitution or frame shift is not a general property of carcinogens.

To determine if the ability to induce chromosomal rearrangement is a general property of carcinogens, we will consider those carcinogens (excluding metals) selected for review by Hollstein *et al.* (1979) on the basis of their having been examined in several different tests systems. Of those tests specifically sensitive to chromosomal rearrangements, Hollstein *et al.* have included results from SCE tests, chromosome aberration tests, and micronucleus tests. In order to make the analysis as complete as possible, we have examined recent literature for test results on those compounds that Hollstein *et al.* indicated had not been tested in a given test system. The carcinogens and relevant test systems are presented in Table V. For our analysis, we are particularly interested in positive results, because only if a compound has been thoroughly tested in systems sensitive to all types of chromosomal rearrangement and found to be negative in all tests can it reasonably be concluded that the compound is unable to induce chromosomal rearrangement.

Of the 61 carcinogens presented in Table V, 45 are Ames test positive and 16 are Ames test negative. Of the 45 Ames test positive compounds, 34 are also positive in at least one of the chromosomal rearrangement tests; 11, to the best of our knowledge, have not been tested in any of the specific chromosomal rearrangement tests; and 1 has been tested and found to be negative in only one of the tests. Of the 16 Ames test negative compounds, 10 are positive in at least one of the chromosomal rearrangement tests; 4 have not been tested; and 2 are negative in only one of the tests.

Although still incomplete, the data are fully consistent with the hypothesis that the ability to induce chromosomal rearrangement is correlated with carcinogenicity. Particularly encouraging is the finding that every carcinogen that has been thoroughly tested in systems specifically sensitive to chromosomal rearrangement has been found to be positive in at least one test. The incompleteness of the data makes it impossible to ask if carcinogens share a common ability to induce a specific type or class of chromosomal rearrangement and, because an insufficient number of noncarcinogens have been thoroughly tested in test systems sensitive to chromosomal rearrangement, it is not possible to say that all compounds that induce chromosomal rearrangement will have some effect on carcinogenesis.

## 9. CHROMOSOMAL REARRANGEMENT ASSOCIATED WITH CARCINOGENESIS

Chromosomal rearrangements, principally deletions, translocations, and the gain or loss of entire chromosomes, are associated with a variety of human cancers. These rearrangements tend to be specific, sometimes to the extent that a particular rearrangement may be diagnostic of a particular type of cancer. Some examples of human cancers with associated chromosomal

**Table V**
**Results from Various Test Systems with a Group of Commonly Tested Carcinogens**[a]

| | Ames | SCE | Chromosome aberrations | Micronucleus |
|---|---|---|---|---|
| 2-AAF | + | + | − | + |
| N-hydroxy-2-AAF | + | + | − | |
| N-acetoxy-2-AAF | + | + | + | |
| 2-Aminofluorene | | | | |
| β-Naphthylamine | + | +[b] | | − |
| Benzidine | + | | | + |
| Cyclophosphamide | + | + | + | + |
| Nitrogen mustard | + | + | + | |
| Captan | + | | + | |
| Benzo(a)pyrene | + | + | + | − |
| Benz(a)anthracene | + | + | − | |
| 7,12-Dimethylbenz(a)anthracene | + | + | + | + |
| 3-Methylcholanthrene | + | + | + | + |
| Methyl methane sulfonate | + | + | + | + |
| Myleran (busulfan) | + | + | + | − |
| Ethyl methane sulfonate | + | + | + | + |
| Dimethylsulfate | + | + | + | |
| β-Propiolactone | + | + | + | |
| 1,3-Propane sultone | + | + | + | |
| 1,2,3,4-Diepoxybutane | + | + | + | |
| 4-Nitroguinoline-1-oxide | + | + | + | + |
| AF-2 (furylfuramide) | + | | + | − |
| N, N-dimethylnitrosamine | + | + | + | + |
| N, N-diethylnitrosamine | + | + | + | − |
| N-methyl-N-nitro-N-nitrosoguanidine | + | + | + | |
| N-methyl-N-nitrosourea | + | + | + | |
| Aflatoxin B1 | + | + | + | + |
| Mitomycin C | + | + | + | + |
| Hycanthone | + | + | + | + |
| 3-Methyl-4-dimethylaminoazobenzene | + | | + | |
| Trenimon (triazoquone) | + | + | + | + |
| Ethylensimine | + | | + | |
| Thio-TCPA | + | + | + | + |
| Ethidium bromide | + | − | +[c] | |
| 2-Methyl-4-dimethylaminoazobenzene | + | | − | |
| 4-Aminoazobenzene | + | | | |
| 4-Aminobiphenyl | + | | | |
| p-Rosaniline | + | | | |
| Auramine | + | | | |
| ICR-170 | + | | | |
| Benzo(e)pyrene | + | | | |
| Diethylsulfate | + | | | |
| 4-Hydroxyaminoguinoline-1-oxide | + | | | |
| Safrole | + | | | |
| Cycasin | + | | | |

*(continued overleaf)*

**Table V**
**(*Continued*)**

| | Ames | SCE | Chromosome aberrations | Micronucleus |
|---|---|---|---|---|
| Carbon tetrachloride | − | +[d] | | |
| DDE | − | | + | |
| Urethane | − | + | + | + |
| Thioacetamide | − | +[d] | | |
| Thiourea | − | +[d] | | |
| Diethylstilbestrol | − | − | +[e] | |
| L-ethionine | − | | | +[b] |
| Griseofulvin | − | | +[f] | − |
| Phenobarbital | − | +[d] | +[e] | |
| Natulan | − | + | + | + |
| 1,2-Dimethylhydrazine | − | | | |
| 3-Amino-1,2,4-triazole | − | −[d] | | |
| Dieldrin | − | | | |
| Acetamide | − | | | |
| 1-Hydroxysafrole | − | | | |
| 4-Aminoantipyrene | − | | | |

[a]Carcinogens and test system results, except where noted, are from Montesano *et al.*, 1980. Blank spaces indicate no test results available.
[b]de Serres and Ashby, 1981.
[c]M. Ishidate, personal communication.
[d]Athanasious and Kyrtopoulos, 1981.
[e]Ploidy change, Ishidate and Odashima, 1977.
[f]Ploidy change, Larizza *et al.*, 1974.

rearrangements are (1) cervical carcinoma—increased ploidy (Spriggs, 1974); (2) chronic myeloid leukemia—terminal deletion of chromosome 22 (Philadelphia chromosome), often associated with a translocation to chromosome 9 (Mittelman and Levan, 1978); (3) lymphoma—reciprocal 8/14 translocation (Zech *et al.*, 1976); (4) retinoblastoma—13qD deletion (Hashem and Khalifa, 1975); (5) Meningiomas—loss or deletion of chromosome 22 (Mark *et al.*, 1972).

The finding of chromosomal rearrangements associated with human cancers does support the hypothesis that chromosomal rearrangement may be a step in carcinogenesis. However, the failure to find such an association in all cancers can not be taken as evidence against the hypothesis, simply because a rearrangement must involve on the order of $10^6$ base pairs to be detectable by current methods. Cancer cells that do not appear to have suffered any chromosomal rearrangement may have undergone either a rearrangement too small to be detected or any rearrangement of the homologous recombination variety.

Chromosomal rearrangements have also been found to be associated with induced tumors in rodents. These rearrangements appear to be characteristic of the type of tumor and the particular compound or treatment used to induce carcinogenesis (Levan *et al.*, 1977). In addition, chromosomal rearrangement, particularly ploidy change, appears to be associated with *in vitro* cell transformation (Cowell and Wigley, 1980; Saxholm and Digerness, 1980).

Although it is consistent with the idea that chromosomal rearrangement is involved in carcinogenesis, the evidence presented in this section does not prove the hypothesis since the data are equally consistent with the possibility that chromosomal rearrangements are a symptom of cancer rather than a cause.

## 10. CHROMOSOMAL REARRANGEMENTS IN HUMAN CANCER-PRONE SYNDROMES

Perhaps more direct evidence for the involvement of chromosomal rearrangement in carcinogenesis comes from the finding that the nonmalignant somatic cells of patients with certain cancer prone syndromes exhibit an increased incidence of chromosomal rearrangement. The three best characterized syndromes of this type are Bloom's syndrome, Fanconi's anemia, and ataxia telangiectasia. The type of chromosomal rearrangement found in cells of patients with each of these syndromes is characteristic (and diagnostic) of the syndrome and is found in all patients with the syndrome.

Bloom's syndrome is associated with enhanced homologous recombination. Cells of patients with Bloom's syndrome show increased mitotic recombination, detected as quadriradials involving homologous chromosomes (chiasmata) and an elevated frequency of SCEs (Chaganti *et al.*, 1974; Meyer–Kuhn, 1978). Nonhomologous recombination is also somewhat elevated, but much less than homologous.

Fanconi's anemia is associated with enhanced nonhomologous recombination. Cells of patients with Fanconi's anemia show increased reciprocal translocation, detected as quadriradials involving nonhomologous chromosomes or homologous chromosomes with exchanges at nonhomologous sites (Meyer–Kuhn, 1978; Schöder and Germen, 1974; Vogel und Schröder, 1974).

Cells of patients with ataxia telangiectasia show a high frequency of chromosome gaps and breaks (Cohen *et al.*, 1975; Thermen and Meyer–Kuhn, 1976), which probably represent deletions.

Pernicious anemia is another case in which spontaneous chromosomal breakage is associated with an increased likelihood of cancer, however, in this case only those cells which are the target cells for malignancy (i.e., bone marrow cells) show increased chromosomal rearrangements, predominantly chromosome breaks (Schröder and Kurth, 1972). The defect in patients with pernicious anemia can be alleviated by treatment with vitamin B12 and/or folic acid, a treatment which also reduces the incidence of chromosome breaks in the lymphocytes.

There are two human cancer-prone syndromes—*Xeroderma pigmentosum* and retinoblastoma—that do not appear to be associated with an increased incidence of chromosomal rearrangements. However, cells of patients with *Xeroderma pigmentosum*, which are defective in the repair of UV-induced pyrimidine dimers, do show increased UV-induced chromosomal rearrangements (Wolff, 1978), and cells of patients with retinoblastoma frequently have an inherited deletion in one of their chromosomes (Hashem and Khalifa, 1975). Thus, the characteristics of these syndromes are certainly consistent with the hypothesis that chromosomal rearrangement is involved in carcinogenesis (Kinsella and Radman, 1980), although the finding of cancer-prone syndromes not associated with chromosomal rearrangement might not be surprising in view of the multistep nature of carcinogenesis. Such syndromes might simply represent alterations in some step not involving chromosomal rearrangment.

The chromosomal rearrangements associated with human cancer-prone syndromes are clearly not a result of malignancy. However, the evidence is not sufficient to allow the conclusion that chromosomal rearrangement is a step in carcinogenesis, because the possibility that chromosomal rearrangement might simply be a byproduct of an early step in carcinogenesis can not be eliminated.

## 11. CARCINOGENIC CHROMOSOMAL REARRANGEMENT

The most direct evidence that chromosomal rearrangement can be carcinogenic comes from transfection experiments involving artificially created chromosomal rearrangements. DNA isolated from nonmalignant cells and used to transfect other nonmalignant cells caused the latter to undergo transformation, but only if the DNA had first been fragmented (sonication was used in the experiments) (Cooper *et al.*, 1980). *E. coli* and salmon sperm DNA did not cause transformation under similar conditions, so the transformation is not due to some nonspecific effect of DNA fragments. High molecular weight DNA isolated from cells transformed with fragmented DNA was able to transform other cells without fragmentation, indicating that some chromosomal rearrangement had taken place in the course of transformation.

## 12. INDUCTION OF CHROMOSOMAL REARRANGEMENT

If chromosomal rearrangements can be a step in carcinogenesis, an understanding of the mechanism of their induction by carcinogens may be of considerable importance to an understanding of cancer. Carcinogen action leading to the induction of chromosomal rearrangement might occur at two levels. At the level of substrate, a carcinogen might act to increase the number of sites on the DNA susceptible to the action of recombination enzymes already present in the cell. Alternatively, a carcinogen might act to induce or activate various enzymes whose activities stimulate recombination.

There is considerable evidence suggesting that some DNA lesions can act as preferential sites for the initiation of DNA exchange (Radding, 1978). In addition, the results of several experiments suggest that carcinogens— radiation, at least—can act epigenetically to induce recombinational activity. In the fungus, *Ustilago maydis*, radiation-induced recombination appears to require *de novo* protein synthesis, as it is completely blocked by cycloheximide (Holliday, 1975). Recombination among undamaged yeast chromosomes can be increased by fusing the cell with another cell that has been treated with x- or UV-irradiation (Fabre and Roman, 1977).

The mechanism by which radiation induces recombinational activity in *Ustilago* and yeast is not known. However, in corn, it appears that chromosome breakage alone is adequate to induce a genetic transposition system. Chromosomal instability similar to that induced by ionizing radiations (Peterson, 1960) was found to be permanently induced as an apparent consequence of the breaking of dicentric chromosomes in the course of mitotic division (Mc Clintock, 1958).

Thus, it appears that carcinogens can act to induce chromosomal rearrangement by creating or revealing sites on the DNA for recombination or by inducing or activating cellular systems resulting in a stimulation of recombination.

## 13. ROLE OF CHROMOSOMAL REARRANGEMENT IN CARCINOGENESIS

Having considered the evidence that chromosomal rearrangement may be involved in carcinogenesis and the means by which chromosomal rearrangement may be induced, we now consider the role of chromosomal rearrangement in carcinogenesis, i.e., how chromosomal rearrangement might accomplish a step towards malignancy.

It is probably safe to assume that the uncontrolled cell growth characteristic of the malignant state results either from the amplification of control factors that stimulate growth or from the loss of control factors that inhibit growth. These changes in control might result from changes in DNA sequences or from changes in RNA or protein synthesis or processing. If in the process of carcinogenesis, chromosomal rearrangements play a role in altering these controls, then the carcinogenic change must take place at the level of the DNA.

There are at least four mechanisms by which the nonhomologous recombination class of chromosomal rearrangements might affect gene expression: (i) gene inactivation involving sequence alteration of the gene itself (e.g., deletion, insertion, or inversion); (ii) gene activation or inactivation involving transposition of a gene into a region of different transcriptional activity; (iii) gene activation or inactivation involving transposition of a transcriptional control element into the vicinity of the gene in question; and (iv) gene amplification involving translocation or transposition to produce an increased number of copies of a given gene. In bacteria (Calos and Miller, 1980), yeast (Greer and Fink, 1979; Klar *et al.*, 1980), and corn (Mc Clintock, 1950) transposable elements are known to alter gene expression by each of the mechanisms (i), (ii), and (iii). In addition, mammalian immunoglobulin gene maturation has been shown to involve chromosomal rearrangement (Davis *et al.*, 1980).

The homologous recombination class of chromosomal rearrangements might affect carcinogenesis in at least three ways: (a) by allowing the expression of recessive genes by making them homozygous as a result of mitotic recombination; (b) by increasing the copy number of duplicated genes by unequal (but homologous) sister chromatid exchange; or (c) by affecting the pattern of DNA methylation and thus altering gene expression. The pattern of DNA methylation is known to affect gene expression (Razin and Riggs, 1980). If SCEs occur via a process similar to that thought to operate in mitotic recombination, then they would presumably involve the formation of hybrid or heteroduplex DNA, i.e., duplex DNA with one strand derived from each of two different parent molecules. Thus, SCEs involving newly synthesized DNA strands, which are known to be transiently undermethylated (Adams, 1974), could produce regions of duplex DNA with both strands unmethylated (Holliday, 1979).

The ploidy change class of chromosomal rearrangements can allow either the amplification of genes, by increasing ploidy, or the expression of recessive genes, by decreasing ploidy. Thus, all classes of chromosomal rearrangement (Table IV) may affect gene expression and, therefore, carcinogenesis.

## 14. MECHANISM OF CARCINOGENESIS

We conclude this chapter with a proposal concerning some of the steps of carcinogenesis, intended to account for many of the findings to date—in particular the involvement of chromosomal rearrangement—and to provide some testable predictions to help guide future work. The basis of this proposal is the idea that malignancy may be a result of the expression of cellular "cancer genes" which are either not expressed or insufficiently expressed in normal cells because they are linked with a nontranscribing control region.

The existence of cancer genes with control regions is suggested by the results of the transfection experiments described above, in which the need for fragmenting DNA from normal cells may reflect the need to separate the cancer gene from its control region. In cells transformed by the fragmented DNA, the cancer gene is presumably associated with actively transcribing DNA, since the DNA of these cells is able to transform without being fragmented.

Chromosomal rearrangements of the nonhomologous recombination class may cause activation of cancer genes either by transposing the cancer gene to a location with a transcribing control region, or by inserting a transcribing control region into the cancer gene control region or between the cancer gene and its control region. If DNA methylation is involved in the control of cancer genes, then chromosomal rearrangements of the homologous recombination class may affect expression by altering the pattern of methylation, as discussed above. It may also be possible to activate cancer genes by means of sequence alteration in the control region, which could be accomplished either by chromosomal rearrangement or by base substitution or frame shift. However, if the control region is necessary for transcription of the cancer gene, i.e., contains a promoter, sequence alteration may not be possible or else may need to be so specific as to make its occurrence unlikely. Any activation of cancer genes involving chromosomal rearrangement may require the induction of cellular recombination systems. Such induction would represent additional steps in the process of carcinogenesis.

Viral carcinogenesis may involve the activation of cellular cancer genes by virus-mediated chromosomal rearrangement. Some RNA and DNA tumor viruses have been found to carry genes of cellular origin (Duesberg, 1979). If a virus carries a cellular cancer gene, the gene may be expressed in a host cell as a result of being integrated near a transcribing control region or as a result of being associated with a transcribing control region in the viral genome.

The DNA from most transformed cells that have been examined can not cause transformation without being fragmented (Shih et al., 1978; Cooper et al., 1980), indicating that there must be a pathway of carcinogenesis not involving the linking of cancer genes with transcribing control regions. It may be that the control region is a binding site for a repressor. If so, there must be repressor genes in the cell. In such a case, an alternative and clearly multistep pathway of carcinogenesis would be inactivation of repressor genes. Inactivation of a gene could presumably be accomplished by base substitution, frame shift, integration of a virus, or any of the nonhomologous recombination class of chromosomal rearrangements. If one copy of a repressor gene is inactivated, homologous recombination or ploidy change should be able to make the cell homo- or hemizygous for the mutant allele and, after the dilution or inactivation of any repressor molecules remaining in the cell, allow activation of the cancer gene.

It may be that one of the effects of tumor promoters (e.g., TPA) and viral gene products necessary for the maintenance of the transformed state (e.g., RSV src and SV40 and polyoma "T" proteins) is to act as antagonists of the repressor, either by inactivating it more rapidly than it can be synthesized or by repressing the repressor genes. Such action could account for the reversible nature of the effects of some promoters and viral transforming proteins (Bissell and Calvin, 1979; Weinstein, 1980). In the absence of functional repressor genes, effects on repressor would not be reversible, but would hasten the appearance of the malignant state. There may be species or tissue-specific differences in repressor stability or in the number of repressor molecules per cell. Such differences could account for differences in "expression time" observed in the transformation of human and rodent cells treated with carcinogens (Kakunaga, 1977). The differences in expression time may not be related to differences in frequences of chromosomal rearrangement, which for detectable chromosomal rearrangements appear to be similar in the two types of cell (De Boer *et al.*, 1977).

ACKNOWLEDGMENTS

We thank Dr. R. Wagner for helping us write the part of this chapter dealing with chromosomal rearrangement and the mechanism of carcinogenesis, which was submitted for publication elsewhere in an extended form.

## REFERENCES

Abrahamson, S., Bender, M. A., Conger, A. D., and Wolff, S., 1973, Uniformity of radiation-induced mutation rates among different species, *Nature* **245**:460–462.

Adams, R. L. P., 1974, Newly synthesized DNA is not methylated, *Biochim. Biophys. Acta* **335**:365–373.

Arrighi, F. E., and Saunders, G. F., 1973, The relationship between repetitious DNA and constitutive heterochromatin with special reference to man, in *Modern Aspects of Cytogenetics: Constitutive Heterochromatin in Man*, Symposium Medica Hoechst.

Arrighi, F. E., and Hsu, F. C., 1965, Experimental alteration of metaphase chromosome morphology, *Exp. Cell Res.* **39**:305–318.

Athanasiou, K., and Kyrtopoulos, S. A., 1981, Induction of sister chromatid exchanges by nonmutagenic carcinogens, in *Chromosome Damage and Repair* (edited by E. Seeberg) Plenum Press, New York.

Aula, P., and Von Koskull, H., 1976, Distribution of spontaneous chromosome breaks in human chromosomes, *Hum. Genet.* **32**:143–148.

Aurias, A., Prieur, M., Dutrillaux, B., and Lejeune, J., 1978, Systematic analysis of 95 reciprocal translocations of autosomes, *Hum. Genet.* **45**:259–282.

Ayala, F., 1967, Evolution of fitness in irradiated populations of *Drosophila serrata*, *Proc. Natl. Acad. Sci. USA.* **58**:1919–1924.

Aymé, S., Mattei, J. F., Mattei, M. G., Aurran, Y., and Giraud, F., 1976, Nonrandom distribution of chromosome breaks in cultured lymphocytes of normal subjects, *Hum. Genet.* **31**:161–175.

Bak, A. L., Bak, P., and Zeuthen, J., 1979, Higher levels of organization in chromosomes, *J. Theor. Biol.* **76**:205–217.

Barbin, A., Bartsch, H., Leconte, P., and Radman, M., 1981, Studies on the miscoding properties of 1,N6-ethenoadenine and 3,N4-ethenocytosine, DNA reaction products of vinyl chloride metabolites, during *in vitro* DNA synthesis, *Nucleic Acids Res.* **9**:375–387.

Bender, M. A., Griggs, H. G., and Bedford, J. S., 1974, Mechanisms of chromosomal aberration production. III. Chemicals and ionizing radiation, *Mutat. Res.* **23**:197–212.

Beuzer, S., 1962, On the topography of the genetic fine structure, *Proc. Natl. Acad. Sci. USA.* **47**:410–415.

Bessman, M. J., Muzyeska, N., Goodman, M. T., and Schnaar, R. L., 1974, Studies on the biochemical basis of spontaneous mutation, *J. Mol. Biol.* **88**:409–421.

Bhambiani, R., Kuspira, J., and Giblak, R. E., 1973, A comparison of cell survival and chromosome damage using CHO cells synchronized with and without colcemid, *Can. J. Genet. Cytol.* **14**:605–618.

Bissell, M. J., Hatie, C., and Calvin, M., 1979, Is the product of *src* gene a promotor? *Proc. Natl. Sci. USA.* **76**:348–352.

Bodell, W. J., 1977, Nonuniform distribution of DNA repair in chromatin after treatment with methyl methane sulfonate, *Nucleic. Acid. Res.* **4**:2619–2628.

Bostock, C. J., and Sumner, A. T., 1978, Chromosome damage and repair, in *The Eucaryotic Chromosome* (edited by C. J. Bostock and A. T. Sumner) North Holland Publishing Company, Amsterdam, pp. 437–473.

Bourgeois, C. A., 1974, Distribution of mitomycin-C-induced damage in human chromosomes with special reference to regions of repetitive DNA, *Chromosoma* **48**:203–211.

Brinkley, B. R., and Rao, P. M., 1973, Nitrous oxide effects on the mitotic apparatus and chromosome movement in *Hela* cells, *J. Cell Biol.* **58**:96–106.

Brinkley, B. R., and Shaw, H. W., 1970, Ultrastructural aspects of chromosome damage, in *Genetic Concepts and Neoplasma.* A collection of papers presented at the XXIIIth An. Symp. on Fundamental Cancer Research, Williams and Wilkins, Baltimore, pp 313–345.

Brewen, J. G., Preston, R. J., Jones, K. P., and Gosslee, G. E., 1973, Genetic hazards of ionizing radiations: cytogenetic extrapolations from mouse to man, *Mutat. Res.* **17**:245–254.

Brewen, J. G., 1976, Practical evaluation of mutagenicity data in mammals for estimating human risk, *Mutat. Res.* **41**:15–24.

Brøgger, A., 1971, Apparently spontaneous chromosome damage in human leukocytes and the nature of chromatid gaps, *Humangenetik* **13**:1–14.

Brøgger, A., 1975, Is the chromatid gap a folding defect due to protein change? Evidence from mercaptoethanol treatment of human lymphocyte chromosomes, *Hereditas* **80**:131–136.

Brøgger, A., 1977, Nonrandom localization of chromosome damage in human cells and targets for clastogenic action, in *Chromosomes Today, Vol. 6* (edited by A. de la Chapelle and M. Sorsa), Elsevier, New York, pp. 297–306.

Brøgger, A., 1979, Chromosome damage in human mitotic cells after *in vivo* and *in vitro* exposure to mutagens, in *Genetic Damage in Man Caused by Environmental Agents*, (edited by R. Berg), Academic Press, New York, pp. 87–99.

Bruttag, D., and Kornberg, A., 1972, Enzymatic synthesis of deoxyribonucleic acid, XXXVI: A proofreading action for the $3' \rightarrow 5'$ exonuclease activity in deoxyribonucleic acid polymerases, *J. Biol. Chem.* **247**:241–248.

Buckton, K. E., 1976, Identification with G- and R-banding of the position of breakage points induced in human chromosomes by *in vitro* x-irradiation, *Int. J. Radiat. Biol.* **29(5)**:475–488.

Cabral, F., Sobel, M. E., and Gottesman, M. M., 1980, CHO mutants resistant to colchicine, colcemid, or griveofulvin have an altered $\beta$-tubulin, *Cell* **20**:29–36.

Cairns, J., 1981, The origin of human cancers, *Nature* **289**:353–357.

Calos, M. P., and Miller, J. H., 1980, Transposable elements, *Cell* **20**:579–595.

Cann, J. R., and Hirman, N. D., 1975, Interaction of chlorpromazine with brain microtubule subunit protein, *Mol. Pharmacol.* **11**:256–267.

Caspersson, T., Haglund, U., Lindell, B., and Zech, L., 1972, Radiation-induced nonrandom chromosome breakage, *Exp. Cell Res.* **75**:541–543.

Carrano, A. V., 1975, Induction of chromosome aberrations in human lymphocytes by X rays and fission neutrons: Dependence on cell cycle stage, *Radiat. Res.* **63**:403–421.

Cech, T., and Pardue, M. L., (1977), Cross-linking of DNA with trimethylpsoralen is a probe for chromatin structure, *Cell* **11**:631–640.

Chaganti, R. S. K., Schönberg, S., and German, J., 1974, A many-fold increase in sister chromatid exchanges in Bloom's syndrome lymphocytes, *Proc. Natl. Acad. Sci. USA.* **71(11)**:4508–4512.

Chu, E. H. Y., Giles, N. H., and Passano, K., (1962), Types and frequencies of human chromosome aberrations induced by X rays, *Proc. Natl. Acad. Sci. USA.* **48**:522–532.

Cleaver, J. E., 1975, Methods for studying repair of DNA damaged by physical and chemical carcinogens, in *Methods in Cancer Research* (edited by H. Busch) Academic Press, New York, Vol. 11, pp. 123–165.

Cleaver, J. E., 1978, DNA repair and its coupling to DNA replication in eukaryotic cells, *Biochim. Biophys. Acta* **516**:489–516.

Cohen, M. M., Shaham, M., Dagan, J., Shmueli, E., and Kohn, G., 1975, Cytogenetic investigations in families with ataxia telangiectasia, *Cytogenet. Cell Genet.* **15**:338–356.

Comings, D. E., 1978, Mechanisms of chromosome banding and implications for chromosome structure, *Ann. Rev. Genet.* **12**:25–46.

Comings, D. E., 1974, What is a chromosome break? in *Chromosomes and Cancer* (edited by J. Eerman) John Wiley and Sons, New York, pp. 95–113.

Comings, D. E., 1980, Nonhistone proteins of chromosomes and the nucleus, *Abstract of the 2nd Int. Congress on Cell Biology*, Berlin, p. 113.

Cooke, P., Seabright, M., and Wheeler, M., 1978, The differential distribution of x-ray-induced chromosome lesions in trypsin-banded preparations from human subjects, *Humangenetik* **28**:221–231.

Cooper, G. M., Okenquist, S., and Silverman, L., 1980, Transforming activity of DNA of chemically transformed and normal cells, *Nature* **284**:418–421.

Corneo, G., Ginelli, E., and Polli, E., 1968, Isolation of the complementary strands of a human satellite DNA, *J. Mol. Biol.* **33**:331–335.

Coulondre, C. and Miller, J. H., 1977, Genetic studies of the Lac repressor. IV. Mutagen specificity in the Lac *i* gene of *Escherichia coli, J. Mol. Biol.* **117**:577–593.

Cowell, J. K., and Wigley, C. B., 1980, Changes in DNA content during *in vitro* transformation of mouse salivary gland epithelium, *J. Natl. Cancer Inst.* **64**:1443–1448.

Cox, E. C., and Gibson, T. C., 1974, Selection for high mutation rates in chemostats, *Genetics* **77**:169–184.

Crossen, P. E., Drets, M. E., Arrighi, F. E., and Johnston, D. A., 1977, Analysis of the frequency and distribution of sister chromatid exchanges in cultured human lymphocytes, *Hum. Genet.* **35**:345–352.

Davis, M. M., Kim, S. K., and Hood, L., 1980, Immunoglobin class switching: Developmentally regulated DNA rearrangements during differentiation, *Cell* **22**:1–2.

De Boer, P., Van Buul, P. P. W., Van Beek, R., Van Der Hoeven, F. A., and Natarajan, A. T., 1977, Chromosomal radiosensitivity and karyotype in mice using cultured peripheral blood lymphocytes, and comparison with this system in man, *Mutat. Res.* **42**:379–394.

Defais, M., Caillet-Fauquet, P., Fox, M. S., and Radman, M., 1976, Induction kinetics of mutagenic DNA repair activity in *E. coli* following UV-irradiation, *Mol. Gen. Genet.* **148**:125–131.

de Serres, F. J., 1979, Problems associated with the application of short-term tests for mutagenicity in man-screening programs, *Environ. Mutagen.* **1**:203–208.

de Serres, F., and Ashby, J. (eds.), 1981, Short-term tests for carcinogenesis, in *Report of the International Collaborative Program*, Elsevier, New York.

De Weerd-Kasteleyn, G. A., Keijzer, W., Rainaldi, G., and Bootsman, D., 1977, Introduction of SCE in xeroderma pigmentation cells following exposure to UV light, *Mutat. Res.* **46**:163; Abstract of paper on DNA repair mechanisms in mammalian cells, *IInd Int. Workshop, May 1976, Netherlands.*

Deysson, G., 1968, Antimitotic substances, *Int. Rev. Cytol.* **24**:99–143.

Deysson, G., 1976, Recherches sur les inhibiteurs microtubulaires, *J. Eur. Toxicol.* **9**:259–270.

Doubleday, O. P., Lecomte, P., Brandenburger, A., Diver, W. P., and Radman, M., 1982, Replication and mutagenesis of irradiated single-stranded phage DNA, in *Induced Mutagenesis: Molecular Mechanisms and Their Implications for Environmental Protection* (edited by C. Lawrence) Plenum Press, New York, in press.

Doubleday, O. P., Michel-Maenhaut, G., Brandenburger, A., Lecomte, P., and Radman, M., 1981, Inhibition or absence of DNA proofreading exonuclease is not sufficient to allow copying of pyrimidine dimers, in *Chromosome Damage and Repair* (edited by E. Seeberg) Plenum Press.

Drake, J. W., 1973, The genetic control of spontaneous and induced mutation rates in bacteriophage T4, *Genetics (suppl.)* **75**:45–51.

Drake, J. W. and Baltz, R. H., 1976, The biochemistry of mutagenesis in *Annual Review of Mutagenesis*, pp. 11–37.

Drake, J. W., and Koch, R. E., 1976, *Mutagenesis: Benchmark Papers Vol. 4*, Dowden, Hutchinson, and Ross, Inc.

Drake, J. W., 1977, Fundamental mutagenic mechanisms and their significance for environmental mutagenesis, in *Progress in Genetic Toxicology* (edited by D. Scott, B. A. Bridges, and F. H. Bels) Elsevier, Amsterdam, pp. 43–55.

Druckrey, H., 1967, Quantitative aspects in chemical carcinogenesis, in *Potential Carcinogenic Hazards from Drugs*, UICC Monograph Series 7:60–87, Springer-Verlag, Berlin.

Du Bos, C., Veigas-Pequignot, E., and Dutrillaux, B., 1978, Localization of x-ray-induced chromatid breaks using three consecutive stains, *Mutat. Res.* **49**:127–131.

Deusberg, P. H., 1979, Transforming genes of retroviruses, *Cold Spring Harbor Symp. Quant. Bio.* **44**:13–29.

Dustin, P., 1978, *Microtubules*, Springer-Verlag, Berlin.

Dutrillaux, B., Couturier, J., Viegas-Pequignot, E., and Schaison, G., 1977, Localization of chromatid breaks in Fanconi's anemia using three consecutive stains, *Hum. Genet.* **37**:65–71.

Evans, H. J., 1962, Chromosome aberrations induced by ionizing radiations, *Int. Rev. Cytol.* **13**:221–321.

Evans, H. J., 1974, Effects of ionizing radiation on mammalian chromosomes, in *Chromosomes and Cancer*, (edited by J. German) John Wiley and Sons, New York, pp. 191–237.

Evans, H. J., 1977a, Molecular mechanisms in the induction of chromosome aberrations, in *Progress in Genetic Toxicology* (edited by D. Scott, B. A. Bridges, and F. H. Sobels) Elsevier, Amsterdam, pp. 57–74.

Evans, H. J., 1977b, Some facts and fancies relating to chromosome structure in man, in *Advances in Human Genetics* (edited by H. Harris and K. H. Hirschhorn) Vol. 8, Plenum Press, New York.

Evans, J. A., Canning, N., Hunter, A. G. W., Martsolf, J. T., Ray, M., Thompson, D. R., and Hamerton, J. L., 1978, A cytological survey of 14,069 newborn infants, *Cytogenet. Cell Genet.* **20**:96–123.

Fabre, F., and Roman, H., 1977, Genetic evidence for inducibility of recombination competence in yeast, *Proc. Natl. Acad. Sci. USA.* **74**:1667–1671.

Felsenberg, G., 1978, Chromatin, *Nature* **271**:115–122.

Feron, V. J., Grice, H. C., Griesemer, R., and Peto, R., 1980, Report 1:Basic requirements for long-term assays for carcinogenicity, in *Long-Term and Short-Term Screening Assays for Carcinogens: A Critical Appraisal*, IARC Monographs, Suppl. 2, pp. 21–83.

Fox, D. P., 1967, The effects of X rays on the chromosomes of locust embryos. IV. Dose response and variation in sensitivity of the cell cycle for the induction of chromatid aberrations, *Chromosoma* 20:413–441.

Friedrich, U., and Nielsen, J., 1973, Break points in reciprocal autosomal translocations, *Hereditas* 74:141–144.

Funes-Cravioto, F., Yakovienko, K. N., Kuleshov, N. P., and Zhurkov, V. S., 1974, Localization of chemically induced breaks in chromosomes of human leucocytes, *Mutat. Res.* 23:87–105.

Galas, D. J., and Branscomb, A. W., 1978, Enzymatic determinants of DNA polymerase accuracy. Theory of coliphage T4 polymerase mechanisms, *J. Mol. Biol.* 124:653–687.

Galloway, S. H., and Evans, H. J., 1975, Sister chromatid exchange in human chromosomes from normal individuals and patients with ataxia telangiectosia, *Cytogenet. Cell Genet.* 15:17.

Galloway, S. H., and Wolff, S. H., 1979, The relation between chemically induced sister chromatid exchanges and chromatid breakage, *Mutat. Res.* 61:297–307.

Geard, C. R., Colvett, R. D., and Rohrig, N., 1980, On the mechanics of chromosomal aberrations, a study with single and multiple spatially associated protons, *Mutat. Res.* 69:81–99.

Gerber, G. B., Léonard, A., and Jacquet, P., 1980, Toxicity, mutagenicity, and teratogenicity of lead, *Mutat. Res.* 76:115–141.

Giraud, F., Ayme, S., Mattei, J. F., and Mattei, M. G., 1976, Constitutional chromosomal breakage, *Hum. Genet.* 34:125–136.

Glideman, B. W., and Radman, M., 1980, *Escherichia coli* mutator mutants deficient in methylation instructed DNA mismatch correction, *Proc. Natl. Acad. Sci. USA.* 77: 1063–1067.

Goetz, P., Sram, R. J., and Dohnalova, J., 1975, Relationship between experimental results in mammals and man. I. Cytogenetic analysis of bone marrow injury induced by a single dose of cyclophosphamide, *Mutat. Res.* 31:247–254.

Gosden, J. R., Buckland, R. A., Clayton, R. P., and Evans, H. J., 1975, Chromosomal localization of DNA sequences in condensed and dispersed human chromatin, *Exp. Cell Res.* 92:138–147.

Gottesman, S., 1981, Genetic control of the SOS system in *E. coli, Cell* 23:1–2.

Greer, H., and Fink, G., 1979, Unstable transpositions of *his4* in yeast, *Proc. Natl. Acad. Sci. USA.* 76:4006–4010.

Hadlaczky, G., Sumner, A. T., and Ross, A., 1981, Protein-depleted chromosomes. I. Structure of isolated protein-depleted chromosomes, *Chromosoma* 81:537–555.

Haglund, U., and Zech, I., 1979, Simultaneous staining of sister chromatid exchanges and Q-bands in human chromosomes after treatment with methyl methane sulphonate, quinacrine mustard, and quinacrine, *Hum. Genet.* 49:307–317.

Hanawalt, P. C., Cooper, P. K., Ganesan, A. K., and Smith, C. A., 1979, DNA repair in bacteria and mammalian cells, *Annu. Rev. Biochim.* 48:783–836.

Hansmann, I., Röhrborn, G., and Neher, J., 1975, Chromosome aberrations in metaphase. II. Oocytes of Chinese hamsters (*cricetulus grisues*), *Mutat. Res.* 29:218–219.

Hashem, N., and Khalifa, S., 1975, Retinoblastoma: a model of hereditary fragile chromosomal regions, *Hum. Hered.* 25:35–49.

Heddle, J. A., Bodycotte, J., 1970, On the formation of chromosomal aberrations, *Mutat. Res.* 9:117–126.

Herich, R., 1969, The effect of zinc on the structure of chromosomes and on mitosis, *Nucleus* 12:81–85.

Herreros, B., and Gianelli, F., 1967, Spatial distribution of old and new chromated subunits and frequency of chromatid exchanges in induced human lymphocyte endoreduplications, *Nature* 216:286–288.

Hicks, J., Strathern, J. N., and Klar, A. J. S., 1979, Transposable mating types genes in *Saccharomyces cerevisiae, Nature* **282**:478–483.

Holliday, R., 1975, Further evidence for an inducible recombination repair system in *Ustilago maydis, Mutat. Res.* **29**:149–153.

Holliday, R., 1979, A new theory of carcinogenesis, *Br. J. Cancer* **40**:513–522.

Hollstein, M., McCann, J., Angelosanto, F. A., and Nichols, W. W., 1979, Short-term tests for carcinogens and mutagens, *Mutat. Res.* **65**:133–226.

Holmberg, M., and Jonasson, J., 1973, Preferential location of x-ray-induced chromosome breakage in the R-bands of human chromosomes, *Hereditas* **74**:57–68.

Hsu, T. C., 1975, A possible function of constitutive heterochromatin: the bodyguard hypothesis, Symposium No. **14**:Chromosome structure, *Genetics* **79**:137–150.

IARC, 1980, IARC monographs on long-term and short-term screening assays for carcinogens: A critical appraisal, Suppl. 2, Lyon, International Agency for Research on Cancer.

Ishidate, M., Jr., and Odashima, S., 1977, Chromosome tests with 134 compounds on Chinese hamster cells *in vitro*—a screening for chemical carcinogens, *Mutat. Res.* **48**:337–354.

Jacobs, P. A., Buckton, K. A., Cunningham, C., and Newton, M., 1974, An analysis of the break points of structural rearrangements in man, *J. Med. Genet.* **11(1)**:50–64.

Kakunaga, T., 1977, The transformation of human diploid cells by chemical carcinogens, in *Origins of Human Cancer* (edited by Hiatt, H. H., Watson, J. D., and Winsten, J. A.), Cold Spring Harbor Laboratory, New York, pp. 1537–1548.

Kato, H., 1974, Photoreactivation of sister chromatid exchanges induced by ultraviolet irradiation, *Nature* **249**:552–558.

Kim, M. A., 1974, Chromatidaustausch und Heterochromatinveranderungen menschlicher Chromosomenach BUdR-Markierung, *Hum. Genet.* **25**:179–188.

Kinsella, A. R., and Radman, M., 1978, Tumor promotor induces sister chromatid exchanges: Relevance to mechanisms of carcinogenesis, *Proc. Natl. Acad. Sci., USA.* **75**:6149–6153.

Kinsella, A. R., and Radman, M., 1980, Inhibition of carcinogen-induced chromosomal aberrations by an anticarcinogenic protease inhibitor, *Proc. Natl. Acad. Sci. USA.* **77**:3544–3547.

Klar, A. J. S., McIndoo, J., Strathern, J. N., and Hicks, J. B., 1980, Evidence for a physical interaction between the transposed and the substituted sequences during mating-type gene transposition in yeast, *Cell* **22**:291–298.

Kornberg, R. D., 1977, Structure of chromatin, *Annu. Rev. Biochem.* **46**:931–954.

Kucerova, M., and Polivkova, L., 1976, Banding technique used for the detection of chromosomal aberrations induced by radiation and alkylating agents tepa and epichlorohydrin, 1976, *Mutat. Res.* **34**:279–290.

Lacks, S., and Greenberg, B., 1977, Complementary specificity of restriction endonucleases of *Diplococcus pneumoniae* with respect to DNA methylation, *J. Mol. Biol.* **114**:153–168.

Larizza, L., Simoni, G., Tredici, F., and De Carli, L., 1974, Griseofulvin: A potential agent of chromosomal segregation in cultured cells, *Mutat. Res.* **25**:123–130.

Latt, S. A., 1973, Microfluorometric detection of DNA replication in human metaphase chromosomes, *Proc. Natl. Acad. Sci. USA.* **70**:3395–3399.

Latt, S. A., 1974, Localization of sister chromatid exchanges in human chromosomes, *Science* **185**:74–76.

Latt, S. A., Stetten, G., Jürgens, L. A., Buchanan, G. R., and Gerald, P. S., 1975, Induction by alkylating agents of sister chromatid exchanges and chromatid breaks in Fanconi's anemia, *Genetics* **72(10)**:4066–4070.

Laval, J., 1980, Enzymology of DNA repair, in *Molecular and Cellular Aspects of Carcinogen Screening Tests*, (edited by Montesano, R., Bartsch, H., and Tomatis, L.), IARC Scientific Publ., Vol. 27, pp. 55–73.

Lehmann, A. R., 1972, Postreplication repair of DNA in UV-irradiated mammalian cells, *J. Mol. Biol.* **66**:319–337.

Leonard, A., and Lauwerys, P. R., 1980, Carcinogenicity, teratogenicity, and mutagenicity of arsenic, *Mutat. Res.* **75**:49–62.

Levan, A., Levan, G., and Mitelman, F., 1977, Chromosomes and cancer, *Hereditas* **86**:15–30.

Lilley, D. M., and Pardon, J. F., 1979, Structure and function of chromatin, *Ann. Rev. Genet.*, **13**:197–233.

Lindahl, T., 1979, DNA glycosylases, *Progr. Nucl. Acids Res. and Mol. Biol.*, **22**:135–192.

Lindgren, V., 1981, The location of chromosome breaks in Bloom's syndrome, *Cytogenet. Cell Genet.* **29**:99–106.

Loeb, L. A., Weymouth, L. A., Kunkel, T. A., Gopinathan, K. P., Beckman, R. A., and Dube, D. K., 1979, Fidelity of DNA synthesis, *Cold Spring Harbor Symp. Quant. Biol.* **43**:921–927.

Lubs, H. A., and Samuelson, J., 1967, Chromosome abnormalities in lymphocytes from normal human subjects, a study of 3720 cells, *Cytogenetics* **6**:402–411.

Madle, S., and Obe, G., 1980, Methods for analysis of the mutagenicity of indirect mutagens–carcinogens in eukaryotic cells, *Hum. Genet.* **56**:7–20.

Mark, J., Levan, G., and Mitelman, F., 1972, Identification by fluorescence of the G chromosome lost in human meningiomas, *Hereditas* **71**:163–168.

Marsland, D., 1966, Antimitotic effects of colchicine and hydrostatic pressure, synergistic action on the cleaving eggs of *Lytechinus variegatus, J. Cell Physiol.* **67**:333–338.

Mattei, M. G., Ayme, S., Mattei, J. F., Aurran, Y., and Giraud, F., 1979, Distribution of spontaneous chromosome breaks in man, *Cytogenet. Cell Genet.* **23**:95–102.

McCann, J., Choi, E., Yamasaki, E., and Ames, B. N., 1975, Detection of carcinogens as mutagens in the *Salmonella*–microsome test: assay of 300 chemicals, *Proc. Natl. Acad. Sci. USA.* **72**:5135–5139.

McClintock, B., 1950, The origin and behavior of mustable loci in maize, *Proc. Natl. Acad. Sci. USA.* **36**:344–355.

Meselson, M., and Russell, K., 1977, Comparison of carcinogenic and mutagenic potency, in *Origins of Human Cancer* (edited by Hiatt, H. H., Watson, J. D., and Winsten, J. A.), Cold Spring Harbor Laboratory, New York, pp. 1473–1481.

Meyer–Kuhn, E., 1978, Mitotic chiasmata and other quandriradials in mitomycin C-treated Bloom's syndrome lymphocytes, *Chromosoma* **66**:287–297.

Mitelman, F., and Levan, G., 1978, Clustering of aberrations to specific chromosomes in human neoplasms. III. Incidence and geographic distribution of chromosome aberrations in 856 cases, *Hereditas* **89**:207–232.

Montesano, R., Bartsch, H., and Tomatis, L. (eds.), 1980, Long-term and short-term screening assays for carcinogens, a critical appraisal, IARC Monographs, Suppl. 2, IARC, Lyon.

Morad, M., and Elzawahri, M., 1977, Nonrandom distribution of cyclophosphamide-induced chromosome breaks, *Mutat. Res.* **42**:125–130.

Morad, M., Jonasson, J., and Lindsten, J., 1973, Distribution of mitomycin-C-induced breaks on human chromosomes, *Hereditas* **74**:273–282.

Morgan, W. F., and Crossen, P. E., 1977, The frequency and distribution of sister chromatid exchanges in human chromosomes, *Hum. Genet.* **38**:271–278.

Moutschen, J., 1979, Introduction à la toxicologie génétique, *Masson*, Paris.

Nakagome, Yasvo and Chiyo, 1976, Nonrandom distribution of exchange points in patients with structural rearrangements, *Am. J. Hum. Genet.* **28**:31–41.

Natarajan, A. T., Obe, G., Zeeland, A. A., Palitti, F., Meijers, M., and Verdegaal-Immerzeel, A. M., 1980, Molecular mechanisms involved in the production of chromosomal aberration. II. Utilization of neurospora endonuclease for the study of aberration production by X rays in $G_1$ and $G_2$ stages of the cell cycle, *Mutat. Res.* **69**:293–305.

Nielsen, J., and Rasmussen, K., 1976, Distribution of break points in reciprocal translocations in children ascertained in population studies, *Hereditas* **82**:73–78.

Obe, G., and Luers, H., 1972, Inter- and intrachromosomal distribution of achromatic lesions and chromatic breaks in human chromosomes, *Mutat. Res.,* **16**:337–339.

Oksala, T., and Therman, E., 1974, Mitotic abnormalities and cancer, in *Chromosomes and Cancer* (edited by J. Eerman) John Wiley and Sons, New York, pp. 239–263.

Ostergren, G., 1951, Narcotized mitosis and the precipitation hypothesis of narcosis, in *Méchanisme de la Narcose (Colloques Internationeaux du Centre National de la Recherche Scientific),* Vol. 26, p. 77.

Olsson, M., and Lindahl, T., 1980, Repair of alkylated DNA in *E. Coli*: methyl group transfer from $O^6$-methyl guanine to a protein cysteine residue, *J. Biol. Chem.* **225**:10569–10571.

Pathak, S., Stock, A. D., and Lusby, A., 1975, A combination of sister chromatid differential staining and Giemsa banding, *Experientia* **31**:916–917.

Paulson, J. R., and Laemmli, U. K., 1977, The structure of histone-depleted metaphase chromosomes, *Cell* **12**:817–828.

Perry, P., and Evans, S., 1974, New Giemsa method for the differential staining of sister chromatids, *Nature* **251**:156–158.

Peterson, P. A., 1960, The plae green mutable system in maize, *Genetics* **45**:115–126.

Peto, R., Roe, F. J. C., Lee, P. N., Levy, L., and Clack, J., 1975, Cancer and aging in mice and men, *Br. J. Cancer* **32**:441.

Peto, R., 1977, Epidemiology, multistage models, and short-term mutagenicity tests, in *Origins of Human Cancer* (edited by Hiatt, H. H., Watson, J. D., and Winsten, J. A.), Cold Spring Harbor Laboratory, New York, pp. 1403–1428.

Radding, C. M., 1978, Genetic recombination: strand transfer and mismatch repair, *Annu. Rev. Biochem.* **47**:847–880.

Radman, M., 1977, On the mechanism and genetic control of mutation: an approach to carcinogenesis, *Colloques Internationaux du CNRS.* **256**:213–306.

Radman, M., Villani, G., Boiteux, S., Defais, M., Caillet–Fauquet, P., and Spadari, S., 1977, On the mechanism and genetic control of mutagenesis induced by carcinogenic mutagens, in *Origins of Human Cancer*, (edited by Hiatt, H., Watson, J. D., and Winsten, J.), Cold Spring Harbor Laboratory, pp. 903–921.

Radman, M., Villani, G., Boiteux, S., Kinsella, A. R., Glickman, B. W., and Spadari, S., 1979, Replicational fidelity: mechanisms of mutation avoidance and mutation fixation, *Cold Spring Harbor Symp. Quant. Biol.* **43**:937–946.

Radman, M., 1980, Is there SOS induction in mammalian cells? *Photochem. Photobiol.* **32**:823–830.

Radman, M., Wagner, R. E., Glickman, B. W., and Meselson, M., 1980, DNA methylation, mismatch repair and genetic stability, in *Progress in Environmental Mutagenesis,* (edited by Alačevič, M.), Elsevier, Amsterdam, pp. 121–130.

Ramel, C., 1969, Genetic effects of organic mercury compounds. I. Cytological investigations on allium roots, *Hereditas* **61**:208–230.

Ramel, C., 1972, Genetic effects, in *Mercury in the Environment, A. Toxicological Appraisal* (edited by Friberg, L., and Vostel, J.) CRC Press, pp. 169–181.

Razin, A., and Riggs, A. D., 1980, DNA methylation and gene function, *Science* **210**:604–610.

Read, J., 1959, Radiation biology of *Vicia faba* in relation to the general problem, *Int. J. Radiol.* **9**:53–65.

Regan, J. D., and Setlow, R. B., 1974, Two forms of repair in the DNA of human cells damaged by chemical carcinogens and mutagens, *Cancer Res.* **34**:3318–3325.

Revees, B. R., and Margoles, C., 1974, Preferential location of chlorambucil induced breakage in the chromosomes of normal human lymphocytes, *Mutat. Res.* **26**:205–208.

Revell, S. H., 1959, The accurate estimation of chromatid breakage and its relevance to a new interpretation of chromatid aberrations induced by ionizing radiation, *Proc. R. Soc. London Ser. B* **150**:563–589.

Revell, S. H., 1963, Chromatid aberrations—the generalized theory, in *Radiation-Induced Chromosome Aberrations*, by S. Wolff, Columbia University Press, New York, pp. 41–72.

Revell, S. H., 1966, Evidence for a dose-squared term in the dose-response curve for real chromatid discontinuities induced by X rays and some theoretical consequences thereof, *Mutat. Res.* **32:**34–53.

Rinkus, S. J., and Legator, M. S., 1979, Chemical characterization of 365 known or suspected carcinogens and their correlation with mutagenic activity in the *Salmonella typhimurium* system, *Cancer Res.* **39:**3289–3318.

Rodman, T. C., Flehinger, B. J., and Rohlf, F. J., 1980, Metaphase chromosome associations: Colcemid distorts the pattern, *Cytogenet. Cell Genet.* **27:**98–110.

Röhrborn, G., and Hansmann, I., 1971, Induced chromosome aberrations in unfertilized oocytes of mice, *Humangenetik* **13:**184–198.

Roobal, A., Golle, K., and Pogron, C. I., 1977, Evidence that griseofulvin binds to a microtubule associated protein, *FEBS Letters* **75:**149–158.

Roth, L. E., 1967, Electron microscopy of mitosis in amebae. III. Cold and urea treatments: A basis for tests of direct effects of mitotic inhibitors on microtubule formation, *J. Cell Biol.* **34:**47–59.

Rupp, W. D., Wilde, C. E., III, Reno, D. L., and Howard-Flouders, P., 1971, Exchanges between DNA strands in UV-irradiated *E. coli, J. Mol. Biol.* **61:**25–44.

San Roman, C., and Bobrow, M., 1973, The sites of radiation-induced breakage in human lymphocyte chromosomes, determined by quinacrine fluorescence, *Mutat. Res.* **18:**325–331.

Sasaki, M. S., 1977, Sister chromatid exchange and chromatid interchange as possible manifestation of different DNA repair processes, *Nature* **269:**623–625.

Sasaki, M. S., 1973, DNA repair capacity and susceptibility to chromosome breakage in xeroderma pigmentosum cells, *Mutat. Res.* **20:**291–293.

Sathaich, V., and Venkat Reddy, P., 1973, Chromosome spreading by zinc ethylene pindithiocarbamate "zinc ciba," *Curr. Sci.* **42:**143–144.

Savage, J. R. K., Bigger, T. R. L., and Watson, G. E., 1974, Location of quinacrine mustard-induced chromatid exchange points in relation to ASG bands in human chromosomes, *Chromosomes Today* **5:**281–291.

Savage, J. R. K., 1976, Classification and relationship of induced chromosomal structural changes, *J. Med. Genet.* **13:**103–122.

Sawada, M., and Ishidate, M., 1978, Colchicine-like effect of diethylstilbestrol (DES) on mammalian cells *in vitro, Mutat. Res.* **57:**175–182.

Sax, K., 1938, Chromosome aberrations induced by X rays, *Genetics* **23:**494–516.

Saxholm, H. J., and Digernes, V., 1980, Progressive loss of DNA and lowering of the chromosomal mode in chemically transformed C3H/10T½ cells during development of their oncogenic potential, *Cancer Res.* **40:**4254–4260.

Schaap, T., Sagi, M., and Cohen, M. M., 1980, Chromosome-specific patterns of mitomycin-C-induced rearrangements in human lymphocytes, *Cytogenet. Cell Genet.* **28:**240–250.

Schalet, A. P., and Sankaranarayanan, 1976, Evolution and reevaluation of genetic radiation hazards in man, *Mutat. Res.* **35:**341–370.

Scheid, W., and Traut, H., 1971, On the nature of a chromatic lesions ("gaps") induced by X rays in chromosomes of *Vicia faba, Z. Naturforsch.* **26B:**1384–1385.

Schnedl, W., Pumberger, W., Czaker, R., Wagenbichler, P., and Schwarzacher, M. G., 1976, Increased SCE events in the human late replicating, *Hum. Genet.* **32:**199–202.

Schroeder, T. M., and Kurth, R., 1971, Spontaneous chromosomal breakage and high incidence of leukemia in inherited disease, *Blood* **37:**96–112.

Schroeder, T. M., and German, J., 1974, Bloom's syndrome and Fanconi's anemia: Demonstration of two distinctive patterns of chromosome disruption and rearrangement, *Humangenetik* **25:**299–306.

Schubert, J., and Rieger, R., 1981, Sister chromatid exchanges and heterochromatin, *Hum. Genet.* **57**:119–130.

Schwarzacher, H. G., 1979, V. structural differences along the chromosomes (chromosome banding) in *Handbuch der Microscopischen Anatomie des Menschen: 1/3 Chromosomen*, Springer-Verlag, Berlin, pp. 33–48.

Scott, D., and Evans, H. J., 1967, X-ray-induced aberrations in *Vicia faba*: changes in response during the cell cycle, *Mutat. Res.* **4**, 579–599.

Scott, D., Fox, M., and Fox, B. W., 1975, Differential induction of chromosome aberrations in mammalian cell lines, *Mutat. Res.* **29**:201–202.

Scott, D., 1980, Molecular mechanisms of chromosome structural changes, in *Progress in Environmental Mutagenesis* (edited by M. Alačevič), Elsevier, Amsterdam, pp. 101–113.

Seabright, M., 1973, High-resolution studies on the pattern of induced exchanges in the human karotype, *Chromosoma* **40**:333–346.

Shafer, D. A., 1973, Binding human chromosomes in culture with actonomicyn D., *Lancet* **1**:828–829.

Shih, C., Shilo, B. Z., Goldfarb, M. P., Dannenberg, A., and Wienberg, R. A., 1979, Passage of phenotypes of chemically transformed cells via transfection of DNA and chromatin, *Proc. Natl. Acad. Sci. USA.* **76**, 5714–5718.

Shiraishi, Y., and Sandberg, A. A., 1977, The relationship between sister chromatid exchanges and chromosome aberrations in Bloom's syndrome, *Cytogenet. Cell Genet.* **18**:13–23.

Silverman, M., Zieg, J., Hilmen, M., and Simon, M., 1979, Phase variation in *Salmonella*: Genetic analysis of a recombinational switch, *Proc. Natl. Acad. Sci. USA.* **76**:391–395.

Smyth, D. R., and Evans, H. J., 1976, Mapping of sister chromatid exchanges in human chromosomes using C-banding and autoradiography, *Mutat. Res.* **35**:139–154.

Sperling, K., Wegner, R. D., Riehm, H., and Obe, G., 1975, Frequency and distribution of sister chromatid exchanges in a case of Fanconi's anemia, *Humangenetik* **27**:227–230.

Spriggs, A. I., 1974, Cytogenetics of cancer and precancerous states of the cervix uteri, in *Chromosomes and Cancer* (edited by J. German) John Wiley and Sons, New York, pp. 423–450.

Stich, H. F., and San, R. H. C., 1973, DNA repair synthesis and survival of repair deficient human cells exposed to the K-region epoxide of Benz (α) anthracene (36979), *Proc. Soc. Exp. Biol. Med.* **142**:155–158.

Stoll, Cl., 1980, Nonrandom distribution of exchange points in patients with reciprocal translocations, *Hum. Genet.* **56**:89–93.

Thrasher, J. D., 1973, The effects of mercuric compounds on dividing cells, in *Drugs and the Cell Cycle* (edited by Zimmerman, A. E., Perdille, G. M., and Cameron, I. L.), Academic Press, New York, pp. 25–48.

Tice, R., Chaillet, J., and Schneider, E. L., 1975, Evidence derived from sister chromatid exchanges of restricted rejoining of chromatid subunits, *Nature* **256**:642–644.

Van Buul, P. P. W., and Natarajan, A. T., 1980, Chromsomal radiosensitivity of human leucocytes in relation to sampling time, *Mutat. Res.* **70**:61–69.

Van de Putte, P., Cramer, S., and Giphart-Gassler, M., 1980, Invertible DNA determines host specificity of bacteriophage Mu, *Nature* **286**:218–222.

Veatch, W., and Okada, S., 1969, Radiation-induced breaks of DNA in cultured mammalian cells, *Biochem. J.* **9**:330–346.

Verschaeve, L., and Susanne, C., 1978, Chromosome banding produced after mercury chloride treatment in culture, *Acta Anthropogenet.* **2(4)**:1–8.

Verschaeve, L., Kirsch-Volders, M., Hens, L., and Susanne, C., 1978, Chromosome distribution studies in phenyl mercury acetate exposed subjects and in age-related controls, *Mutat. Res.* **57**:335–347.

Verschaeve, L., Driesen, M., Kirsch-Volders, M., Hens, L., and Susanne, C., 1979, Chromosome distribution studies after inorganic lead exposure, *Hum. Genet.* **49:**147–158.

Vogel, F., and Schroeder, T. M., 1974, The internal order of the interphase nucleus, *Humangenetik* **25:**265–297.

Von Koskull, H., and Aula, P., 1973, Nonrandom distribution of chromosome breaks in Fanconi's anemia, *Cytogenet. Cell Genet.* **12:**423–434.

Wang, R. W. J., Rebhun, L. I., and Kupchan, S. H., 1976, Antimitotic and antitubulin activity of the tumor inhibitor steganicin, *J. Cell Biol.* **70:**335.

Weinstein, D., Mauer, J., Katz, M., and Kazmer, S., 1973, The effects of caffeine on chromosomes of human lymphocytes: Nonrandom distribution of damage, *Mutat. Res.* **20:**441–443.

Weinstein, I. B., 1980, Cell culture systems for studying multifactor interactions in carcinogenesis, in *Mechanisms of Toxicity and Hazard Evaluation* (edited by Holmstedt, B., Lauwerys, R., Mercier, M., and Roberfroid, M.) Elsevier, Amsterdam, pp. 149–164.

Wilson, L., Cresweld, K. M., and Cher, D., 1975, The mechanism of action of vinblastine. Binding of (acetyl-[3]H) vinblastine to embryonic chick brain tubulin and tubulin from sea urchin sperm tail outer doublet microtubules, *Biochemistry* **14:**5586–5592.

Witkin, E. M., 1976, Ultraviolet mutagenesis and inducible DNA repair in *E. coli, Bacteriol. Rev.* **40:**869–907.

Wolff, S., Bodycote, J., and Painter, R. B., 1979, SCE induced in Chinese hamster cells by UV-irradiation of different stages of the cell cycle: The necessity for cells to pairs through S. *Mutat. Res.* **25:**73–81.

Wolff, S., Rodin, B., and Cleaver, J. E., 1977, Sister chromatid exchanges induced by mutagenic carcinogens in normal and xeroderma pigmentosum cells, *Nature* **265:**347–349.

Wolff, S., 1978a, Chromosomal effects of mutagenic carcinogens and the nature of the lesions leading to SCE, in *Mutagen-Induced Chromosome Damage in Man* (edited H. J. Evans and D. C. Lloyd), Edinburgh University Press, Edinburgh, pp. 208–215.

Wolff, S., 1978b, Relation between DNA repair, chromosome aberration, and sister chromatid exchanges, in *DNA Repair Mechanisms*, (edited by P. C. Hanawalt, E. C. Friedberg, and C. F. Fox), Academic Press, New York, pp. 751–760.

Wright, A. S., 1980, The role of metabolism in chemical mutagenesis and chemical carcinogenesis, *Mutat. Res.* **75:**215–241.

Wun, K. L., and Sutherland, J. C., 1977, Photoreactivating enzyme from *E. coli*: Appearance of new absorption on binding to vitranblet-irradiated DNA, *Biochemistry* **16:**921–924.

Zech, L., Haglund, U., Nilsson, K., and Klein, G., 1976, Characteristic chromosomal abnormalities in biopsies and lymphoid-cell lines from patients with Burkitt and non-Burkitt lymphomas, *Int. J. Cancer* **17:**47–56.

Zimmerman, F. K., 1971, Induction of mitotic gene conversion by mutagens, *Mutat. Res.* **11:**327–337.

*Chapter 2*

# Carcinogenicity, Mutagenicity, and Teratogenicity of Industrially Used Metals

## A. Léonard, G. B., Gerber, P. Jacquet, and R. R. Lauwerys

## 1. GENERAL CONSIDERATIONS

### 1.1. Risks and Their Assessment

Modern industrial development has brought about a worldwide spread of toxic metals in the environment, and hitherto unknown symptoms of intoxication have been recognized, whereas certain other types, quite common about 100 years ago (such as intoxication caused by the use of lead and mercury in certain crafts) have virtually disappeared. In general, the problem of pollution by metals has shifted from a local to a worldwide scale as an ever increasing amount of metals is released in the environment, and attention has focused more and more on insidious long-term effects on man and his environment (Table I).

In this respect, it is useful to distinguish between (a) stochastic risks for which the probability of occurrence is a function of dose and which may, therefore, arise without a threshold, and (b) nonstochastic risks for which the severity of an effect depends on the dose and for which a threshold may exist. This distinction is crucial for setting exposure limits in public health, since, to prevent nonstochastic risks, it suffices to lower exposure levels well below the threshold, whereas stochastic risks such as mutagenesis, cancer induction, and perhaps also allergic and teratogenic effects must be limited by keeping all justifiable exposure as low as is reasonably achievable. This review concentrates on the stochastic effects of mutagenesis, carcinogenesis, and terato-

A. Léonard, G. B. Gerber, and P. Jacquet • Department of Radiobiology, CEN-SCK, B-2400 Mol, Belgium. R. R. Lauwerys • Medical and Industrial Toxicology Unit, University of Louvain, B-1200 Brussels, Belgium. This work was supported by Contract No. 140-76-12 Env. B and Contract No. 229-76-12 Env. B of the European Communities Research Program.

Table I
**Annual Productions of Industrially Used Metals**

| Metal | Annual production (tons) |
|---|---|
| Arsenic | 50,000 |
| Beryllium | 150 |
| Cadmium | 14,000 |
| Chromium | >8,000,000 |
| Lead | >4,000,000 |
| Mercury | 10,000 |
| Nickel | 600,000 |
| Cobalt | 30,000 |

genesis, and touches upon other aspects only as far as needed for the understanding of the above alterations.

The need for establishing dose response curves arises, particularly for stochastic effects, since animal experiments yield data at a reasonable expenditure only for relatively high incidence levels, whereas our concern for public health obliges us to take account also of responses which occur at an incidence of $10^{-3}$ or less and thus are not detected in such experiments. Dose–response relationships, which for stochastic effects are generally linear or quadratic, are often difficult to extrapolate to the low dose range, especially when an effect, such as cancer, is caused also by other agents than that under consideration.

Indeed, man in today's industrial society lives in an environment charged with a multitude of potentially toxic agents. It is not surprising that these agents, including heavy metals, can interact, sometimes yielding smaller, antagonistic, sometimes larger, synergistic effects than expected from the sum of individual actions. Moreover, many metals which are toxic at higher levels fulfill an essential role at lower ones. A well-known example of an interaction between different metallic agents is the protection afforded by selenium against testicular damage by cadmium. Such interactions may not only be caused by a competitive action at the biological target, but also by interference in metabolism of the toxic agent, in hormonal regulation, promotion of tumors, etc. In addition, species, sex, age, nutrition, and many other factors influence the outcome of an exposure.

## 1.2. Metabolism and Toxicity

The risks to man from the release of a metal depend not only on its inherent toxicity, but also on its transfer into the environment and its uptake and metabolism by man. To exemplify extremes: On the one hand, alkali metals form mostly soluble salts, spread easily through the environment, are readily taken up by the organism, and distribute through all organs, but they are also readily excreted. On the other hand, actinide compounds are mostly insoluble at neutral pH, move but little through the environment, and are poorly absorbed, but—once take up by a tissue such as bone—they are retained for long periods of time.

Metals can enter the body by several routes: Intestinal absorption depends on solubility and transport characteristics, and is of the order of a few percent for most toxic metals, but can be much lower for certain ones, e.g., $Cr < 1\%$, actinides $<0.01\%$. Material inhaled into the lungs is often taken up to a larger extent than that which is ingested (e.g., lead up to 50%), since it stays on site for a longer time. Certain insoluble compounds may exert their most deleterious effects directly in the lungs (e.g., Cr, Ni, Be dusts). Uptake by the skin is important for liposoluble compounds and under conditions of prolonged contact (e.g., Ni, Cr).

Distribution in the body depends on the compound in question: Heavy metals often accumulate in the liver and kidneys. A few, such as Mn, have an affinity for the central nervous system or the pancreas. Many elements are deposited in bone and may remain there for long periods of time, e.g., the alkaline earths, lead, the actinides, etc. Unless it can act on bone itself, such material in the skeleton may be inert from a toxicological point of view, although it will continue to supply the body with small amounts of the toxin.

Heavy metals are excreted via the feces and frequently by the way of the salivary glands or bile, where part may be reabsorbed, or via urine, hair, skin (e.g., As), sweat, and in some cases via the lungs (metallic Hg). The ratio of excretion of urine to feces depends on the metal and may differ for different oxidation stages.

## 1.3. Mechanisms of Metal Toxicity

Inherent toxicity of a metal, i.e., its toxic effect when it has entered the body, depends on properties specific for each element, such as electrochemical behavior, solubility, ability to chelate with biomolecules, and the stability of such chelates. Our theoretical understanding of the reactions between metals and biomolecules is still insufficient to predict in detail which particular structures are most susceptible to such reactions. Many metallic salts exert a general cytotoxic action, causing denaturation of macromolecules, but the crucial factors in toxic action are usually specific reactions with certain chemical groups in biomolecules, or with certain sites in tissues or organelles. One can cite as examples the reaction of mercury with sulfhydryl groups, and for a more specific reaction, that of lead with delta-aminolevulinic acid dehydratase. In other instances, a toxic metal may enter in competition with an essential metal (e.g., Ca, Zn, Mg), which is required as an enzymatic cofactor or needed to stabilize the structure of a biomolecule. The reaction of metal ions with nucleic acids are of particular interest in this respect (and eventually also in DNA synthesis and repair), since they probably account for the stochastic effects of mutagenesis and carcinogenesis. One can distinguish "soft" and "hard" metal ions on the basis of their reactions with different ligands (Jacobson and Turner, 1980). Hard ions, e.g., Mg, or Ca, bind to phosphate groups and tend to stabilize the double helix. Soft ions, e.g., Hg, Ag, bind to bases and decrease the stability of the helix. Nickel, cobalt, and zinc are considered as intermediary.

## 1.4. Mutagenesis: Tests and Their Interpretation

The increasing awareness of the possible consequences of industrial pollution has greatly enhanced the number of publications dealing with mutagenic properties of metals in recent years. The results were summarized in several reviews (Flessel, 1978; Léonard, 1978; Kazantzis and Lilly, 1979). In order to evaluate such data in terms of relevance for genetic risks to man, the many test systems which range from *in vitro* experiments on microorganisms to *in vivo* observations in man must be briefly reviewed as to their capability to detect gene mutations and chromosome aberrations.

The two principal systems used in bacteria are the Rec-assay in *Bacillus subtilis* and the reversion assay in *E. coli* or in *Salmonella typhimurium*. Positive results in the Rec-assay usually indicate a covalent binding to DNA, or a chemical breakage of DNA, but the mode of action is obscure and perhaps unrelated to genetic damage. On the contrary, the reversion assay is more indicative for genetic damage since it detects frameshift mutations and base-pair substitutions and often parallels the carcinogenic potential of a compound.

A few tests in yeast and mammalian cells also aim to detect gene mutation, but the great majority of tests in eukaryotes assess the capability to induce structural or numerical chromosome aberrations. It should be pointed out that the alterations in DNA thought to be responsible for induction of malignancy are gene mutations, so that cytogenetics provide only an indication, but no proof of an induction of gene mutations and carcinogenic properties of a chemical. The fact that such a correlation must not exist follows also from observations on metals: Mercury readily induces chromosome aberrations in plants, but is not carcinogenic in animals or man.

Chromosome aberrations and segregation of chromosomes after treatment with metals have often been studied in plants and, according to Kihlman (1975), there exists a good correlation between the ability of some chemicals to induce chromosome aberrations in plants and in mammalian cells, but as shown by the data on mercury, this may not be true for metals. Chromosome aberrations induced in peripheral blood lymphocytes of man are widely used as a biological indicator for exposure to ionizing radiation, and the possibility of using the same system to obtain a record of exposure to other mutagens appeared attractive. Consequently, many publications have appeared reporting an increase in structural or numerical aberrations in persons exposed professionally or accidentally to metals. Many of these positive reports are highly questionable because inappropriate techniques were used. The culture must proceed for the correct amount of time, and at least 500 metaphases per individual should be scored. This corresponds roughly to the sampling of one cell per $500 \times 10^6$ blood lymphocytes (circulating and recirculating ones; Trepel, 1976). Particular attention must be devoted to the choice of adequate control groups. It would be best to compare cell samples from the same individuals before and after exposure and to match them with a nonexposed population, but in practice this can rarely be realized. Difficulties also arise in studies where a population may be exposed to a mixture of potential mutagens, as is frequently the case under conditions of industrial exposure (Evans, 1976; Kilian and Picciano, 1976; Evans and O'Riordan, 1975).

## 1.5. Carcinogenesis: Mechanisms and Evaluation

General principles of carcinogenesis as well as the tests to recognize carcinogenic properties of an agent are treated in detail in another chapter of this book; at this place, it suffices to point out certain aspects particular to carcinogenesis by heavy metals. Development of tumors is a multistep process in which induction must usually be followed by various factors promoting growth of the transformed cells. It should be kept in mind that an increase in tumor incidence may also be caused by an action on promoting factors and that this is often the case when large interspecies differences are found. One should not forget either that the probability that a tumor arises depends on concentrations at the target sites. Certain insoluble compounds of chromium, nickel, and beryllium are much more carcinogenic than the soluble compounds of these metals. This may be due to a high concentration gradient present for a long time near the target cells. It may also be related to the physicochemical and surface properties of this material, or to a selective action on certain cells with which it enters into contact. The extent mechanisms of carcinogenesis by metals remain, however, to be elucidated.

Information on carcinogenic properties of a metal originates from epidemiological studies, from experimental investigations in animals, or from mutagenic tests in microorganisms. A positive outcome of the *Salmonella typhimurium* or similar tests is a strong indication that a substance has carcinogenic properties but represents no proof; nor is a negative finding a definite counterproof. When tumors are observed in several species and/or several tissues, an agent must be considered as carcinogenic even if human data are not yet available. It is much more difficult to judge the relevance of isolated tumors in one organ and in a single species, e.g., the renal tumors in rats after lead administration. In general, such observations should raise suspicion and give cause for further studies, but if they are remaining isolated observations, it should not require the full spectrum of action needed for a carcinogenic agent.

Epidemiological studies on cancer induction in man suffer from the same drawbacks as those on chromosome aberrations in circulating lymphocytes: Exposure is rarely confined to only one agent, and appropriate controls are difficult to find. Such control groups are, however, usually larger for carcinogenesis than for genetic changes since death registers can be utilized.

## 1.6. Action on the Developing Organism

The developing organism is particularly susceptible to the action of certain heavy metals. All phases of development can be affected, as is illustrated for lead below. Failure of pregnancy or death can follow exposure prior to implantation (until day 5.5 in the mouse, day 6.5 in man). Malformations occur mainly when the agent acts during the period of major organogenesis (until day 13 in the mouse, day 60 in man). Later, during fetal growth and even post partum, more subtle changes in development, particularly in the CNS, can occur as is exemplified by the action of lead on the CNS of children. At all stages, maternal factors, hormonal equilibrium, and placental function play a role. The action of metals after implantation is determined by their capacity to reach the fetus. A few metal ions cross the placenta readily, but for the majority there exists a certain placental barrier; a few do not cross at all, or only in organically bound form (e.g., Cr).

Experimental data have been obtained in rodents and chickens, although the effect of metals on the developing organism has been less well studied than carcinogenesis. Failure of pregnancy or preimplantation and postimplantation death are readily ascertained. Detected malformations usually involve the skeleton or gross malformations of the central nervous system and the eye, but more sensitive tests, especially in the central nervous system, are desirable. Epidemiological data are often unreliable, but some older studies where pregnant women had still continued to work in a contaminated environment, or where certain agents were used as abortifacient have provided useful information.

## 2. ARSENIC

### 2.1. Exposure, Occurrence, and General Toxicity

Since ancient times arsenic has been widely used in medicine, for paints, and, sometimes, as a fashionable poison. Today it still finds application in agriculture for rodenticides, fungicides, insecticides, food additives, preservatives, and, to a much smaller extent than formerly, in medicine and in paints.

Most food contains but little arsenic (<0.25 mg/kg). Fish contains from 1 to 10 mg/kg (Fowler *et al.*, 1979) and crustacea and shellfish up to 100 mg/kg. In marine organisms, arsenic occurs as relatively atoxic organo-arsenicals of still unknown structure (NAS, 1977). Surface waters contain usually less than 10 $\mu$g/liter of, mainly inorganic, arsenic (Fowler *et al.*, 1979), but may attain levels of more than 1 mg/liter in certain areas with thermal activity (Table II). Arsenic in ground water also varies considerably from below 10 $\mu$g/liter to more than 1 mg/liter in certain areas (Fowler *et al.*, 1979). In air, arsenic exists in various forms, but most is present as particles of the trioxide (EPA, 1978), and has been released from combustion of fuels or from local industrial sources. In urban areas of the U.S., air concentrations from below 10 to 750 ng/m$^3$ have been measured (Sullivan, 1969). Near smelters, values up to 1600 ng/m$^3$ were observed (Fowler, 1977). Another source of arsenic is tobacco treated with arsenic-containing pesticides. Concentrations

## Table II
### Reported Levels of Several Metals in Food, Water and Ambient Air

| Metal | Food (daily intake) | Water | Ambient air |
|---|---|---|---|
| Arsenic | <10 $\mu$g | Surface and ground water <10$\mu$g/liter–1 mg/liter | Rural air <10 ng/m$^3$ Urban air <10 ng–750 ng/m$^3$ |
| Beryllium | 20 $\mu$g | Surface water <1 $\mu$g/liter | Rural air <0.1 ng/m$^3$ Urban air <3 ng/m$^3$ |
| Cadmium | 20 $\mu$g | Surface water <2 $\mu$g/liter Drinking water <5 $\mu$g/liter | Rural air <3 ng/m$^3$ Urban air <5 ng/m$^3$ |
| Chromium | 0.03–0.2 mg | Surface water <20 $\mu$g/liter Drinking water <20 $\mu$g/liter | Rural air <10 ng/m$^3$ Urban air <10–300 ng/m$^3$ |
| Lead | 200–300 $\mu$g | Drinking water <50 $\mu$g/liter | Rural air <500 ng/m$^3$ Heavy traffic up to 14,000 ng/m$^3$ |
| Mercury | 1–20 $\mu$g (up to 300 $\mu$g) | Surface water <200 ng/liter Ground water <50 ng/liter | Rural air <2–3 ng/m$^3$ Urban air up to 50 ng/m$^3$ |
| Nickel | 250 $\mu$g | Surface water <20 $\mu$g/liter Drinking water <20 $\mu$g/liter | Rural air <70 ng/m$^3$ Urban air <80 ng/m$^3$ |

in U.S. tobacco are presently below 10 $\mu$g/g, of which about 10–20% are volatilized in the smoke.

Over 60% of soluble inorganic and organic arsenic compounds are absorbed from the gastrointestinal tract. Airborne arsenic particles deposited in the respiratory tract and the gas arsine seem to be rapidly taken up from the lung but their absorption rates are not known in man. Inorganic trivalent arsenic is oxidized *in vivo* to pentavalent, which then can be methylated to monomethylarsonic acid and, especially, to cacodylic acid. The reverse reaction, i.e., conversion of organic arsenic to inorganic, does not seem to be important *in vivo*. Most arsenic derivatives are rapidly excreted in the urine (about 50% in 2 days), but some accumulate in various tissues, mainly in the liver, kidneys, bone, and skin.

Acute exposure to arsine gas can cause serious hemolysis, sometimes complicated by renal insufficiency. Acute exposure to other arsenic compounds may lead to a severe inflammation of the gastrointestinal tract after ingestion and to grave damage of the respiratory system after inhalation.

Chronic intoxication by arsenic is characterized by lesions of the skin and mucous membranes, by peripheral neuritis, by hematologic disturbances, occasionally by liver dysfunction and cardiovascular disorders, as well as by skin, lung, and liver cancer, and possibly by leukemia.

## 2.2. Mutagenesis

Arsenite at high concentrations arrests mitosis (Dustin and Grégoire, 1933), an effect attributed to its action on sulfhydryl enzymes. Arsenite also affects DNA synthesis and repair, presumably by binding to the thiols of DNA polymerase (Webb, 1966), or by incorporation into nucleotides in place of phosphate during DNA synthesis (Petres and Berger, 1972). A summary of the results of mutagenicity tests with As, based on the recent review by Léonard and Lauwerys (1980b), is compiled in Table III.

In contradiction to the observations of Andersen *et al.* (1972) and Loefroth and Ames (1978) on *Salmonella typhimurium*, and the negative findings of Ficsor and Nii Lo Piccolo (1972) on *E. coli*, certain results of Nishioka (1974, 1975) and Moreau and Devoret (1977) suggest that arsenic derivatives may produce gene mutations in microorganisms. Recent additional experiments by Rossman *et al.* (1977) on *E. coli* and on V79 Chinese hamster cells indicate that positive results in the Rec-assay are no proof for mutagenic acitivity, and that arsenic is incapable of inducing gene mutations.

Qualitative tests on plants or on mammalian cells *in vitro* revealed clearly the clastogenic potential of arsenic, and showed that trivalent compounds were more effective in causing chromosome breaks than pentavalent ones.

The genetic risk of arsenic to mammals has been studied only by Sram and Beneko (1974), who failed to find an increase in dominant lethals after a single administration of 250 mg sodium arsenite/kg. Negative results were also obtained after chronic administration of 10 or 100 mg/liter in the drinking water of male mice from weaning to an age of 8 weeks, over 4 generations. Animals given arsenic for several generations yielded more dominant lethals after treatment with TEPA (*tris*-l-aziridinyl-phosphine oxide) than those on a normal diet, and the authors suggest that this may reflect an inhibition by arsenic of the enzyme's ability to repair genetic damage.

For the reasons cited in the introduction, the observations on persons exposed to arsenic for medical or professional purposes cannot be considered as evidence of the ability of arsenic to induce chromosome aberrations in human somatic cells *in vivo*.

## 2.3. Carcinogenesis

Experimental and epidemiological data on the carcinogenic potential of arsenic are contradictory. On the one hand, there exists no reliable evidence that arsenic produces tumors in experimental animals. On the other hand, epidemiological studies demonstrated clearly that arsenic is a carcinogen in man (for review, see Sunderman, 1977a; Kazantzis and Lilly, 1979; Léonard and Lauwerys, 1980b).

Recent studies confirmed this conclusion of the extensive review by Neubauer (1946), based on case reports dating back to 1891. An increase in respiratory cancer has been observed following occupational exposure in the smelting industry (Axelsson *et al.*, 1978; Hill and Faning, 1948; Kuratsune *et al.*, 1975; Milham and Strong, 1974; Ott *et al.*, 1974; Pinto *et al.*, 1977), in gold mines in Rhodesia (Osburn, 1969), and among persons spraying arsenicals in agriculture (Blejer and Wagner, 1976; Friedrich, 1972; Roth 1958; Zachariae, 1972). Malignant neoplasms of the lymphatic and hemopoietic tissues have also been found in exposed workers (Axelsson *et al.*, 1978; Oswald and Goerttler, 1971). Skin cancers, hyperpigmentation, and keratosis, as well as cancers of the lungs, liver, and gastrointestinal tract are seen in persons drinking beverages contaminated with arsenic, such as drinking water containing as much as 0.8–2.6 ppm arsenic in Taiwan or Argentina (Arguello *et al.*, 1938; Bergoglio, 1964; Terada *et al.*, 1960; Yoshikawa *et al.*, 1960), or beer and wine (Satterlee, 1960). Therapy with arsenic, often used in the past, has also been associated with the development of precancerous skin lesions, multiple epitheliomatosis, and bronchial carcinoma (Goldman, 1973; Lander *et al.*, 1975; Minkowitz, 1964; Novey and Martel, 1969; Regelson *et al.*, 1968; Robson and Jelliffe, 1963).

Except for the increase in lymphocytic leukemia and malignant lymphoma

## Table III
## Summary of the Mutagenicity Tests Performed with Arsenic Compounds

| Material | Test | Compound | Result | Reference |
|---|---|---|---|---|
| Lysogen WP2s($\lambda$) | Induction of $\lambda$ prophage | $NaAsO_2$ | – | Rossman et al. (1980) |
| Bacillus subtilis | Rec-assay | $AsCl_3$ | + | Nii Lo Piccolo (1972) |
|  |  | $NaAsO_2$ | + | Nishioka (1974, 1975) |
|  |  | $(CH_3)_2AsS_2CNH_2$ | + |  |
|  |  | $CH_3AsNa_2O_3$ | – | Shirasu et al, (1976) |
|  |  | $CH_3AsCaO_3$ | – |  |
| Escherichia coli | Interference with DNA repair | $NaAsO_2$ | + | Rossman et al. (1975) |
|  | Reversion assay | $NaAsO_2$ | + | Nishioka (1974, 1975) |
|  |  |  | ± | Moreau and Devoret (1977) |
|  |  | $NaAsO_2$ | – | Ficsor and Nii Lo Piccolo (1972) |
|  |  | $AsHNa_2O_4$ | – | Nii Lo Piccolo (1972) |
|  |  | $CH_3(CH_2)_7NH_4AsCH_3O_3$ | – | Rossman et al. (1980) |
|  |  | $CH_3(CH_2)_{11}NH_4AsCH_3O_3$ |  |  |
| Salmonella typhimurium | Reversion assay | $NaAsO_2$ | – | Löfroth and Ames (1978) |
|  |  | $AsHNa_2O_4$ | – |  |
|  |  | $CH_5AsO_3$ | – | Andersen et al. (1972) |
|  |  | $CH_4AsNaO_3$ | – |  |
| Pennisetum typhoides | Pollen sterility | $C_2H_7AsO_2$ | + | Powell and Taylorson (1967) |
| Beta vulgaris | Pollen sterility | $C_2H_7AsO_2$ | – | Hecker et al. (1972) |
| Zea mais | Chromosomal aberrations | $CH_3C_6H_4AsO_3$ | + |  |
|  |  | $ClC_6H_4AsO_3$ | + | El-Sadek (1972) |
|  |  | $HO_2C_6H_4AsO_3$ | + |  |
| Allium cepa | Chromosomal aberrations | $CH_3ClC_6H_3AsO_3$ | + | Nygren (1949) |
| Drosophila melanogaster | Increase of crossover | $AsHNa_2O_4$ | + | Ahmed and Walker (1972) |
|  |  |  |  | Walker and Bradley (1969) |

| Test system | Compound | Effect | Reference |
|---|---|---|---|
| Mammals *in vitro* | | | |
| Effect on DNA and protein synthesis | $NaAsO_2$ | + | Nakamuro and Sayato (1981) |
| | $AsCl_3$ | + | |
| | $As_2O_3$ | + | |
| | $Na_2HAsO_4$ | + | |
| | $H_3AsO_4$ | + | |
| | $As_2O_5$ | + | |
| Genic mutations | $NaAsO_2$ | − | Rossman *et al.* (1980) |
| Sister chromatid exchanges | $Na_2HAsO_4$ | + | Zanzoni and Jung (1980) |
| Chromosome aberrations | $NaAsO_2$ | + | King and Lunford (1950) |
| | $KAsO_2$ | + | |
| | $AsCl_3$ | + | Nakamuro and Soyato (1981) |
| | $As_2O_3$ | + | Oppenheim and Fishbein (1965) |
| | $As_2O_5$ | + | Paton and Allison (1972) |
| | $H_3AsO_4$ | + | Petres (1972) |
| | $Na_2HAsO_4$ | + | Petres and Berger (1972) |
| | $R \cdot AsO_3H_2$ | + | Petres *et al.* (1970) |
| | $R_2 \cdot AsO(OH)$ | + | Petres *et al.* (1974) |
| | $R \cdot NH(CH_2)_3AsO_3H_2$ | + | |
| Mammals *in vivo* | | | |
| Dominant lethals | $NaAsO_2$ | +? | Sram and Beneko (1974) |
| Humans *in vivo* | | | |
| Chromosome aberrations in somatic cells | $NaAsO_2$ | + | Beckman *et al.* (1977) |
| | | | Happle and Hoehn (1973) |
| | | | Nordenson *et al.* (1978) |
| | | | Petres *et al.* (1970) |

claimed by Oswald and Goerttler (1971) to occur after subcutaneous injection of sodium arsenite into pregnant mice, all attempts to demonstrate the carcinogenity of arsenic in experimental animals have given negative results. As pointed out above, arsenic must, therefore, be considered as a cocarcinogen which may act via a suppression of host resistance (Stone, 1969), inhibition of DNA repair (Jung, 1971; Jung and Trachsel, 1970; Rossman *et al.*, 1977), or interaction with selenium (Dubois *et al.*, 1940; Frost, 1967, 1970; Levander and Argrett, 1969; Levander and Bauman, 1966; Moxon and Dubois, 1939; Neubauer, 1946; Osward and Goerttler, 1971).

## 2.4. Teratogenesis

Organic arsenicals have been claimed not to pass the placenta readily, but to be stored in placental tissues (Eastman, 1931), whereas inorganic arsenic enters the fetus of the mouse (Gerber *et al.*, 1982), rat (Morris *et al.*, 1938), hamster (Ferm, 1977; Hanlon and Ferm, 1977), and man (Lugo *et al.*, 1969).

Methyl arsenate caused spina bifida in chicks (Ancel 1946); inorganic arsenic elicited stunting, micromelia, abdominal edema, and dose-related death (Birge and Roberts, 1976). Low doses of arsenite administered in drinking water to mice (Schroeder and Mitchener, 1971b), or in food to sheep (James *et al.*, 1966), did not affect fertility or provoke malformations. Injection of 25 mg/kg of arsenate to hamsters during the stage of neurulation (day 8) engendered exencephaly (Ferm and Carpenter, 1968a; Ferm, 1977), which may result from a specific effect on the embryonic cephalic mesoderm (Ferm, 1972; Hanlon and Ferm, 1977). Exencephaly was also observed in mice after administration of 45 mg/kg arsenate on days 6–12 (Hood, 1972; Hood and Bishop, 1972). Injection later during organogenesis provoked other malformations in hamsters, e.g., cleft palate and lip, micro or anophthalmia, ear and genitourinary defects, and renal agenesis (Holmberg and Ferm, 1969; Ferm *et al.*, 1971). Simultaneous administration of selenium (Holmberg and Ferm, 1969) reduced the teratogenic action of arsenic in hamsters, and treatment with BAL protected mice (Hood and Piken, 1972). Renal agenesis and other anomalies also occured in rats (Burk and Beaudoin, 1977). Trivalent arsenic given to rats at day 9 is more toxic than is pentavalent, and at a dose of 30 mg/kg, caused 100% mortaility, apparently as a result of the action of arsenic on mesodermic and neuroectodermic cells of the fetus (Takeuchi, 1979).

Aside from a case of a woman poisoned with arsenic during pregnancy who gave birth to a small baby that died soon thereafter, no data on the effects of arsenic on human development are available. It must be concluded that, although malformations have only been observed after injections into animals, arsenic at high doses should be considered a potential teratogenic agent in man.

## 3. BERYLLIUM

### 3.1. Exposure, Occurrence, and General Toxicity

The main uses of beryllium and its compounds are in electrical and electronic industries, nuclear reactors, the aerospace industry, and production of beryllium alloys, mainly with copper. For nonoccupationally exposed persons, food appears to be the main source of beryllium. Reeves (1979) estimated that the average daily intake is $20\mu g$. Beryllium concentrations in surface waters are usually below 1 $\mu g$/liter.

Beryllium in air originates mainly from the combustion of coal. Atmospheric concentrations of beryllium are usually below 0.1 $ng/m^3$ and 3 $ng/m^3$ in rural and urban air, respectively (IARC, 1980). Higher concentrations, up to 100 $ng/m^3$, have been found near beryllium processing plants (Sussman et al., 1959). Smokers are, in addition, exposed to beryllium in cigarette smoke.

Few data are available on absorption of beryllium salts by the lungs and gastrointestinal tract. Oral absorption of soluble beryllium salts is below 20%. Absorption of soluble beryllium salts from the lungs may be higher, whereas insoluble salts are retained in the lungs for long periods of time. Absorbed beryllium is mainly deposited in bone and liver. Very little beryllium is excreted into urine, but due to its long halflife, has been detected as late as 10 years after exposure.

Acute exposure to beryllium causes mainly an irritative or allergic dermatitis and an acute pneumonitis. Chronic intoxication is manifested by a granulomatous, interstitial pneumonitis (beryllosis).

### 3.2. Mutagenesis

Relatively few studies have been carried out so far to assess the mutagenic potential of beryllium. $BeSO_4$ enhances the binding of nucleic acids (DNA and RNA) to cell membranes, a property which could be of significance in the carcinogenic activity of a substance (Kubinski et al., 1976). $BeCl_2$ produces some infidelity of in vitro DNA synthesis (Sirover and Loeb, 1976), but in contrast to $BeSO_4$ gave negative results in the Rec-assay (Nishioka, 1975). Beryllium can induce mutations at the hypoxanthine-guanine phosphoribosyl transferase (HGPRTase) locus in Chinese hamster V79 cells (Miyaki et al., 1977), an observation which is of particular interest in view of the close relationship between the carcinogenic properties of a substance and its ability to induce gene mutations in mammalian cells.

### 3.3. Carcinogenesis

The possible carcinogenic risks of beryllium are disputed. Mancuso (1970) and Hasan and Kazemi (1974) observed a significant increase in respiratory cancers among beryllium workers, but these results were not confirmed by Bayliss (1972) who investigated the causes of death in 3900 persons who had been occupationally exposed to beryllium. A recent study by Wagoner *et al.* (1980) reported 47 lung cancers observed against 34 expected among 3055 workers exposed to beryllium at the Kawecki plant at Reading, Pa. This study has, however, recently been seriously criticized by one of the coauthors [Bayliss, see Smith (1981)] "disavowing it and charging that his colleagues used inappropriate statistics." Indeed, if the statistics had included the period between 1968 and 1975, the expected incidence would have been 38, a value not significantly different from 47. Although beryllium is considered to be an established carcinogen for occupational exposure in Sweden and the German Federal Republic, the issue is not yet settled, and the small number of studies performed so far, all of which are at the borderline of significance, make a final appraisal difficult.

Animal experiments on beryllium carcinogenesis have been reviewed by Sunderman (1977a), Kazantzis and Lilly (1979), and Reeves (1979), and indicate that several beryllium compounds, such as beryllium oxide, sulfate, phosphate, and zinc beryllium salts can cause malignant tumors, e.g., osteosarcoma after intravenous injection (Cloudman *et al.*, 1949; Hoagland *et al.*, 1950; Sissons, 1950; Jones *et al.*, 1954; Gardner and Heslington, 1946; Barnes *et al.*, 1960; Kelly *et al.*, 1961), respiratory tumors after intrabronchial implantation (Vorwald *et al.*, 1966), or inhalation (Dutra *et al.*, 1951; Reeves and Vorwald, 1967; Reeves *et al.*, 1967).

## 4. CADMIUM

### 4.1. Exposure, Occurrence, and General Toxicity

Cadmium is used in metallurgy for protective coatings, in the manufacture of pigments, in alkaline batteries, in photo detectors, in certain plastic stabilizers (Cadmium Association, 1980), and is also released as a by-product in the smelting of zinc. Industrial use of cadmium dates back only a century and has continued to expand since then (Lauwerys, 1978). Intake of cadmium from food, the principal source of cadmium in the body beside smoking, amounts to about 20 $\mu$g/day with a range from 10 to 50 $\mu$g or more. Children living near sources of cadmium emission may ingest significant amounts in dirt (Buchet *et al.*, 1980). Cadmium concentrations in uncontaminated surface water and drinking water are low, less than 2$\mu$g/liter and 5 $\mu$g/liter, respectively. Galvanized pipes used for plumbing may represent a potential source of cadmium. Rural and even urban air contain little cadmium ($<$3 ng/m$^3$ and $<$5 ng/m$^3$, respectively) and do not contribute much to cadmium exposure except near emission sources, where levels of 500

$ng/m^3$ can be attained. A cigarette contains from 0.9 to 2.3 $\mu g$ of cadmium, of which 10% is inhaled. Smoking thus implies a significant cadmium exposure.

Cadmium is poorly absorbed from the intestine—of the order of 5% or less—but its long half-life of more than one year gives rise to an appreciable accumulation in the body. Absorption of cadmium from the lungs depends on the solubility of the compound. Cadmium in tissues is bound to metallothionein, which may represent an attempt of the body to detoxify this metal, but also accounts for its long retention. Accumulation occurs mainly in the liver and kidneys, and excretion is preferentially into urine. When the kidney has become damaged, more cadmium is excreted into urine.

The principal acute manifestations of cadmium intoxication in man are gastrointestinal disturbances following ingestion, and chemical pneumonitis following inhalation of cadmium oxide fumes. In animals, acute administration of cadmium can also produce toxic effects in other organs (cardiovascular system, kidneys, liver, nervous system, hemopoietic system, pancreas, immunological system, and the reproductive system).

Long-term human exposure to cadmium has been linked to the development of various signs and symptoms, in particular to lung insufficiency, renal damage, osteomalacia, and anemia. Cadmium, perhaps in association with dietary and other factors, is usually also considered to be responsible for cases of ostemalacia and renal disturbances found in elderly women in Japan (Itai-itai Byo disease). A few studies suggested that cadmium may be carcinogenic in man. Animals given cadmium for longer periods of time also displayed other types of tissue damage or functional disturbances, e.g., hypertension.

## 4.2. Mutagenesis

A summary of data on mutagenesis by cadmium (Table IV), based on the recent, exhaustive review by Degraeve (1981), shows that the potential of cadmium to cause gene mutations or chromosome aberrations has been assayed in numerous test systems. In spite of the fact that some recent results (Mandel and Ryser, 1981; Lemontt et al., 1981) suggest that toxic doses of cadmium salts ($CdCl_2$) could induce gene mutations in microorganisms (Salmonella typhimurium) and yeast, the most obvious effects that can be ascribed to cadmium were the findings of chromosome damage in plants. No information is, however, available regarding the mechanisms by which such effects in plants could occur and, as pointed out above, observations with metals in plants may not be relevant for mutagenicity testing in mammals. Indeed, almost all experiments carried out on mammalian cells in vivo or in vitro following acute or chronic exposure yielded negative results. The chromosome aberrations reported in persons professionally or accidentally

Table IV

**Summary of the Mutagenicity Tests Performed with Cadmium Compounds**

| Material | Test | Compound | Result | Reference |
|---|---|---|---|---|
| *Bacillus subtilis* | Rec-assay | $CdCl_2$ | + | Kanematsu et al. (1980) |
| | | $CdSO_4$ | + | |
| | | $Cd(NO_3)_2$ | + | Nishioka (1975) |
| *Escherichia coli* | Reversion assay | $CdCl_2$ | − | Kanematsu et al. (1980) |
| | | $CdSO_4$ | − | |
| | | $Cd(NO_3)_2$ | − | Venitt and Levy (1974) |
| *Salmonella typhimurium* | Reversion assay | $CdCl_2$ | − | Bruce and Heddle (1979); Heddle and Bruce (1977) |
| | | | ? | Kalinina and Polukhina (1977) |
| | | | ? | Polukhina et al. (1977) |
| | Reversion assay (host-mediated assay) | $CdCl_2$ | + | Mandel and Ryser (1981) |
| | Reversion assay | $CdCl_2$ | + | Kalinina et al. (1977) |
| | | $CdS_4N_2C_2H_4$ | + | Hedenstedt et al. (1979) |
| *Saccharomyces cerevisiae* | Gene mutation | $CdCl_2$ | − | Putrament et al. (1977) |
| | | $CdCl_2$ | + | Lemontt et al. (1981) |
| Plant material | Gene mutation | Lead plant | ? | Lower et al. (1978) |
| | | $CdCl_2$ | + | Reddy and Vaidyanath (1978 a,b) |
| | C-mitosis | $CdCl_2$ | + | Clain and Deysson (1976) |
| | | $CdBr_2$ | + | Degraeve (1969, 1971) |
| | Stickiness | $CdI_2$ | + | Glaess (1955, 1956a, 1956b) |
| | | $Cd(NO_3)_2$ | + | Levan (1945) |
| | | | | Moutschen et al. (1965) |
| | | | | Oehlkers (1953) |
| | Chromosome aberrations | $CdSO_4$ | + | Ruposhev (1976a, 1976b) |
| | | $Cd(CH_3COO)_2$ | + | Ruposhev and Garina. (1976, 1977) |
| | | | | Von Rosen (1953, 1954a, 1954b) |
| *Drosophila melanogaster* | Gene mutations | $CdCl_2$ | − | Ramel and Friberg (1974) |
| | | | − | Sorsa and Pfeifer (1973) |
| | | | − | Inoue and Watanabe (1978) |
| | Dominant lethals | $CdCl_2$ | + | Vasudev and Krishnamurthy (1979) |

| | | | | |
|---|---|---|---|---|
| *Poeciloceurs pictus* | Chromosome aberrations | $CdCl_2$ | + | Kumaraswamy and Sekarasetty (1977) |
| Mammalian cells *in vitro* | Chromosome aberrations | $CdCl_2$ | − | Deknudt (1978) |
| | | | | Deknudt and Deminatti (1978) |
| | | | | Nishimura and Umeda (1978) |
| | | | | Paton and Allison (1972) |
| | | | | Umeda and Nishimura (1979) |
| | | | | Zasukhina et al. (1975, 1976) |
| | | $CcCl_2$ | + | Deaven and Campbell (1980) |
| | | | | Voroshilin et al. (1978) |
| | | $Cd(CH_3COO)_2$ | − | Majone and Rensi (1979) |
| | | | | Shiraishi et al. (1972) |
| | | CdS | + | Bauchinger and Röhr (1976) |
| | | $CdSO_4$ | + | Röhr and Bauchinger (1976) |
| Mammals *in vivo* | Structural aberrations in somatic cells | $CdCl_2$ | − | Deknudt (1978) |
| | | | − | Deknudt and Gerber (1979) |
| | | | − | Vilkina et al. (1979) |
| | | | + | Felten (1978) |
| | Micronucleus test | $CdCl_2$ | − | Bruce and Heddle (1979) |
| | | | − | Heddle and Bruce (1977) |
| | Numerical aberrations | $CdCl_2$ | + | Doyle et al. (1974) |
| | Sperm abnormalities | $CdCl_2$ | − | Bruce and Heddle (1979) |
| | | | | Heddle and Bruce (1977) |
| | Spermatocyte test | $CdCl_2$ | − | Gilliavod and Léonard (1975) |
| | | | | Léonard et al. (1975) |
| | F₁ translocation test | $CdCl_2$ | − | Gilliavod and Léonard (1975) |
| | | | | Léonard et al. (1975) |
| | Dominant lethals | $CdCl_2$ | − | Sutou et al. (1980) |
| | Mouse oocytes | | | |
| | Structural aberrations | $CdCl_2$ | − | Shimada et al. (1976) |
| | Numerical aberrations | $CdCl_2$ | − | Shimada et al. (1976) |
| | Chromosome aberrations | Occupational exposure | − | Bui et al. (1975) |
| | | | | O'Riordan et al. (1978) |
| | Chromosome aberrations | Occupational exposure | + | Bauchinger et al. (1976) |
| | | | | Deknudt et al. (1973) |
| | | | | Deknudt and Léonard (1975) |
| | | | | Shiraishi and Yosida (1972) |

exposed cannot be accepted as proof for a mutagenic action of cadmium for the reasons outlined above (inadequate methods and/or simultaneous expoxure to other potential mutagens).

## 4.3. Carcinogenesis

Certain epidemiological investigations suggested that occupational cadmium exposure may increase the risk of prostate cancer, but the number of persons studied is too small to be conclusive (Kazantzis and Lilly, 1979). Potts (1965) reported three deaths from prostate cancer among 74 workers with at least 10 years exposure to cadmium oxide. Concentrations ranged from 0.6 to 236 mg/m$^3$ until 1949, but diminished to below 0.5 mg/m$^3$ by 1950 and 0.1 mg/m$^3$ by 1956. This survey was enlarged by Kipling and Waterhouse (1967), who observed 4 cases of prostate cancer (including the three from Potts) among a cohort of 248 workers exposed for at least one year; the expected frequency was 0.58. It is, however, noteworthy that no prostate cancers were observed in rats given cadmium sulfate orally or by subcutaneous injection for several months (Levy *et al.*, 1973; Levy and Clack, 1975; Levy *et al.*, 1975). Liver and kidney concentrations of cadmium in these rats were of the same order of magnitude as those in the exposed workers. The observation that persons suffering from lung cancer display high cadmium levels in the liver, kidneys, and blood (Morgan, 1970), and that cancers are seen in persons simultaneoulsy exposed to cadmium and nickel, or to cadmium, nickel and arsenic (Kjellstroem *et al.*, 1979; Lemen *et al.*, 1976), are obviously no proof for a carcinogenic action of cadmium in man.

Intramuscular or subcutaneous injection to experimental animals of metallic powder, sulfide, oxide, sulfate, or chloride of cadmium can elicit local rhabdomyosarcoma and fibrosarcoma (Kazantzis and Lilly, 1979 and Degraeve, 1981). Interstitial cell tumors develop in the testis far from the site of injection, but according to Kazantzis and Lilly (1979), this could be an effect secondary to the necrosis caused by cadmium in the interstitial cells. It is noteworthy that zinc protects against the necrotic action of cadmium on the testis (Gunn *et al.*, 1964).

## 4.4. Teratogenesis

Cadmium does not pass readily through the placental barrier of mice (Berlin and Ullberg, 1963) or hamsters (Dencker, 1975) during the late stages of pregnancy, although it apparently does so at an earlier time, since radioactive cadmium could be found in the hamster embryo 24 hours after injection on day 8 (Ferm *et al.*, 1969). Human placenta is also less transmissible for cadmium than it is for most other heavy metals (Henke *et al.*,

1970; Piscator, 1971; Finklea *et al.*, cited in Task groups on metal accumulation, 1973; Lauwerys *et al.*, 1978; Roels *et al.*, 1978).

The teratogenic action of cadmium has been studied in chickens and rodents. Intravitelline application of cadmium in eggs caused malformations in the caudal part of the chicken, whereas supravitelline application resulted in embryonic death (Ribas and Schmidt, 1973). Injection of 2 mg/kg to hamsters on day 8 of gestation provoked facial abnormalities (cleft lips and palate) and, less often, exencephaly and anophthalmia (Ferm and Carpenter, 1967a; 1968b); the former abnormalities apparently resulted from a direct action of cadmium on the mesodermic tissue (Mulvihill *et al.*, 1970). Following injection during a later period of gestation, abnormalities of the limbs and fusion of ribs were observed (Ferm, 1971; Gale and Ferm, 1973). The many experiments performed on rats yielded variable results. Oral administration caused some anomalies of the genito-urinary tract and of the heart (Nolen *et al.*, 1972; Scharpf *et al.*, 1972), but was much less toxic than injection, since more than half of the fetuses survived an oral administration by intubation of 80 mg/kg/day from days 6 to 19 of pregnancy. Intravenous or intraperitoneal injection of 1–2 mg/kg to rats on days 9–11 elicited hydrocephaly, microphthalmy and anophthalmy (Barr, 1973; Samarawickrama and Webb, 1979), except in the Holtzman strain, where only stunting of the head region was observed (Parzyk *et al.*, 1978). Abnormalities, such as micrognathy or small lung size, were most frequent after s.c. injection of 12 mg on day 14 or 15 (Chernoff, 1973), but it should be recalled in this context that at this time of gestation, the placenta is barely permeable to cadmium, and that some effects may also result from an impaired supply of nutrients due to cadmium-induced damage of the placenta (Chiquoine, 1965; Parizek, 1963).

Continuous administration of drinking water containing 5 ppm of cadmium to mice resulted in fetal and maternal death after three generations (Schroeder *et al.*, 1964). A larger dose (10 ppm) caused malformations such as twisting of the tail (Schroeder and Mitchener, 1971b). Injection of cadmium in mice gave similar malformations to those in hamsters (Ishizu *et al.*, 1973; Pierro and Haines, 1976; Keino *et al.*, 1975ab). It also increased mortality and impaired motility in the offspring (Keino and Yamamura, 1974). The toxic effects of cadmium on the hamster embryo are alleviated by treatment with zinc (Ferm and Carpenter, 1967a), lead (Ferm, 1969), or selenium (Holmberg and Ferm, 1969). Pretreatment with cadmium or mercury also protects the embryo from cadmium (Semba *et al.*, 1974, 1977; Ferm and Layton, 1979; Layton and Ferm, 1980), perhaps by inducing synthesis of metallothioneins, which may bind cadmium before it can pass the placenta. As pointed out by Layton and Ferm (1980), such a situation may prevail in a human population chronically exposed to heavy metals. In conclusion, there is no doubt that cadmium in high doses is teratogenic in animals, but so far no observations in man have been reported.

## 5. CHROMIUM

### 5.1. Exposure, Occurrence, and General Toxicity

Chromium is used extensively in metallurgy for the production of alloys and stainless steels, in electroplating and coatings, in paints, for tanning, and for the production of sodium chromate and dichromate (NAS, 1974). Intake via food ranges from 0.03 to 0.2 mg/day. In drinking water, usually less than 10 $\mu$g/liter are found. Chromium content in rural air rarely exceeds 10 ng/m$^3$; in urban air, it ranges from less than 10 to 300 ng/m$^3$ (Kretzschmar *et al.*, 1980), but inhalation contributes little to the body's chromium.

Trivalent chromium is essential as a constituent of the glucose tolerance factor. Little inorganic chromium ($<$1%) is absorbed from the gastrointestinal tract. Organically bound chromium is more readily taken up (Mertz, 1969). Absorption of inhaled chromium dust is also small, but depends on the solubility of the compound. Chromium does not pass through intact skin but can enter at minor cuts or when prolonged contact causes sensitization. In the blood, Cr(III) is bound to siderophilin, while Cr(VI) binds to globin. Chromium is concentrated in the liver and kidneys and is excreted into urine with a relatively short half-life (Mertz, 1969).

Acute ingestion of chromium salts is rare and causes severe gastrointestinal inflammation followed by liver and kidney necrosis. Chronic exposure to hexavalent chromium has been associated with contact dermatitis (cement eczema), irritation and ulceration of the nasal mucosa and, more rarely, with occupational asthma. Allergy toward chromium is found in about 10% of all persons with skin diseases. An increased prevalence of lung cancers has been reported in workers exposed to insoluble chromate.

### 5.2. Mutagenesis

Hexavalent chromium has given positive results in the majority of assay systems, whereas trivalent chromium seemed generally inactive. The ultimate mutagen, i.e., that which binds to the genetic material is, however, Cr(III), which is produced by intracellular reduction from Cr(VI), although it cannot enter the cell *per se*. Trivalent chromium complexes with many ligands in the cell, but accumulates mainly in the nuclear fraction (about 50%). Recent results by Petrilli and De Flora (1978a, 1978b) demonstrate clearly the poor uptake and consequent genetic inactivity of trivalent chromium. All trivalent compounds tested [CrK(SO$_4$)$_2$, CrCl$_3$, and Cr(NO$_3$)$_2$] yielded negative results in reversion assays with *Salmonella typhimurium*, but were positive after oxidation with KMnO$_4$.

Table V summarizes the qualitative and quantitative mutagenic tests which have been carried out using chromium, and which are discussed in more detail in the review by Léonard and Lauwerys (1980a). Venitt and Levy (1974), based on experiments with *E coli*, had concluded that chromates belong to the class of mutagens producing transition mutations, but, as shown in Table V, it is evident from most experiments that chromium can induce chromosome aberrations as well as gene mutations. Competition between calcium and chromium for binding sites at nucleic acids may contribute to the clastogenic properties of chromium (Anghileri, 1973).

The ability to induce chromosome aberrations *in vivo* in mammals has been tested in only a few experiments. Confirming observations of Bigaliev *et al.* (1974), Wild (1978) determined a dose-response relationship for induction of micronuclei by $K_2Cr_2O_7$ in mouse bone marrow. After a dose of $2 \times 48.5$ mg/kg i.p. 15.0% micronuclei were found, after $2 \times 24.25$ mg/kg 9.6% and after $2 \times 12.12$ mg/kg 4.8%. A similar relation was found by Fabry (1980) with 18% micronuclei 30 hours after 50 mg/kg and 23% after 75 mg/kg. No micronuclei were obtained with the highly carcinogenic salt $CaCrO_4$ (75 and 150 mg/kg), but this could be due to the low solubility of this compound. The potential genetic hazards of chromium are underlined by the observation that, when an unspecified chromium compound was added at a concentration of 1 ppm to a Se-deficient but vitamin E supplemented diet, spermatogenesis was arrested in rats (Wu *et al.*, 1971). Indeed, highest concentrations of $^{51}Cr$ Chromate injected into rats were found in testis and epididymis (Hopkins, 1965).

## 5.3. Carcinogenesis

It is well documented by epidemiological observations and animal experiments that chromium derivatives, particularly the slightly soluble hexavalent ones, can cause cancer at the sites of deposition. In man, these are mainly in the respiratory tract, while in animals they are near injection sites. This restricted localization of tumors could be due to the fact that only chromium persisting at the site of deposition can provide a continuous flow into the cells, and also that the mutagenic property is lost when chromate is reduced by the microsomal fraction of certain organs (Petrilli and De Flora, 1978a; Gruber and Jenette, 1978).

Epidemiological surveys made since 1930 in Germany, Switzerland, the U.S.A., Great Britain, and Scandinavia demonstrated that workers in industries producing chromate and, to a lesser extent, those manufacturing pigments, display a greater risk of cancer of the lungs, larnyx, and nasal cavities (for review, see Sunderman, 1976; Kazantzis and Lilly, 1979; Leonard and Lauwerys, 1980a). The increase in risk reported varied from 3 to 38 times, and the latency period from 10.5 to 27 years. The risk is lower and possibly absent (Axelsson *et al.*, 1980) in workers of the ferro-chromium industry and inconclusive for those in electroplating. Several histological types of

## Table V
## Mutagenicity Tests Performed with Chromium Compounds

| Species | Test | Compound | Result | References |
|---|---|---|---|---|
| Bacteriophage T4 | | $CaCrO_4$ | − | Corbett et al. (1970) |
| Bacillus subtilis | Rec-assay | $CrCl_3$ | − | |
| | | $CrO_3$ | + | Kanematsu et al. (1980) |
| | | $K_2Cr_2O_4$ | + | Nakamuro et al. (1978) |
| | | $K_2Cr_2O_7$ | + | Nishioka (1974, 1975) |
| | | $Cr(CH_3COO)_3$ | + | |
| Escherichia coli | Reversion assay | $K_2Cr_2O_7$ | + | Kanematsu and Kada (1978) |
| | | $Na_2CrO_4$ | + | Kanematsu et al. (1980) |
| | | $K_2CrO_4$ | + | Green et al. (1976) |
| | | $CaCrO_4$ | + | Nestmann et al. (1979) |
| | | $PbCrO_4$ | + | Nishioka (1975) |
| | | $Cr_2(SO_4)_3$ | − | Tindall et al. (1978) |
| | | | | Venitt and Levy (1974) |
| Salmonella typhimurium | Reversion assay | $Cr_2(CrO_4)_3$ | + | Cooper et al. (1981) |
| | | $Na_2Cr_2O_7$ | + | De Flora (1978) |
| | | $K_2Cr_2O_7$ | + | Löfroth and Ames (1978) |
| | | $K_2CrO_4$ | + | Nestman et al. (1979) |
| | | $CrO_3$ | + | Petrilli and De Flora (1977; 1978 a,b) |
| | | $ZnCrO_4$ | + | Tamaro et al. (1975) |
| | | $PbCrO_4$ | + | Tindall et al. (1978) |
| | | $K_2Cr_2O_7$ | + | Kanematsu et al. (1980) |
| | | $CrK(SO_4)_2CrCl_3$ | − | De Flora (1978) |
| | | $Cr(NO_3)_3$ | − | Petrilli and De Flora (1977; 1978b) |
| Schizasaccharomyces | Gene conversion | $K_2Cr_2O_7$ | + | Bonatti et al. (1976) |
| Saccharomyces cerevisae | Recombination | $PbCrO_4$ | + | Nestmann et al. (1979) |
| Vicia faba | Mitotic aberrations | $Cr(NO_3)_2$ | + | Gläss (1955, 1956 a,b) |
| Drosophila melanagoster | Puff formation | $CrCl_3$ | + | Nikiforov et al. (1970) |

| System | Endpoint | Compound | Result | Reference |
|---|---|---|---|---|
| Mammalian cells *in vitro* | Gene mutations | $K_2Cr_2O_7$ | + | Fradkin et al. (1975) |
| | | $K_2CrO_4$ | + | Newbold et al. (1979) |
| | | $ZnCrO_4$ | + | Tindall and Hsie (1980) |
| | | $CaCrO_4$ | + | Tsuda and Kato (1977) |
| | | $(CH_3COO)_3Cr$ | − | |
| | | $PbCrO_4$ | − | |
| | Chromosome damages and/or SCE | $K_2Cr_2O_7$ | + | Douglas et al. (1980) |
| | | $CrO_3$ | + | MacRae et al. (1979) |
| | | $K_2CrO_4$ | + | Mayone (1977) |
| | | $PbCrO_4$ | + | Nakamuro et al. (1978) |
| | | | | Newbold et al. (1979) |
| | | | | Tsuda and Kato, (1976, 1977) |
| | | | | Umeda and Nishimura (1979) |
| | | $Cr(CH_3COO)_3$ | ± | Nakamuro et al. (1978) |
| | | $Cr(NO_3)_2$ | ± | |
| | | $CrCl_3$ | ± | |
| | | $Cr_2(SO_4)_3$ | − | |
| | | $CrCl_3$ | − | MacRae et al. (1979) |
| | | $CrCl_2$ | − | Tsuda and Kato (1977) |
| Mammals *in vivo* | | | | |
| Mouse somatic cells | Chromosome aberrations | $K_2Cr_2O_7$ | + | Bigaliev et al. (1974) |
| | | | | Wild (1978) |
| | | | | Fabry (1980) |
| | | $CaCrO_4$ | − | Fabry (1980) |
| | | $Cr(NO_3)_3$ | − | |
| Human somatic cells (professional exposure) | Chromosome aberrations | | + | Bigaliev et al. (1977) |

carcinoma were observed in man, including squamous cell, round cell, anaplastic, and adenocarcinoma. Cancer of the skin has not been observed in chromate workers, although such chromium exposure can cause dermatitis and ulcers of the skin and nasal cavities. The initial results of studies on carcinogenesis by chromium in animals were negative. Later, however, tumors were produced by several investigators after administration in muscle, bronchia, and pleura of chromite ore roast or calcium chromate (Hueper, 1958; Hueper and Payne, 1959; Payne, 1960; Roe and Carter, 1969; Laskin *et al.*, 1970; Kuschner and Laskin, 1971), of chromium trioxide (Hueper and Payne, 1959), strontium or lead chromate (Furst *et al.*, 1976), and chromic oxide (Drizhkov and Federova, 1967). Inhalation of calcium chromate dust (13 mg/m$^3$) produced pulmonary adenomas in mice exposed 35 hours per week during their life time, i.e., under conditions comparable to occupational exposure (Nettesheim and Hammons, 1971).

### 5.4. Teratogenesis

Experiments with labeled and unlabeled chromium(III) indicate that almost no inorganic chromium passes the placenta (Visek *et al.*, 1953; Mertz *et al.*, 1969; Gerber and Maes, 1983). Significant amounts of chromium are, however, present in fetal tissues (Mertz, 1969). Indeed, chromium in organic form appears readily to cross the placental barrier. In view of the limited chromium transfer under conditions of toxic exposure, it appears unlikely that this metal can affect the embryo, and the embryotoxic effect and malformations reported (Gale, 1974, 1978; Gale and Bunch, 1979; Iijima *et al.*, 1975) may, in fact, have been due to an action on the mother or on the placenta.

## 6. LEAD

### 6.1. Exposure, Occurrence, and General Toxicity

Lead, a metal known since the dawn of civilization, has many industrial uses, i.e., for the production of lead batteries, alloys, pigments, and alkylated compounds. Mainly tetraethyl lead is used as an antiknock agent in gasoline. Workers in these industries, as well as those occupied in lead smelters or in cutting and welding metals covered with lead-based paint, run the greatest risk of overexposure to lead. The total amount of lead released into the environment has reached unprecedented levels. Therefore, our main concern today is the high level of environmental contamination by lead, which could harm the developing organism in particular.

For the general population, diet represents the main source of lead, from which about 200–300 μg/day are ingested daily by an adult (WHO, 1977).

Other sources of oral intake may also be of importance for certain groups of the general population. Young children living in old houses in which lead-based paints had been used may ingest significant amounts of lead, sometimes resulting in encephalopathy. Children residing in areas where the soil and diet contain large amounts of lead (e.g., around smelters) may also ingest excessive amounts of lead.

Less than 50 $\mu$g/liter of lead are usually present in drinking water, but soft water conducted through leaden pipes may infuse water with several milligrams of lead per liter. Air concentration in rural areas is below 500 ng/$m^3$, but in areas of heavy traffic or near smelters, concentrations up to 14,000 ng/$m^3$ may be attained (Lafontaine et al., 1977; WHO, 1977). The chemical composition of lead particles in air is still incompletely characterized; they contain chlorides, bromides, oxides, etc. A cigarette contains about 10 $\mu$g of lead, of which about 2% are transferred to the mainstream smoke (WHO, 1977).

Intestinal absorption of lead is about 5% in adults, and somewhat higher in children. Lead released into the atmosphere is effectively absorbed from the lung (up to 50%). Although lead is readily excreted into urine, it is also accumulated in the skeleton, and high concentrations may occur in the liver and kidneys. Organic lead compounds can enter the central nervous system. Absorption and retention of lead are greatly influenced by dietary factors, particularly calcium.

Symptoms and mechanisms of lead intoxication have been studied in detail (for review Gerber et al., 1980, Nriagu, 1978). Heme synthesis is strongly inhibited by lead. In the central nervous system, the metabolism of neurotransmitters may be affected. Acute lead intoxications are rare. Chronic symptoms relate mainly to the hemopoietic system, the nervous system, the kidneys, and the gastrointestinal tract. Anemia from impaired heme synthesis and increased destruction of red cells occurs after high doses of lead. In the adult, lead affects mainly the peripheral nervous system. Children who eat lead paint (pica) can suffer from lead encephalopathy with convulsions, coma, and eventually, permanent brain damage. There has also been increasing concern and dispute that small exposure to lead may cause mental retardation in children.

## 6.2. Mutagenesis

The experimental data do not furnish an unequivocal proof that lead is mutagenic in mammals (Gerber et al., 1980 for review). Although lead affects the fidelity of DNA synthesis, cell proliferation, and in vivo DNA synthesis, negative results were obtained in all test systems utilized to assess its capacity to induce gene mutations in prokaryotes and eukaryotes (Table VI). The positive results obtained by Maxild et al. (1978) in the Salmonella microsome test, of Lower et al. (1978), on plants and of Lower (1975) on Drosophila

**Table VI**

**Mutagenicity Tests Performed with Lead Compounds**

| Species | Test | Compound | Result | References |
|---|---|---|---|---|
| T4 | | $PbCl_2$ | − | Corbett et al. (1970) |
| Bacillus subtilis | Rec-assay | $PbCl_2$ | − | Nishioka (1975) |
| | | $Pb(CH_3COO)_2$ | − | Nishioka (1975) |
| Salmonella typhimurium | Reversion assay | Arc welding | ? | Maxild et al. (1978) |
| Platymonas | Gene mutations | $PbCl_2$ | − | Hessler (1974, 1975) |
| Rice | Gene mutations | $PbCl_2$ | ± | Reddy and Vaidyanath (1978 a,b) |
| Zea mays and | Gene mutations | Lead plant | ? | Lower et al. (1978) |
| Tradescantia | Pollen abortion | | | |
| Allium cepa | C-mitosis | $(C_2H_5)_2PbCl_2$ | + | Ahlberg et al. (1972) |
| | | $(C_2H_5)_3PbCl$ | + | Ramel (1973) |
| | | $(CH_3)_3PbCl$ | + | |
| | | $Pb(NO_3)_2$ | + | Levan (1945) |
| Drosophila melanogaster | Gene mutations | Lead plant | ? | Lower (1975) |
| | Chromosome loss | $PbCl_2$ | − | Ramel (1973) |
| Mammalian cells in vitro | SCE | $(C_2H_5)_3PbCl$ | + | Ahlberg et al. (1972) |
| | Chromosome aberrations | $Pb(CH_3COO)_2$ | + | Stella et al. (1979) |
| | | $Pb(CH_3COO)_2$ | − | Schmid (1972) |
| | | | − | Deknudt and Deminatti (1978) |
| | | | + | Schwanitz et al. (1970) |
| | | | + | Bauchinger and Schmid (1972) |
| | | | + | Beek and Obe (1974) |
| | | | + | Obe et al. (1975) |
| Mammals in vivo | Micronucleus test | $Pb(CH_3COO)_2$ | − | Jacquet et al. (1977 b) |
| | | | − | Heddle and Bruce (1977) |

| Category | Compound | Result | Reference |
|---|---|---|---|
| Chromosome aberrations | Pb(CH₃COO)₂ | + | Muro and Goyer (1969) |
| | | − | Léonard et al. (1972) |
| | | + | Deknudt et al. (1977) |
| | | + | Jacquet et al. (1977 b) |
| | | − | Deknudt and Gerber (1979) |
| | | + | Jacquet and Tachon (1981) |
| Sperm abnormalities | Pb(CH₃COO)₂ | + | Heddle and Bruce (1977) |
| | | + | Wyrobek and Bruce (1978) |
| Fertility | Pb(CH₃COO)₂ | − | Eyden et al. (1979) |
| | | − | Kennedy and Arnold (1971) |
| | | +? | Léonard et al. (1972) |
| Man *in vivo* (occupational exposure) | Chromosome aberrations | − | Varma et al. (1974) |
| | | − | Sperling et al. (1970) |
| | | − | Bauchinger et al. (1972) |
| | | − | Schmid et al. (1972) |
| | | − | O'Riordan and Evans (1974) |
| | | − | Bui et al. (1975) |
| | | − | Bauchinger et al. (1977) |
| | | + | Forni and Secchi (1972), Forni et al. (1976) |
| | | + | Schwanitz et al. (1970, 1975) |
| | | + | Deknudt et al. (1973, 1977) |
| | | + | Deknudt and Léonard (1975) |
| | | + | Bauchinger et al. (1976) |
| | | + | Calugar and Sandulescu (1977) |
| Sperm abnormalities | | + | Norderson et al. (1978) |
| | | + | Lancranjan et al. (1975) |

*melanogaster* are not conclusive because the organisms were simultaneously exposed to several metals so that it cannot be decided which one had been responsible for the effects observed. Persons exposed occupationally or accidentally to lead have usually also been exposed to other potential mutagens, and this probably explains the increase in structural chromosome aberrations found in somatic cells from these persons. Indeed, experiments *in vitro* on mammalian cells also showed no or only a slight increase in structural chromosome aberrations, mostly achromatic lesions. Investigations on laboratory animals given lead also did not provide clear evidence for clastogenic properties of lead. Thus, Jacquet *et al.* (1977b) and Heddle and Bruce (1977) could not observe micronuclei in mice after an i.p. injection of 50 mg/kg lead acetate, and Léonard *et al.* (1972) detected no aberrations in bone marrow cells of mice given 1 g/liter of lead in their drinking water for 9 months. Similar findings were reported by Deknudt and Gerber (1979) for male mice kept on a diet containing 0.5% of lead for one month, whereas Jacquet *et al.* (1977b) detected a slight dose-dependent increase in gaps when 0, 0,25, 0.5, or 1% of dietary lead were given to mice for one month. Deknudt *et al.* (1977a) reported an increase in gaps and fragments in Cynomolgus monkeys (*Macaca irus*), receiving 1.5, 6, or 15 mg of lead acetate in the diet six days per week for 16 months, but no fragments were observed in a follow-up of the same material (Jacquet and Tachon, 1981). Muro and Goyer (1969) observed gaps and chromatid aberrations in cultured bone marrow cells from mice kept on 1% of lead for 2 weeks, but the culture time of 4 days was too long to give meaningful results.

One must conclude, therefore, that lead is not mutagenic, does not have clastogenic properties and does not affect the fertility of male and female mice (Kennedy and Arnold, 1971; Léonard *et al.*, 1972). Certain results (Heddle and Bruce, 1977; Wyrobek and Bruce, 1978; Eyden *et al.*, 1978) obtained with lead acetate given intraperitoneally to mice indicate, however, that lead may induce abnormalities in sperm-shape with a doubling dose of about 80 mg/kg. Alterations in sperm morphology were also reported in workers from a plant manufacturing storage batteries (Lancranjan *et al.*, 1975). Most likely, these effects reflect the general cytotoxic action of lead.

### 6.3. Carcinogenesis

No significant excess of cancers has been found among workers professionally exposed to lead (Dingwall-Fordyce and Lane, 1963; Cooper and Gaffey, 1975; Cooper, 1976).

Renal tumors (adenoma and adenoma carcinoma) were reported following high doses of lead given orally or by subcutaneous injection as lead phosphate or lead acetate to rodents (Boyland *et al.*, 1962; Coogan, 1973; Van Esch and Kroes, 1969; Zollinger, 1953). An increased incidence of lymphoma was observed in animals treated with tetraethyl lead (Epstein and Mantel, 1968) and, according to Zawirska and Medras (1972), prolonged feeding of lead acetate could cause interstitial cell tumors in rat testis. Nevertheless, one may conclude that proof is lacking that lead represents a carcinogenic risk in man.

## 6.4. Teratogenesis

The effects of lead on the developing embryo have recently been reviewed (Gerber *et al.*, 1980). Lead crosses the placental barrier less readily than mercury but more readily than cadmium (Lauwerys *et al.*, 1978), and lead concentrations in cord blood are lower than in maternal blood (Harris and Holley, 1972). Lead is also transferred to the fetus of hamsters (Carpenter *et al.*, 1973), mice (McClain and Becker, 1970; Gerber *et al.*, 1981), and goats (McLellan *et al.*, 1974).

It has been known since the last century that women working in the lead industry suffered from menstrual disorders, were often sterile, and had spontaneous abortions (Paul, 1860; Oliver, 1911; Nogaki, 1958); lead was sometimes used as abortifacient (Hall, 1905; Taussig, 1936). Abnormalities such as retarded growth and neurological symptoms were reported after accidental lead intoxication during pregnancy (Angle and McIntire, 1964; Palmisano *et al.*, 1969). A higher rate of mental retardation was noted in children from women living in areas with a water supply from leaden pipes (Beattie *et al.*, 1975).

Lead injected to chick embryos during day 2 causes, in addition to death (Fabre and Girault, 1957), abnormalities of the head (cranioschisis, ruptured brain, and shortened neck) (Catizone and Gray, 1941; Gilani, 1973). Injection on days 3 or 4, or later, can give rise to hydrocephalus and meningoceles (Hirano and Kochen, 1973; De Gennaro, 1978), perhaps via an action on blood vessels, alterations in permeability and subsequent hemmorrhage.

Mice treated with dietary lead (0.125% or more) starting at fertilization (vaginal plug) have a reduced number of pregnancies (Jacquet *et al.*, 1975). Such an interference with implantation could have resulted from a retarded cell division (Jacquet *et al.*, 1976) due to a toxic effect of lead on the embryo, also seen in culture (Streffer *et al.*, 1978). It could also be related to a hormonal imbalance of the mothers (Jacquet *et al.*, 1977), which also leads to an early regression of the corpora lutea. Indeed, the embryos still can reach the blastocyst stage, but do not form trophoblastic giant cells and do not implant (Jacquet, 1977; Wide and Nilsson, 1977).

Malformations after injection of lead were reported in hamsters (Ferm and Carpenter, 1967b; Ferm and Ferm, 1971), rats (McClain and Becker, 1975), and mice (Jacquet and Gerber, 1979). In hamsters, they involve abnormal caudal and sacral vertebrae, and are enhanced when lead is combined with cadmium (Ferm, 1969). The malformation may arise as a result of edema separating the caudal neural tube and the adjacent paraxial mesenchyme and ectoderm (Carpenter and Ferm, 1977). In mice, anterior vertebrae can become fused, and this effect is more marked when the mice are kept on a low calcium diet (Jacquet and Gerber, 1979), whereas in rats, malformations of the posterior end of the fetus occur (McClain and Becker, 1975).

Retardation in fetal and postnatal growth and fetal death have been observed in the above species and also in sheep (James *et al.*, 1966), dogs (Azar *et al.*, 1972), and guinea pigs (Weller, 1975). In mice, heme synthesis, particularly incorporation of iron, is reduced (Jacquet *et al.*, 1977b; Gerber and Maes, 1978); placental blood flow and uptake of substrate are also affected (Gerber *et al.*, 1978).

In conclusion, lead reduces fertility and presents a certain teratogenic risk at high exposure levels. Lead exposure during pregnancy should be especially restricted because of its possible neurotoxic action on the developing central nervous system.

## 7. MERCURY

### 7.1. Exposure, Occurrence, and General Toxicity

Mercury finds extensive use in electrical equipment (batteries, relays, etc.), in metallurgy, in catalysts, in fungicides, and in the laboratory. The level of mercury in the environment has consequently increased and, in some areas, has attained critical levels for the population. On the other hand, some of the classical sources of poisoning with inorganic mercury have almost disappeared, i.e., its use in medicine, in the manufacture of mirrors and hats, and as a suicidal agent. Exposure to mercury vapors and to mercuric–mercury aerosols is a hazard in chloralkali plants. In addition, mercury vapor can be inhaled in dental offices and in the manufacture of laboratory glassware and of electrical equipment. Mercury in the environment exists as elemental, mercuric, and organic mercury, the latter being formed principally by bacteria. Most food contains less than 50 $\mu$g/kg mercury, mainly as methylmercury (Bouquiaux, 1974), but concentrations in fish may be much higher, up to 20 mg/kg, depending on the degree of water pollution. Seeds treated with an organomercurial fungicide have given rise to accidental contamination of human and animal food in Iran and Iraq. Mercury concentration in ground and surface water is usually below 50 and 200 ng/liter, respectively; that in air ranges from a few ng/m$^3$ up to 50 ng/m$^3$, depending on the degree of urbanization (WHO, 1976), but the chemical form under which mercury occurs in water and air has not been fully characterized.

Metallic mercury enters the body mainly via inhalation of vapors; it is virtually not absorbed upon ingestion. Inorganic mercury salts are poorly absorbed (about 5%) after oral administration. The organic mercurials which are liposoluble can be absorbed by all routes. The principal sites of mercury deposition are the kidneys and the central nervous system after exposure to mercury vapor, the kidneys after exposure to inorganic mercury salts and to aryl or alkoxy mercury derivatives, and the central nervous system after exposure to alkyl mercury compounds. The latter are highly cumulative and are excreted through the bile. Inorganic mercury is mainly excreted via the urine and feces.

Excessive acute exposure vapors causes an inflammation of the respiratory tract. Acute intoxication by inorganic mercury salts is characterized by a severe irritation of the gastrointestinal tract followed by renal necrosis.

The target organs after chronic exposure to mercury vapor and aryl and alkoxy alkyl mercury compounds are the central nervous system and the kidney. The central nervous system is the main site of action of alkyl mercury. An outbreak of alkyl mercury (Minamata disease) occurred in Japan due to the consumption of fish contaminated with methyl mercury.

## 7.2. Mutagenesis

The mutagenicity of mercury compounds was first noted in 1937 and has been reviewed extensively by Ramel (1972) and by Léonard et al. (1981) (Table VII). Production of C-mitosis, which can result in aneuploidy and polyploidy, is the most noticeable mutagenic effect of mercury observed in eukaryotes. Such a specific and restricted action may explain the negative results obtained in experiments on prokaryotes and the contradictory observations with respect to the clastogenic potential of mercury. The induction of C-mitosis could result from the high affinity of mercury for sulfhydryl groups in the spindle apparatus. The cytotoxicity of organomercurials is, however, probably not only due to an action on sulfhydryl enzymes. Electronmicroscopic-histochemical observations indicate that mercury is bound to plasma membranes, liposomes, endoplasmic reticulum, the Golgi complex, mitochondria, and the nuclear envelope (Chang and Hartmann, 1972). Such membrane structures appear more sensitive towards the effects of methylmercury than metabolic activities such as DNA, RNA, and protein synthesis (Gruenwedel and Friend, 1978). Degenerative changes in cells thus could be due to damage to such sulfhydryl rich membranes (Kasuya, 1972, 1975). Observations on plants suggest, however, that organic mercury may also act directly on genetic material, producing chromosome fragmentation, somatic mutations and pollen sterility, but the mechanism of action of these changes remains unknown. In all test systems, organic mercury appears much more potent than inorganic compounds.

## Table VII
## Summary of the Mutagenicity Tests Performed with Mercury Compounds

| Species | Test | Compound | Result | Reference |
|---|---|---|---|---|
| *Bacillus subtilis* | Rec-assay | $C_8H_8HgO_2$ | − | Shirasu et al. (1976) |
| | | $C_6H_5HgCl$ | − | |
| | | $C_{33}H_{24}Hg_2O_2S_2$ | − | |
| *Salmonella typhimurium* | Reversion assay | $C_3H_6HgO_2$ | − | Heddle and Bruce (1976)<br>Bruce and Heddle (1979) |
| Plant material | Gene mutations | ? | | Reddy and Vaidyanath (1978a,b) |
| | C-mitosis | Organic mercury | + | Ahmed and Grant (1972) |
| | | Inorganic mercury | + | Bruhin (1955) |
| | | | | Fahmy (1951) |
| | | | | Fiskesjo (1969) |
| | | | | Kostoff (1939, 1940) |
| | | | | Levan (1945, 1971) |
| | | | | Macfarlane (1950, 1951) |
| | | | | Ramel (1969, 1973) |
| | Chromosome anomalies | | | Levan (1971) |
| | Somatic mutations | Organic mercury | + | Macfarlane (1950, 1951) |
| | Pollen sterility | | | Ramel (1969) |
| *Drosophila melanogaster* | Effect on mitosis and female meiosis | Organic mercury and inorganic mercury | + | Mathews and Al-Doori (1976) |
| | | | + | Ramel (1969, 1970) |
| | | | | Ramel and Magnusson (1969) |
| | Sex-linked lethal | $CH_3HgCl$ | + | Ramel (1969) |
| | | $C_2H_5HgCl$ | + | Mathews and Al-Doori (1976) |
| Silkworm | Effects on female meiosis | $CH_3HgCl$ | − | Tazima (1974) |
| Mammalian cells *in vitro* | C-mitosis | $C_6H_5ClHg$ | + | Ochi and Tonomura (1975);<br>Umeda et al. (1969) |
| | | $C_2H_5ClHg$ | + | |
| | | $C_4H_{10}NO_2SHg$ | + | Umeda et al. (1969) |

| Endpoint | Compound | | Reference |
|---|---|---|---|
| Chromosome breakage | $C_4HgClHg$ | + | Okada and Oharazawa (1967) |
| | $C_2H_5PO_4Hg$ | + | Fiskesjo (1970); |
| | $CH_3HgCl$ | + | Ochi and Tonomura (1975) |
| | $C_3H_8OHgCl$ | + | Fiskesjo (1970) |
| | $HgCl_2$ | + | Umeda et al. (1969) |
| | $CH_3HgCl$ | + | Kato (1976) |
| **Mammals in vivo** | | | Kato et al. (1976) |
| Experimental animals | | | |
| Micronucleus test | $C_3H_6HgO_2$ | − | Heddle and Bruce (1977); Bruce and Heddle (1979) |
| Chromosome anomalies | $HgCl_2$ | − | Poma et al. (1981) |
| Structural chromosome anomalies | Contaminated fish | + | Skerfving et al. (1970; 1974) |
| | | + | Kato et al. (1976) |
| | Mixture | + | Verschaeve et al. (1976) |
| | Mercury amalgam | + | Verschaeve and Susanne (1978) |
| Human lymphocytes | $C_8H_8HgO_2$ | + | Verschaeve et al. (1978) |
| | Metallic mercury | − | Verschaeve et al. (1979) |
| | | + | Popescu et al. (1979) |
| Mitotic chromosome association | Mercury salts (inhalation) | + | Verschaeve et al. (1978) |
| Sperm abnormalities | $C_3H_6HgO_2$ | − | Heddle and Bruce (1977); Bruce and Heddle (1979) |
| Dominant lethality | $CH_3HgCl$ | − | Ramel (1967) |
| | $CH_3HgCl$ | ? | Khera (1973) |
| | $C_2H_6Hg$ | ? | Varma et al. (1974) |
| Mammalian germ cells | $C_4H_6HgO_4$ | − | |
| Anomalies in oocytes | $C_2H_6Hg$ | − | Jagiello and Lin (1973) |

No evidence for a clastogenic potential of mercury is provided by the few experiments carried out in mammals *in vivo*. Methylmercury acetate gave negative results in the micronucleus test in the mouse (Heddle and Bruce, 1977; Bruce and Heddle, 1979), and Poma *et al.* (1981) failed to detect chromosome aberrations in spermatogonia and bone marrow cells of mice given a single i.p. injection of 2, 4, or 6 mg Hg $Cl_2$/kg body weight. Organic mercury is poorly taken up by the testis, epididymes, and seminal vesicles (only about 1% of the administered dose) (Mehra and Kanwar, 1980), and it is thus not surprising that Ramel (1967) and Lee and Dixon (1973) could not observe more dead implants in the mouse dominant lethal assay with methyl mercury dicyan diamide, methyl mercury hydroxyde, or mercuric chloride (0.1–1 mg/kg). Positive results with the dominant lethal test were reported by Khera and Tabacova (1973) after daily administration of 1, 2, or 5 mg/kg Hg$^{++}$ as methyl mercury chloride and by Varma *et al.* (1974) in mice injected with 50 mg/kg of dimethylmercury, but the small number of animals utilized makes these data open to criticism.

Mercuric acetate (25 $\mu$g/ml) and dimethylmercury (10 $\mu$g/ml) caused severe damage *in vitro* to the nuclei of mouse oocytes (Jagiello and Lin, 1973), but no immediate or delayed effect could be found when 2–10 $\mu$g/kg of mercuric acetate or 1400 $\mu$g/kg dimethylmercury were given *in vivo*. These doses appear, however, very low compared to those administered by Khera and Tabacova (1973) and Varma *et al.* (1974) discussed above. In assessing the risk of mercury to female germ cells it is also noteworthy that sea urchin eggs treated with para-chloromercuriphenyl sulfonic acid (PCMPS) or Na salicyl-g-hydroxy-mercuri-b-methoxy-propylamide *o*-acetic acid (ML, Mersalyl), and then inseminated can be penetrated by more than one sperm. This polyspermy may be related to changes in sulfhydryl groups of the egg membrane.

Several authors reported an increase in structural chromosome aberrations in peripheral blood lymphocytes of persons exposed to mercury, but an inference as to the clastogenic potential of mercury is difficult for the reasons already discussed. In this respect, a recent study by Verschaeve *et al.* (1979) is revealing. They failed to detect any significant increase in structural and numeric chromosome aberrations in peripheral blood lymphocytes from 28 workers exposed to mercury vapours in a chloralkali plant, although their urinary mercury levels were significantly higher than those of the controls. These authors now believe that their previous positive results after exposure to different mercury compounds (Verschaeve *et al.*, 1976), to mercury amalgam in dental work (Verschaeve and Susanne, 1978) and to phenyl mercury acetate (Verschaeve *et al.*, 1978) had been due to a simultaneous exposure to other environmental mutagens. Such an interference and/or inadequate methodology could also explain the positive results in persons who had high mercury levels in blood, probably as a result of consuming contaminated fish (Kato *et al.*, 1976; Skerfving *et al.*, 1970, 1974). An altered position at metaphase of particular chromosomes involved in nucleolar organization has been observed in lymphocytes of persons exposed to mercury (Verschaeve *et al.*, 1978), an effect which, according to the authors, could be due to a greater density in this region of molecules carrying sulfhydryl groups or to an inhibition of specific enzymes regulating nucleolar activity.

## 7.3. Carcinogenesis

No positive data that mercury could be carcinogenic in man has appeared to date. Animal experiments also provided negative results, with the exception of an observation by Druckrey *et al.* (1957) that spindle cell sarcomas containing fine drops of mercury appeared two years after intraperitoneal injection of metallic mercury.

## 7.4. Teratogenesis

Mercury can pass the placenta, although a certain barrier exists which seems to depend on the chemical form and the dose. At a dietary concentration of less than 0.05 ppm, mercury concentrations in the mouse embryo are higher than in the mother; at higher concentrations, the reverse is the case (Child, 1973). Methyl mercury infused into pregnant Rhesus monkeys reaches the fetus rapidly, although the concentration ratio of fetal to maternal blood never exceeds 0.1 (Reynolds and Pitkin, 1975). Many investigations demonstrated that alkyl mercury passes the placenta more readily than inorganic or aryl mercury, resulting in higher concentrations in the fetus than in the mother of rodents (Garrett *et al.*, 1972; Yamaguchi and Nunotani, 1974; Mansour *et al.*, 1975; Kelman *et al.*, 1980) and cats (Morikawa, 1961). Ethyl mercury seems to be more efficiently transferred to the fetus than methyl mercury. Vapors of elementary mercury enter the fetus more readily than injected mercury salts (Greenwood *et al.*, 1972). The human placenta is also readily permeable to methylmercury (Bakir *et al.*, 1973; Skerfving, 1974; Baglan *et al.*, 1974; Wannag and Skjaerasen, 1975, Koos and Longo, 1976, Lauwerys *et al.*, 1978; Roels *et al.*, 1978).

The brain of the rat fetus concentrates mercury more than that of the mother (Yang *et al.*, 1972; Null *et al.*, 1973; Garcia *et al.*, 1974; King *et al.*, 1976; Wannag, 1976). Transfer via the milk also results in high mercury concentrations in the brain (Yang *et al.*, 1973), but, after treatment ceases, the decrease may also be more rapid (Casterline and Williams, 1972).

Central nervous system damage was noted in newborns of mothers suffering from Minamata disease, even when the mother was asymptomatic (Marsh *et al.*, 1977; Harada, 1978). Whereas lesions in the adult central nervous system are limited to the granular layer of the cerebellum and some areas of the cerebrum, they involve the entire cortex of fetuses and infants and are particularly pronounced in fetuses, indicating that the damage is the more severe and widespread the earlier the exposure (Chang, 1977). The consequences of fetal Minamata disease are often not fully manifest at birth, except for a reduction in head size; cerebral palsy and mental defects in learning and behavior develop only later (Weiss and Doherty, 1975). Malformations, other than central nervous system damage, have not been observed in man (Dales, 1972).

Several studies have been carried out on the effects of organic mercury on developing experimental animals. Organic mercury causes a decrease in the weight of trout alevins (Christensen, 1975), as well as death, reduced growth, and impaired learning of avian embryos (Spann *et al.*, 1972; Kojima cited in Earl and Vish, 1980; Rosenthal and Sparber, 1972). Organic mercury is more toxic to the developing chicken than inorganic mercury (Kuwahara, 1970). Whereas feeding of rats with 12 $\mu$g/kg of methyl mercury seemed without adverse effects on the offspring (Newborne *et al.*, 1972), a much higher dose (8 mg/kg) of phenyl mercury reduced litter size drastically (Piechoka, 1968). After injection of organic mercury, embryonic deaths but no malformations were seen in rats (Mottet, 1974) and mice (Ramel, 1967). Most observers agree, however, that injection of a few mg/kg of organic mercury causes malformations (cleft palate, jaw and facial defects) in mice (Murakami *et al.*, 1956; Spyker and Smithberg, 1972; Su and Okita, 1976a; Olson and Massaro, 1977; Fujita *et al.*, 1979), hamsters (Gale and Ferm, 1971; Harris *et al.*, 1972) and dogs (Earl *et al.*, 1973). In the rat, different types of malformations, mainly of the genitourinary organs, were reported (Nolen *et al.*, 1972; Scharpf *et al.*, 1973; Chang and Sprecher, 1976), and ultrastructural damage to the fetal liver occurred after administering as little as 5–10 ppm of methyl mercury in the drinking water from 1 month before mating until the end of pregnancy (Ware *et al.*, 1974; Fowler and Woods, 1977).

Fetal development of the brain is also impaired in experimental animals by organic mercury. High doses of ethyl or methyl mercury cause an atrophy of the external granular layer of the cerebellum in cat fetuses (Morikawa, 1961; Khera, 1973). In rodents, the changes observed after treatment during organogenesis were similar to those seen in adults and, in contrast to the observations in man, usually did not involve the cortical plate (Matsumoto *et al.*, 1967; Khera and Tabacova, 1973; Inouye *et al.*, 1972; Nonaka, 1969) so that degeneration in these species appears to commence only when the brain has reached a certain state of maturity. As in man, subtle changes in behavior may be found in experimental animals, even in the absence of gross lesions in the fetal and maternal brain (Fujita, 1969; Spyker and Chang, 1974; Su and Okita, 1976b). In conclusion, animal data indicate that organic mercury can cause gross malformations, but as these have been observed usually only after injection, the relevance for man is uncertain. The principal risk of mercury to the developing organism, as with lead, is its neurotoxic action, which can cause permanent brain damage by interfering with normal brain development.

## 8. NICKEL

### 8.1. Exposure, Occurrence, and General Toxicity

Nickel is used in metallurgy for alloys, in electroplating, in enamels, in nickel-cadmium batteries, and as a catalyst. Food is the main source of nickel for nonoccupationally exposed persons. The average daily intake from food has been estimated at 250 $\mu$g; the concentration in drinking water is usually below 20 $\mu$g/liter (NAS, 1975). Nickel content in rural and suburban air is usually below 70 and 80 ng/m$^3$, respectively, but near nickel emitting sources can attain 200 ng/m$^3$. Nickel in air originates mainly from automobile exhaust and the burning of oil and coal. Cigarettes contain an average of 2.3 $\mu$g of nickel (Sunderman and Sunderman, 1961). The hazards of nickel exposure to the general population resemble those of chromium and involve mainly the allergic potential of nickel. Occupational exposure to nickel can induce tumors in the nasal sinuses and the lung.

Nickel salts are poorly absorbed from the gastrointestinal tract (about 5%). Aerial intake is significant only under conditions of occupational exposure; the removal of material from the lung depends on its solubility and is slow for metallic or oxidic nickel, faster for soluble nickel salts and most rapid for nickel carbonyl. Nickel attains high concentrations in the skeleton, liver, and kidneys, and is bound to the $a_1$ macroglobulin "nickeloplasmin" in blood. Nickel is mainly excreted into urine and, compared to other heavy metals with the exception of chromium, has a relatively short half-life of less than one week.

Only acute exposure to nickel carbonyl can elicit generalized severe symptoms, such as headache, delirium, dyspnea, pulmonary edema, and even death; orally ingested nickel salts are almost harmless. The principal chronic hazards of nickel to man, beside its carcinogenic action discussed below, is its ability to provoke sensitization reactions, the "nickel itch" dermatitis. Nickel is responsible for about 5% of all eczema in man, and about 10% of a tested population is potentially allergic to nickel.

## 8.2. Mutagenesis

Nickel(II) salts react readily with DNA and affect DNA and protein synthesis more than RNA synthesis. They may also modify the transcription (Miyaki *et al.*, 1977; Sirover and Loeb, 1976; Nishimura and Umeda, 1979).

The results of the mutagenicity studies have been reviewed in detail by Léonard *et al.* (1981) and are summarized in Table VIII. On the basis of the data actually available, it seems impossible to decide with certainty whether nickel is mutagenic or not. Nickel failed to induce gene mutations in microorganisms and gave negative results in the Rec-assay with *Bacillus subtilis*. Nickel may, however, have some mutagenic activity on mammalian cells. Recent results by Miyaki *et al.* (1977) showed a slight increase in the incidence of gene mutations in cells treated with $NiCl_2$, and cell transformation was induced by $Ni_3S_2$ (Waksvik *et al.*, 1980) and $NiSO_4$ (Rivedal and Sanner, 1980). Moreover, $NiS_4$ (Wulf, 1980) and $Ni_3S_2$ (Waksvik *et al.*, 1980) can produce SCE in mammalian cells *in vitro*, but these *in vitro* studies did not indicate that nickel is clastogenic for mammalian chromosomes. Nishimura and Umeda (1979) observed, however, an increase in chromosome aberrations during the recovery period following treatment with $NiCl_2$, $Ni(CH_3COO)_2$, $K_2Ni(CN)_4$, and NiS.

## 8.3. Carcinogenesis

Occupational nickel exposure can cause cancer of the lungs and nasal sinuses. An increase up to 900 times of nasal cancers and up to 10 times of lung cancers had been observed in workers of nickel refineries, but improvements in the refining process have markedly reduced these values (Doll, 1958; Doll *et al.*, 1970). Earlier, nickel carbonyl was thought to be the tumorigenic agent, but now dusts of nickel oxide and sulfide produced during calcination are considered also to be responsible for cancer induction (IARC, 1976). Information on cancer induction is less extensive for other conditions of exposure, such as welding, electroplating, grinding, and production of catalysts. Cancers of the larynx, stomach, kidney, and sarcoma of soft tissues have also been attributed to nickel exposure although this is not proven (review Kazantzis and Lilly, 1979; Léonard *et al.*, 1981; Sunderman, 1976). Various factors, such as exposure to arsenic, polycyclic carbons, and smoking habits may increase the carcinogenic risk of nickel (see the above reviews).

Experimental studies in animals have demonstrated that only water-insoluble nickel compounds have carcinogenic potential, and that malignant tumors develop after a latency period of several months, usually either at the site of application or, more rarely, elsewhere. Sarcomas have been observed in muscle and testis, but lung tumors have been most often induced. Of all nickel

**Table VIII**

**Summary of the Mutagenicity Test Performed with Nickel Salts**

| Species | Test | Compound | Result | References |
|---|---|---|---|---|
| Bacteriophage | T4 inactivation | $NiSO_4$ | + | Corbett et al. (1970) |
| | Gene mutation | $NiSO_4$ | − | Nishioka (1975) |
| Bacillus subtilis | Rec-assay | $NiCl_2$ | − | Shirasu et al. (1976) |
| | | $NiS_4N_2C_5H_8$ | − ⎫ | |
| | | $NiS_4N_2C_6H_{12}$ | − ⎭ | |
| Escherichia coli | Reverse mutations | $NiCl_2$ | − | Green et al. (1976) |
| Salmonella typhimurium | Reverse mutations | $NiCl_2$ | − | Bulselmaier et al. (1972) |
| Vicia faba | Cellular effects | $Ni(NO_3)_2$ | + | Glaess (1955, 1956a,b) |
| | | $NiCl_2$ | + ⎫ | Komczynnski et al. (1963) |
| | | $NiSO_4$ | ? ⎭ | |
| Mammalian cells in vitro | Gene mutations | $NiCl_2$ | + | Miyaki et al. (1977) |
| | Cell transformation | $Ni_3S_2$ | + | Waksvik et al. (1980) |
| | | $NiSO_4$ | + | Rivedal (1980) |
| | SCE | $Ni_3S_2$ | + | Wulf (1980) |
| | | $NiSO_4$ | + | Waksvik et al. (1980) |
| | Chromosome aberrations | $NiS$ | + ⎫ | Swieringa and Boersma (1968); Umeda and Nishimura (1979) |
| | | $Ni$ | − ⎫ | |
| | | $NiO$ | − | |
| | | $NiCl_2$ | ? ⎬ | Paton and Allison (1972) |
| | | $Ni(CH_2COO)_2$ | ? | |
| | | $K_2Ni(CN)_4$ | + ⎭ | Umeda and Nishimura (1979) |
| Human lymphocytes | Chromosome aberrations | $Ni_3S_2$ | ⎫ | |
| in vivo | | $NiO$ | gaps ⎬ | Waksvik et al. (1980) |
| | | $NiCl_2$ | | |
| | | $NiSO_4$ | ⎭ | |

compounds so far tested, nickel subsulfide appears to be most effective in causing cancer in a dose-dependent manner.

### 8.4. Teratogenesis

Nickle can cross the placental barrier of mice (Lu *et al.*, 1976; Jacobsen *et al.*, 1978; Gerber and Maes, 1981) or rats (Sunderman *et al.*, 1978), and enters the mouse embryo from day 5–8 of pregnancy (Lu *et al.*, 1979; Olsen and Jonsen, 1979) but not before. In man, the concentration of nickel in fetal tissue is about the same as in the adult (McNeely *et al.*, 1971; Stack *et al.*, 1976; Casey and Robinson, 1978).

Nickel can cause death and various anomalies in chick embryos (Ridgway and Karnofsky, 1952; Gilani and Marano, 1980). Administration of nickel to pregnant rats in food or drinking water does not produce malformations, but increases fetal and postnatal mortality and reduces growth (Schroeder and Mitchener, 1971b; Ambrose *et al.*, 1976; Nadenko *et al.*, 1979). Parenteral administration of nickel to mice and hamsters during organogenesis provoked various general malformations (Ferm, 1972; Lu *et al.*, 1979). Interestingly, parenteral administration of nickel to mice before implantation caused malformations such as exencephaly (Storeng and Jonsen, 1980, 1981). Similar defects, as well as cystic lung disease, were found following inhalation of nickel by hamsters before implantation (Sunderman *et al.*, 1979). Since exencephaly is usually caused by application of teratogens later during organogenesis, a delay of 1–2 days between injection and teratogenic activity of nickel seems to occur as a result of a retarded transfer via the placenta. This is also suggested by the observation that eye malformations (anophthalmia and microphthalmia) arise in rats after nickel inhalation on days 7 and 8 (Sunderman *et al.*, 1980), and after irradiation on day 9 or 10. In conclusion, nickel appears to be teratogenic, but this could play a role for man only after inhalation exposure to relatively soluble nickel compounds.

## 9. OTHER METALS

### 9.1. Mutagenesis

The literature available on other metals is scanty and insufficient to estimate their genetic hazards, and only a few examples of such studies will be quoted.

Cobalt in the form of $CoCl_2$ provided negative results in the Rec-assay in *Bacillus subtilis* (Nishioka, 1975), but this salt as well as $Co(OH)_3$, $CoSO_4$, and $2CoCO_3 \cdot 3Co(OH)_2$ gave positive results in the same test system in experiments by Kanematsu et al. (1980). $CoCl_2$ produced gene mutations in yeast mitochondria (Prazmo et al., 1975) and in mammalian cells in vitro (Miyaki et al., 1979). On the other hand, Paton and Allison (1972) could not observe chromosome aberrations in mammalian cells treated with $Co(NO_3)_2$ in vitro.

The Rec-assay on Bacillus subtilis (Nishioka, 1975) yielded negative results for $FeCl_2$, $FeCl_3$, $K_3Fe(CN)_6$ and $K_4Fe(CN)_6$.

Iron(II) as well as iron (III) enhanced, however, the clastogenic properties of ascorbate in mammalian cells (Stich et al., 1979).

Lithium was inactive in the Rec-assay (Nishioka, 1975), and did not produce chromosome aberrations in mammalian cells in vitro (Friedrick and Neilssen, 1969; Timpson and Price, 1971) or in man in vivo (Genest and Villeneuve, 1971; Jarvik et al., 1971).

Manganese salts [$MnCl_2$, $Mn(NO_3)_2$, $MnSO_4$, $Mn(CH_3COO)_2$] are apparently potent mutagens. Positive results were obtained in the Rec-assay with Bacillus subtilis (Nishioka, 1975), bacteriophage (Orgel and Orgel, 1965), yeast (Prazmo et al., 1975; Putrament et al., 1977) and E. coli (Demerek et al., 1975).

Recent results suggest that platinum can induce gene mutations in mammalian cells (Taylor et al., 1979) and in Salmonella typhimurium (Beck and Fisch, 1980; Lecointe et al., 1979; Suraikina et al., 1979).

Nakamuro et al. (1976) reported positive results for the Rec-assay with $H_2SeO_4$, $Na_2SeO_2$ and $SeO_2$ and negative ones with $H_2SeO_4$ and $Na_2Se$. All five compounds produced chromosome aberrations in mammalian cells in vitro. The negative results of Paton and Allison (1972) may be due to the low doses of $Na_2SeO_3$ and $Na_2SeO_4$ employed.

Zinc in the form of $ZnCl_2$ failed to induce gene mutations in E. coli (Venitt and Levy, 1974) or dominant or sex recessive lethals in Drosophila melanogaster (Carpenter and Ray, 1969). Zinc appears, however, to be clastogenic as shown by the chromosome aberrations observed in mammalian cells in vitro (Pilinskaya, 1971; Deknudt and Deminatti, 1978), in experimental animals in vivo (Deknudt and Gerber, 1979), and in occupationally exposed persons (Pilinskaya, 1970, 1974).

## 9.2. Carcinogenesis

Much speculation, but little actual epidemiological and experimental data, are available concerning the carcinogenic potential of other metals. Injection of cobalt powder (including that from chromium–cobalt alloys of protheses), as well as of cobalt oxide and sulfide can induce sarcoma at the site of injection (Gilman, 1962; Heath et al., 1971). Cobalt is considered a suspected carcinogen in the work environment in Sweden (Norseth, 1977), but no epidemiological information sustains this claim.

Hematite (iron oxide) has been suspected as causing lung cancers in miners in Cumberland (Boyde *et al.*, 1970) and Sweden (Joergensen, 1973), but other factors such as smoking, and exposure to radon daughters cannot be clearly separated in these surveys. Iron therapy seemed unrelated to development of sarcoma, although local sarcoma could be induced by injection of iron complexes (see review, Kazantzis and Lilly, 1979), and the significance of other tumors provoked by iron appears doubtful.

Injection of $ZnCl_2$ can elicit teratomas after local injection into the testis (review, Sunderman, 1976), and this was indeed the first observation that metals could be carcinogenic (Michalowsky, 1926). However, no other experimental system or epidemiological observations indicate that zinc could be carcinogenic in man.

## 9.3. Teratogenesis

Information on metals others than those treated above is limited. Deficiency of certain trace metals such as copper, manganese, and zinc can cause malformations (reviewed in Hurley, 1981), and deficiency of selenium can affect reproductive capacity (Harr, 1978). It is of interest that, conversely, high doses of copper and selenium can also cause malformations.

Cobalt injection induces cleft lips and palate in mice (Kasirsky *et al.*, 1967).

Copper salts are poorly absorbed from the intestinal tract, but pass the placental barrier when injected intraperitoneally to hamsters on day 8 of gestation, and can provoke malformation of the head as well as resorption of fetuses (Ferm and Hanlon, 1974a). Copper sulfate (10 mg/kg/day) added to the diet of pregnant ewes for a period of 45–146 days caused abortion in one of four animals (James *et al.*, 1966).

Lithium was found to be teratogenic in chickens, frogs, toads, mice, and rats (Loevy, 1973). On the other hand, only three malformed children were born from 60 lithium-treated mothers, a percentage not significantly above that found in a nontreated population (Shou and Amdisen, 1971).

Selenium crosses the placental barrier (Westfall *et al.*, 1938; Hadjimarkos *et al.*, 1959) and increases the rate of fetal death in mice (Schroeder and Mitchener, 1971b), rats (Rosenfeld and Beath, 1954), and pigs (Wahlstrom and Olson, 1959). Malformations after selenium treatment were observed in chickens (Franke *et al.*, 1936; Gruenwald, 1958; Kury *et al.*, 1967), but not in rats (Westfall *et al.*, 1938) and hamsters (Holmberg and Ferm, 1969). However, when pregnant ewes grazed on seleniferous ranges, deformities of the eyes and the extremities, and hypoplasia of the reproductive organs were observed in the surviving lambs (Rosenfeld and Beath, cited in Earl and Vish, 1980). No adverse effects on pregnancy were noted in women preparing bacteriological media with selenite powder (Robertson, 1970), and the rate of neonatal death did not differ significantly between areas with high and low selenium content in the environment (Shamberger, 1971).

Thallium has been reported to cause delayed maturation of the cartilage in chickens (Ridgway and Karnofsky, 1952; Hall 1972), and rats (Nogami and Terashima, 1973).

Zinc crosses the hamster placenta (Ferm and Hanlon, 1974b; Ferm and Carpenter 1968b) but, even at large doses, was found unable to induce malformations in guinea pigs, sheep, or man (James *et al.*, 1966; Earl and Vish, 1980).

## 10. CONCLUSIONS

The metallurgical industry contributes most to the dispersion of metals in our environment, and this has become a matter of increasing concern, since several metals have been shown to have mutagenic, carcinogenic, or teratogenic potential.

For certain of these metals, such as beryllium and cobalt, the risk of excessive exposure is usually restricted to persons occupationally exposed or living near sources of emission, whereas for other metals, such as arsenic, lead, cadmium, and mercury, such exposure can extend to large parts of the general population.

Although there are now available more than 100 systems to test mutagenic properties, data are still insufficient to decide whether certain metals are mutagenic or not. Doubtless, hexavalent chromium, which is reduced in the cell to the trivalent state, must be considered as a potent mutagen. Arsenic, mainly in the form of its trivalent compounds, has clastogenic properties but apparently is unable to induce gene mutations. Most of the relatively few studies carried out on beryllium yielded positive results. A few data suggest that toxic doses of cadmium can induce gene mutations in microorganisms and chromosome aberrations in plants, but in mammals cadmium does not seem to act as a mutagen. Likewise, experimental data do not furnish a clear proof that lead is mutagenic in mammals, and the only evident effect of mercury is the production of C-mitosis. Nickel failed to induce gene mutations in microorganisms but may have mutagenic activity in mammalian cells. The information actually available thus allows us to classify the metals according to their mutagenic potential about as follows: $Cr > Be > As > Ni > Hg > Cd > Pb$.

Experimental studies in mammals and epidemiological observations in man have been utilized to assess the carcinogenic properties of metals. Although so far arsenic has not been shown to produce tumors in experimental animals, epidemiological studies on industrial and farm workers or persons treated for medical reasons strongly suggest that arsenic is a human carcinogen. Whereas the observations on beryllium exposure in man are still a matter of some controversy, data on animals indicate that this metal represents a carcinogenic hazard to man. A variety of chromium derivatives has produced cancer in animals, and an increase in incidence of respiratory cancers has been observed in persons occupationally exposed to chromium. Likewise, occupational nickel exposure can cause cancer of the lung and the nasal sinuses, whereas in experimental animals only insoluble nickel compounds engendered tumors, usually at the site of application. Lead has produced tumors in animals, but epidemiological data do not suggest that lead, mercury or cadmium should be considered as human carcinogens. Taking in account the number of persons potentially exposed, one can classify metals according to their carcinogenic risks as follows: As $>$ Cr $>$ Ni $>$ Be $>$ Pb $=$ Cd $=$ Hg, the latter three metals being practically not carcinogenic in man.

Information on the teratogenic risks is derived almost exclusively from experiments on animals, mainly rodents; no epidemiological data are available, as was the case with carcinogenesis and mutagenesis. Moreover, the conditions of such experimental exposure (injection of high doses) usually differ greatly from those under which man may be exposed, so that extrapolation to man is difficult. Arsenic injected at high doses provokes malformations in rodents. Arsenic could thus be a potential teratogen in man. Cadmium, even at low doses of chronic exposure, is teratogenic in animals and should also be considered so in man. Chromium, due to its poor transplacental transfer, does not represent a teratogenic risk to man under prevailing conditions of exposure. Lead is embryotoxic to the human embryo, can delay growth, and interfere with the development of the central nervous system. Malformations have been observed in animals but so far not in man. Consequently, lead must be considered a risk to the developing organism. Likewise, organic mercury causes central nervous system damage after exposure *in utero*. Malformations were seen in animals but not in man. Mercury, thus, is a serious hazard during pregnancy. Animal experiments suggest that nickel can cause malformations and may do so also in man. Most likely, the greatest risk to human development originates from the toxicity of mercury and lead in the developing central nervous system. The risk of malformations seems greatest for cadmium followed by arsenic, nickel, and chromium.

## REFERENCES

Ahlberg, J. C., Ramel, C., and Wachtmeister, C. A., 1972, Organolead compounds shown to be genetically active, *Ambio* **1**:29–31.

Ahmed, M., and Grant, W. F., 1972, Cytological effects of the mercurial fungicide Panagen 15 on Tradescantia and *Vicia faba* root-tip, *Mutat. Res.* **14**:391–396.

Ahmed, Z. U., and Walker, G. W. R., 1972, Studies on the effect of urethane, selenocystine and sodium monohydrogenarsenate on crossing over in the X-chromosome of *Drosophila melanogaster*, *Can. J. Genet. Cytol.* **14**:719.

Ambrose, A. M., Larson, P. S., Borzelleca, J. F., and Hennigar, G. R. Jr., 1976, Long term toxicologic assessment of nickel in rats and dogs, *J. Food Sci. Technol.* **13**:181–187.

Ancel, P., 1946, Recherche expérimentale sur la spina bifida, *Arch. Anat. Microsc. Morphol. Exp.* **36**:45–68.

Andersen, K. J., Leigthy, E. G., and Takahashi, M. T., 1972, Evaluation of herbicides for possible mutagenic properties, *J. Agric. Food Chem.* **20**:649–656.

Anghileri, L. J., 1973, Calcium metabolism in tumors; its relationship with chromosome complex accumulation, *Oncology*, **27**:30–44.

Angle, C. R., and McIntire, M. S., 1964, Lead poisoning during pregnancy, *Amer. J. Dis. Child.* **108**:436–439.

Arguello, R. A., Cenget, D. D., and Tello, E. E., 1938, Cancer y arsenicismo regional endemico en Cordoba, Rep. Argent., *Dermatofisiol. (Buenos Aires)* **22**:461–487.

Axelsson, O., Dahlgren, E., Jansson, C. D., and Rehnlund S. O., 1978, Arsenic exposure and mortality: A case-referent study from a Swedish copper smelter, *Br. J. Ind. Med.* **35**:8–15.

Axelsson, O., Rylander, R., and Schmidt, A., 1980, Mortality and incidence of tumours among ferrochromium workers, *Br. J. Ind. Med.* **37**:121–127.

Azar, A., Trochimowicz, H. J., and Maxfield, M. E., 1972, Review of lead studies in animals carried out at Haskell Laboratory; Two year feeding study and response to hemmorhage study, *Proc. Inter. Symp. Environ. Health Aspects of Lead*, Amsterdam, pp. 199–209.

Baer, R. L., Ramsey, D. L., and Biondi, E., 1973, The most common contact allergens 1968–1970, *Arch. Dermatol.* **108**:74–78.

Baglan, R. J., Brill, A. B., Schulert, A., Wilson, D., Larsen, K., Dyer, N., Mansour, M., Schaffner, W., Hoffman, L., and Davies, J., 1974, Utility of placental tissue as an indicator of trace element exposure to adult and fetus, *Environ. Res.* **8**:64–70.

Bakir, F., Damluji, S. F., Amin-zaki, L., Murtadha, M., Klalidi, A., Al-Rawi, N. Y., Tikriti, S., Dhahir, H. I., Clarkson, T. W., Smith, J. C., and Doherty, R. A., 1973, Methylmercury poisoning in Iraq: An interuniversity report, *Science* **181**:230–241.

Barnes, J. M., Denz, F. A., and Sissons, H. A., 1950, Beryllium bones sarcomata in rabbits, *Br. J. Cancer* **4**:212–222.

Barr, M., 1973, The teratogenicity of cadmium in two stocks of Wistar rats, *Teratology* **7**:237–242.

Bauchinger, M., and Rohr, G., 1976, Chromosome analysis in cell cultures of Chinese hamsters after application of CdSO₄, *Mutat. Res.* **38**:102–103.

Bauchinger, M., and Schmid, E., 1972, Chromosomenanalysen in Zellkulturen des Chinesischen Hamsters nach Applikation von Bleiazetat, *Mutat. Res.* **14**:95–100.

Bauchinger, M., Schmid, E., and Schmidt, D., 1972, Chromosomenanlyse bei Verkehrspolizisten mit erhoehter Bleilast, *Mutat. Res.* **16**:407–412.

Bauchinger, M., Schmid, E., Einbrodt, H., and Dresp, J., 1976, Chromosome aberrations in lymphocytes after occupational exposure to lead and cadmium, *Mutat. Res.* **40**:57–62.

Bauchinger, M., Dresp, J., Schmid, E., Englert, N., and Krause, C., 1977, Chromosome analysis of children after ecological lead exposure, *Mutat. Res.* **56**:75–80.

Bayliss, D., 1972, Expected and observed deaths by selected causes occurring to beryllium workers, in *Nat. Inst. Occup. Health and Safety*. Criteria for a recommended standard: Occupational exposure to beryllium, pp. IV–22 to IV–23, Tables VII–X, Washington D.C., U.S. Dept. Health, Education, and Welfare.

Beattie, A. D., Moore, M. R., and Goldberg, A., 1975, Role of chronic low-level lead exposure in the etiology of mental retardation, *Lancet* **1**:589–598.

Beaudoin, A. R., 1974, Teratogenicity of rhodium arsenate in rats, *Teratology* **19**:153–158.

Beck, D. J., and Fish, J. E., 1980, Mutagenicity of platinum coordination complexes in *Salmonella typhimurium*, *Mutat. Res.* **77**:45–54.

Beckman, G., Beckman, L., and Nordenson, I., 1977, Chromosome aberrations in workers exposed to aresneic, *Environ. Health Perspect.* **19**:145–148.

Beek, B., and Obe, G., 1974, Effect of lead acetate on human leucocyte chromosomes in vitro, *Experientia* **30**:1006–1007.

Bergoglio, R. M., 1964, Mortalidad por cancer en zonas de aquas arsenicales de la provincia de Cordoba, Republica Argentina, *Prensa Med. Argent.* **51**:994–998.

Berlin, M., and Ullberg, S., 1963, The fate of $Cd^{109}$ in the mouse, *Arch. Environ. Health* **7**:686–693.

Bigaliev, A. B., Elemesova, M. S., and Bigalieva, R. K., 1974, Chromosome aberrations induced by chromium compounds in somatic cells of mammals, *Tsitol. Genet.* **10**:222–224.

Bigaliev, A. B., Turebaev, M. N., Bigalieva, R. K., and Elemesova, M. S., 1977, Cytogenetic examination of workers engaged in chrome production, *Genetika* (Moscow) **10**:222–224.

Birge, W., and Roberts, O. W., 1976, Toxicity of metals to chick embryos, *Bull. Environ. Contam. Toxicol.* **16**:319–324.

Blejer, H., and Wagner, W., 1976, Case study for inorganic arsenic-ambient level approach to the control of occupational cancerogenic, *Ann. N. Y. Acad. Sci.* **271**:179–186.

Bonatti, S., Meini, M., and Abbondandolo, A., 1976, Genetic effects of potassium dichromate in *Schizosacchoromyces pombe*, *Mutat. Res.* **38**:147–150.

Bouquiaux, J., 1974, Mercury and cadmium in the environment. First results of an inquiry on a European scale, in *C. E. C. European Symposium on the Problems of Contamination of Man and his Environment by Mercury and Cadmium*, CID, Luxembourg 3–5 July, pp. 23–46.

Boyd, J. T., Doll, R., Faulds, J. S., and Leiper, J., 1970, Cancer of the lung in iron ore (hematite) miners, *Br. J. Ind. Med.* **27**:97–105.

Boyland, E., Dukas, C. E., Grover, P. L., and Mitchley, C. B. V., 1962, The induction of renal tumors by feeding lead acetate to rats, *Br. J. Cancer* **16**:283–288.

Bruce, W., and Heddle, J., 1979, The mutagenic activity of 61 agents as determined by the micronucleus, *Salmonella* and sperm abnormality assays, *Can. J. Genet. Cytol.* **21**:319–334.

Bruhin, A., 1955, Ueber polyploidisierende Wirkung eines Samenbeizmittels, *Phytopathol. Z* **23**:381.

Buchet, J. P., Roels, H., Lauwerys, R., Bruaux, P., Claeys–Thoreau, F., Lafontaine, R., and Verduyn, G., 1980, Repeated surveillance of exposure to cadmium, manganese, and arsenic in school age children living in rural, urban and nonferrous smelter areas in Belgium, *Environ. Res.* **22**:95–108.

Bui, T. H., Lindsten, J., and Nordberg, G. F., 1975, Chromosome analysis of lymphocytes from cadmium workers and Itai-itai patients, *Environ. Res.* **9**:187–195.

Bulselmaier, von. W., Roehrborn, G., and Propping, P., 1972, Mutagenitaets Untersuchungen mit Pesticiden im Host-mediated assay und mit dem Dominanten Letaltest an der Maux, *Biol. Zentralbl.* **91**:311–325.

Burk, D., and Beaudoin, A. R., 1977, Arsenate induced renal agenesis in rats, *Teratology* **16**:247–260.

Cadmium Association, 1980, Cadmium production, properties and uses, Technical note on cadmium, London.

Calugar, A., and Sandulescu, G., 1977, Investigations on chromosome aberrations in subjects exposed to lead in their occupation, *Rev. Med. Chir.* (*Bucarest*) **81**:87–92.

Carpenter, S. J., 1974, Placental permeability of lead, *Environ. Health Perspect.* **7**:129–131.

Carpenter, S. J., and Ferm, V. H., 1977, Embryopathic effects of lead in the hamster: A morphological analysis, *Lab. Invest.* **37**:369–385.

Carpenter, S. J., Ferm, V. H., and Gale, T. F., 1973, Permeability of the golden hamster placenta to inorganic lead: Radioautographic evidence, *Experientia* **29**:311–313.

Casey, C. E., and Robinson, M. F., 1978, Copper, manganese, zinc, nickel, cadmium, and lead in human foetal tissues, *Br. J. Nutr.* **39:**639–646.

Casterline, J. L., and Williams, C. H., 1972, Elimination pattern of methylmercury chloride from blood and brain of rats (dams and offspring) after delivery, following oral administration of its chloride salt during gestation, *Bull. Environ. Contam. Toxicol.* **7:**292–295.

Catizone, O., and Gray, P., 1941, Experiments on chemical interference with early morphogenesis of the chick, *J. Exp. Zool.* **87:**71–82.

Chang, L. W., 1977, Neurotoxic effects of mercury, a review, *Environ. Res.* **14:**329–373.

Chang, L. W., and Hartman, H. A., 1972, Electron microscopic histochemical study on the localization and distribution of mercury in the nervous system after mercury intoxication, *Exp. Neurol.* **35:**122–137.

Chang, L. W., and Sprecher, J. A., 1976, Degenerative changes in the neonatal kidney following *in utero* exposure to methylmercury, *Environ. Res.* **11:**392–406.

Chernoff, N., 1973, Teratogenic effects of cadmium in rats, *Teratology* **8:**29–32.

Child, E. A., 1973, Kinetics of transplacental movement of mercury fed in a tuna matrix to mice, *Arch. Environ. Health* **27:**50–52.

Chiquoine, A., 1965, Effect of cadmium chloride on the pregnant albino mouse, *J. Reprod. Fertil.* **10:**263–265.

Christensen, G. M., 1975, Biochemical effects of methylmercuric chloride, cadmium chloride and lead nitrate on embryos and alevins of the Brook Trout, Salvelinus fontinalis, *Toxicol. Appl. Pharmacol.* **32:**191–197.

Clain, E., and Deysson, G., 1976, Cytotoxicité du cadmium: étude sur les meristemes radiculaires d'*Allium sativum* L., *C. R. Soc. Biol.* **170:**1151–1155.

Cloudman, A. M., Vinig, D., Barkulis, S., and Nickson, J. J., 1949, Bone changes observed following intravenous injection of beryllium, *Am. J. Pathol.* **25:**810–811.

Coogan, P. S., 1973, Lead-induced renal carcinoma, *Proc. Inst. Med. Chicago* **29:**309.

Cooper, W. C., 1976, Cancer mortality patterns in the lead industry, *Ann. N.Y. Acad. Sci.* **271:**250–259.

Cooper, W. C., and Gaffey, W. R., 1975, Mortality of lead workers, *J. Occup. Med.* **17:**100–107.

Cooper, K., Kelly, J., and Witmer, C., 1981, Effects of salt concentration on mutagenicity and toxicity with Ames *Salmonella* strains, *12th EMS Ann. Meet.*, San Diego, Cal. March 5–8, Abstr. P41.

Corbett, T. H., Heidelberger, C., and Dove, W. F., 1970, Determination of the mutagenic activity to bacteriophage T4 of carcinogenic and noncarcinogenic compounds, *Mol. Pharmacol.* **6:**667–669.

Dales, L. G., 1972, The neurotoxicity of alkylmercury compounds, *Am. J. Med.* **53:**219–232.

Deaven, L., and Campbell, E., 1980, Factors affecting the induction of chromosomal aberrations by cadmium in Chinese hamster cells, *Cytogenet. Cell Genet.* **26:**251–260.

De Flora, S., 1978, Metabolic deactivation of mutagens in the Salmonella micro-test, *Nature(London)* **27:**455–456.

De Gennaro, L. D., 1978, The effects of lead nitrate on the central nervous system of the chick embryo. I. Observations of light and electron microscopy, *Growth* **42:**141–155.

De Graeve, N., 1969, Contribution a l'étude des mécanismes d'action des agents d'alkylation. Modifications des effets du methane sulfonate d'ethyl sur less chromosomes de l'orge, Doctorate Thesis (Univ. Liege) p. 456.

De Graeve, N., 1971, Modification des effets du methane sulfonate d'ethyl au niveau chromosomique. I. Les ions métalliques, *Rev. Cytol. Biol. Veg.* **34:**233–244.

De Graeve, N., 1981, Carcinogenic, teratogenic and mutagenic effects of cadmium, *Mutat. Res.* **80:**115–135.

Deknudt, Gh., 1978, Mutagenicity of heavy metals, *Mutat. Res.* **53:**176.

Deknudt, Gh., and Deminatti, M., 1978, Chromosome studies in huamn lymphocytes after *in vitro* exposure to metal salts, *Toxicology* **10:**67–76.

Deknudt, Gh., and Gerber, G. B., 1979, Chromosome aberrations induced by heavy metals in bone marrow cells of mice fed a normal or calcium-deficient diet supplemented with different heavy metals, *Mutat. Res.* **68**:163–168.

Deknudt, Gh., and Léonard, A., 1975, Cytogenetic investigations on leucocytes in workers from a cadmium plant, *Environ. Physiol. Biochem.* **5**:319–327.

Deknudt, Gh., Léonard, A., and Ivanov, B., 1973, Chromosome aberrations observed in male workers occupationally exposed to lead, *Environ. Physiol. Biochem.* **3**:132–138.

Deknudt, Gh., Colle, A., and Gerber, G. B., 1977a, Chromosomal aberrations in lymphocytes from monkeys poisoned with lead, *Mutat. Res.* **454**:77–83.

Deknudt, Gh., Manuel, Y., and Gerber, G. B., 1977b, Chromosomal aberrations in workers professionally exposed to lead, *J. Toxicol. Environ. Health* **3**:885–891.

Demerek, M., Bertani, G., and Flint, H., 1951, A survey of chemicals for mutagenic action on E. coli, *Am. Nat.* **85**:119–136.

Dencker, L., 1975, Possible mechanisms of cadmium fetotoxicity in golden hamsters and mice: Uptake by the embryo, placenta and ovary, *J. Reprod. Fertil.* **44**:461–472.

Dingwall-Fordyce, I., and Lane, R. E., 1963, A follow-up study of lead workers, *Br. J. Ind. Med.* **20**:313–315.

Doll, R., 1958, Cancer of the lung and nose in nickel workers, *Br. J. Ind. Med.* **15**:217–223.

Doll, R., Morgan, L. G., and Speizer, F. E., 1970, Cancer of the lung and nasal sinuses in nickel workers, *Br. J. Cancer* **24**:623–632.

Doll, R., Mathews, J. D., and Morgan, L. G., 1977, Cancers of the lung and nasal sinuses in nickel workers: A reassessment of the period of risk, *Br. J. Ind. Med.* **34**:102–105.

Douglas, G. R., Bell, R. D. L., Grant, C. E., Wytsma, J. M., and Bora, C., 1980, Effect of lead chromate on chromosome aberration, sister chromatid exchange and DNA damage in mammalian cells in vitro, *Mutat. Res.* **77**:157–163.

Doyle, J. W., Pfander, W., Crenshaw, D., and Snethen, J., 1974, Induction of chromosome hypodiploidy in sheep leucocytes by cadmium, *Interface* **31**:9.

Drizhkov, P. P., and Federova, V. I., 1967, Cancerogenic properties of chromic acid, *Vopr. Onkol.* **13**:57–62.

Druckrey, H., Hamperl, H., and Schmahl, D., 1957, Cancerogene Wirkung von metallischem Quecksilber nach intraperitonealer Gabe bei Ratten, *Z. Krebsforsch.* **61**:511.

Dubois, K. P., Moxon, A. L., and Olson, O. E., 1940, Further studies on the effectiveness of arsenic in preventing selenium poisoning, *J. Nutr.* **18**:477–482.

Dustin, A. P., and Grégoire, C., 1933, Contribution à l'étude de l'action des poisons caryoclastiques sur les tumeurs animales—Premier mémoire: Action du cacodylate de Na et de la trypaflavine sur le sarcome greffé, type Crocker, de la souris, *Bull. Acad. R. Méd. Belg.* **1933**:585–588.

Dutra, F. R., Largent, E. J., and Roth, J. L., 1951, Osteogenic sarcoma after inhalation of beryllium oxide, *AMA Arch. Pathol.* **5**:473–479.

Earl, F. L., and Vish, T. J. 1980, Teratogenicity of heavy metals, in *Toxicity of Heavy Metals in the Environment*, (edited by F. W. Oehme) Marcel Decker Inc., New York and Basel, pp. 617–639.

Earl, F. L., Miller, E., and van Loon, E. J., 1973, in *The Laboratory Animal in Drug Testing*, (edited by A. Spiegel) G. Fischer, Stuttgart p. 233.

Eastman, N. J., 1931, The arsenic content of the human placenta following arsphenamine therapy, *Am. J. Obstet. Gynecol.* **21**:60–64.

El-Sadek, L. M., 1972, Mitotic inhibition and chromosomal aberrations induced by some arylarsonic acids and its compounds in root-tips of maize, *Egypt J. Genet. Cytol.* **1**:218–224.

Environmental Protection Agency (U. S. A.), 1978, Human exposure to atmospheric arsenic, Washington D.C.

Epstein, S. S., and Mantel, N., 1968, Carcinogenicity of tetraethyl lead, *Experientia* **24**:580–581.

Evans, H. J., 1976, Cytological methods for detecting chemical mutagens, in *Chemical Mutagens*, (edited by A. Hollaender) Plenum, New York, vol 4. pp. 1–29.

Evans, H. J., and O'Riordan, N. L., 1975, Human peripheral blood lymphocytes for the analysis of chromosome aberrations in mutagen tests, *Mutat. Res.* **31**:135–148.

Eyden, B. P., Maisin, J. R., and Mattelin, G., 1978, Long-term effects of dietary lead acetate on survival; body weight and seminal cytology in mice, *Bull. Environ. Contam. Toxicol.* **19**:266–272.

Fabre, M. R., and Girault, M., 1957, Contribution a l'étude de l'action des toxiques sur l'embryon de poulet. Application au cas du plomb, *C. R. Acad. Sci. (Paris)* **244**:535–538.

Fabry, L., 1980, Relation entre l'induction de micronoyaux dans les cellules de la moelle par les sels de chrome et leur pouvoir cancérigène, *C. R. Soc. Biol.* **174**:889–892.

Fahmy, F. Y., 1951, Cytogenetic analysis of the action of some fungicide mercurials, Thesis, Univ. of Lund, Sweden.

Farulla, A., Naro, G., Alimena, A., Benvenuti, F., Dolfini, A. M., Lepore, L., Pugliese, D., and Zingarelli, S., 1978, Effeti *in vitro* del vanadio sul cariogramma linfocitario, *Securitas* **63**:252–256.

Felten, T., 1978, A preliminary report of cadmium induced chromsomal changes in somatic and germinal tissues of C57Bl/6J male mice, *Genetics* **88**:s26–s27.

Ferm, V. H., 1969, The synteratogenic effect of lead and cadmium, *Experientia* **25**:56–57.

Ferm, V. H., 1971, Developmental malformations induced by cadmium. A study of timed injections during embryogenesis, *Biol. Neonat.* **19**:101–107.

Ferm, V. H., 1972, The teratogenic effects of metals on mammalian embryos, in *Advances in Teratology*, (edited by D. H. Wodhams) Academic Press, New York, vol. 5, pp. 51–75.

Ferm, V. H., 1974, Effects of metal pollutants upon embryonic development, *Rev. Environ. Health* **1**:237–259.

Ferm, V. H., 1977, Arsenic as a teratogenic agent, *Environ. Health Perspect.* **19**:215–217.

Ferm, V. H., and Carpenter, S., 1967a, Teratogenic effects of cadmium and its inhibition by zinc, *Nature (London)* **216**:1123.

Ferm, V. H., and Carpenter, S., 1967b, Developmental malformations resulting from the administration of lead salts, *Exp. Mol. Pathol.* **7**:208–213.

Ferm, V. H., and Carpenter, S., 1968a, Malformations induced by sodium arsenate, *J. Reprod. Fertil.* **17**:199–201.

Ferm, V. H., and Carpenter, S., 1968b, The relationship of cadmium and zinc in experimental mammalian teratogenesis, *Lab. Invest.* **18**:429–432.

Ferm, V. H., and Ferm, D. W., 1971, The specificity of the teratogenic effect of lead in the golden hamster, *Life Sci.* **10**:35–39.

Ferm, V. H., and Hanlon, D. P., 1974a, Copper toxicity in mammalian embryonic development, *Biol. Reprod.* **11**:97–101.

Ferm, V. H., and Hanlon, D. P., 1974b, Placental transfer of zinc in the Syrian hamster during early embryogenesis, *J. Reprod. Fertil.* **39**:49–52.

Ferm, V. H., and Layton, W. M. Jr, 1979, Reduction in cadmium teratogenesis by prior cadmium exposure, *Environ. Res.* **18**:347–350.

Ferm, V. H., and Saxon, A., 1971, Amniotic fluid volume in experimentally induced renal agenesis and anencephaly, *Experientia* **27**:1066–1068.

Ferm, V. H., Hanlon, D., and Urban, J., 1969, Studies on the permeability of hamster placenta to radioactive cadmium, *J. Embryol. Exp. Morphol.* **22**:107–113.

Ferm, V. H., Saxon, A., and Smith, B. W., 1971, The teratogenic profile of sodium arsenate in the golden hamster, *Arch. Environ. Health* **22**:557–560.

Ficsor, G., and Nii Lo Piccolo, G. M., 1972, Survey of pesticides for mutagenicity by the bacterial-plate assay method, *Environmental Mutagen Society News Letter* **6**:6–8.

Fiskesjo, G., 1969, Some results from Allium tests with organic mercury halogenides, *Hereditas* **62:**314–322.

Fiskesjo, G., 1970, The effects of two organic mercury compounds on human leucocytes in vitro, *Hereditas* **64:**142–146.

Flessel, C., 1978, Metals as mutagens, in *Inorganic and Nutrional Aspects of Cancer*, (edited by G. Shauze) Plenum Press, New York, pp. 117–128.

Forni, A., and Secchi, G. C., 1972, Chromosome changes in preclinical and clinical lead poisoning and correlation with biochemical findings, *Proc. Intern. Symp. Environ. Health Aspects of Lead, Amsterdam*, pp. 473–482.

Forni, A., Cambiaghi, G., and Secchi, G. C., 1976 Initial occupational exposure to lead, *Arch. Environ. Health* **311:**73–75.

Fowler, B. A., 1977, Toxicology of environmental arsenic, in *Advances in Modern Toxicology*, (edited by R. A. Goyer and M. A. Mehlman). Hemisphere Publ. Corp., Washington, vol. 2, pp. 799–822.

Fowler, B. A., and Woods, J. S., 1977, The transplacental toxicity of methylmercury to fetal rat liver mitochondria, *Lab. Invest.* **36:**122–130.

Fowler, B. A., Ishinishi, N., Tsuchiya, K., and Valter, M., 1979, Arsenic, in *Handbook on the Toxicology of Metals*, (edited by L. Friberg, G. F. Nordberg and V. B. Vouk) Elsevier, North Holland Biomedical Press, Amsterdam, pp. 291–313.

Fradkin, A., Janoff, A., Laner, B. P., and Kuischner, M., 1975, In vitro transformation of BHK 21 cells grown in the presence of calcium chromate, *Cancer Res.* **35:**1058–1063.

Franke, K. W., Moxon, A. L., Polcy, W. E., and Tully, W. C., 1936, Monstrosites produced by the injection of selenium salts into hen's eggs, *Anat. Rec.* **65:**15–22.

Friberg, L., Piscator, M., Nordberg, G., and Kjellstroem, T., 1974, *Cadmium In the Environment*, 2nd edition, CRC Press, Cleveland.

Friedrich, E. G., 1972, Vulvar carcinoma in situ in identical twins—an occupational hazard, *Obstet. Gynecol.* **399:**837–841.

Friedrich, U., and Nielsen, J., 1969, Lithium and chromosome abnormalities, *Lancet* **2:**435–436.

Frost, D. V., 1967, Arsenicals in biology—retrospect and prospect, *Fed. Proc.* **26:**194–208.

Frost, D. V., 1970, Tolerances for arsenic and selenium: A psychodynamic problem, *World Rev. Pest Control* **9:**6–28.

Fujita, E., 1969, Experimental studies of organic mercury poisoning; the behavior of the Minamata disease causal agent in maternal bodies and its transfer to their infants via either placenta, or breast milk, *J. Kumamoto Med. Soc.* **43:**47–52.

Fujita, M., Fujimoto, T., and Kiyofuji, E., 1979, Teratogenic effects of a single oral administration of methylmercuric chloride in mice, *Acta Anat.* **104:**356–362.

Furst, A., Schlauder, M., and Sasmore, D. P., 1976, Tumorigenic activity of lead chromate, *Cancer Res.* **36:**1779–1783.

Gale, T. F., 1974, Effects of chromium on the hamster embryo, *Teratology* **9:**1917.

Gale, T. F., 1978, Embryotoxic effects of chromium trioxide in hamsters, *Environ. Res.* **16:**101–109.

Gale, T. F., and Bunch, J. D., 1979, The effect of the time of administration of chromium trioxide on the embryotoxic response in hamsters, *Teratology* **19:**81–86.

Gale, T., and Ferm, V., 1971, Embryopathic effects of mercuric salts, *Life Sci* **10:**1341–1347.

Gale, T., and Ferm, V., 1973, Skeletal malformations resulting from cadmium treatment in the hamster, *Biol. Neonat.* **23:**149–160.

Garcia, J. D., Yang, M. G., Wang, J. H. C., and Bels, P. S., 1974, Translocation and fluxes of mercury in neonatal and maternal rats treated with methylmercuric chloride during gestation. *Proc. Soc. Exp. Biol. Med.* **147:**224–231.

Gardner, L. U., and Heslington, H. F., Osteosarcoma from intravenous beryllium compounds in rabbits, *Fed. Prod.* **5:**221.

Garrett, N. E., Garrett, R. J. B., and Archdeacon, J. W., 1972, Placental transmission of mercury to the fetal rat, *Toxicol. Appl. Pharmacol.* **22**:649–654.

Genest, P., and Villeneuve, A., 1971, Lithium, chromosomes and mitotic index, *Lancet* **1**:1132.

Gerber, G. B., and Maes, J., 1978, Heme synthesis in the lead intoxicated mouse embryo, *Toxicology* **9**:173–179.

Gerber, G. B., and Maes, J., 1983, Metabolism of chromium and nickel in relation to mutagenic and teratogenic risks, in preparation.

Gerber, G. B., Maes, J., and Deroo, J., 1978, Effects of dietary lead on placental blood flow and fetal uptake of *a*-aminoisobutyrate, *Arch. Toxicol.* **41**:125–131.

Gerber, G. B., Léonard, A., and Jacquet, P., 1980, Toxicity, mutagenicity, and teratogenicity of lead, *Mutat. Res.* **76**:115–141.

Gerber, G. B., Maes, J., and Eykens, B., 1982, Transfer of antimony and arsenic to the developing organisms, *Arch. Toxicol.* **49**, 159–168.

Gerber, G. B., Maes, J., Deroo, J., and Jacquet, P., 1981b, Transfer of lead *in utero* in normal and calcium deficient mice, in preparation.

Gilani, S. H., 1973, Congenital anomalies in lead poisoning, *Obstet. Gynecol.* **41**:265–269.

Gilani, S. H., and Marano, M., 1980, Congenital abnormalities in nickel poisoning in chick embryos, *Arch. Environ. Contam. Toxicol.* **9**:17–22.

Gilliavod, N., and Léonard, A., 1975, Mutagenicity tests with cadmium in the mouse, *Toxicology* **5**:43–47.

Gilman, J. P. W., 1962, Metal carcinogenesis. II. A study on the carcinogenic activity of cobalt, copper, iron, and nickel compounds, *Cancer Res.* **22**:158–162.

Glaess, E., 1955, Untersuchungen ueber die Einwirkung von Schwermetallsalzen auf die Wurzelspitzenmitose von *Vicia faba*, *Z. Bot.* **43**:359–403.

Glaess, E., 1956a, Untersuchungen ueber die Einwirkung von Schwermetallsalzen auf die Wurzelspitzenmitose von *Vicia faba*, *Z. Bot.* **44**:1–58.

Glaess, E., 1956b, Die Verteilung von Fragmentationen und achromatischen Stellen auf den Chromosomen von *Vicia faba* nach Behandlung mit Schwermetallsalzen, *Chromosoma* **8**:260–284.

Goldman, A. L., 1973, Lung cancer in Bowen's disease, *Am. Rev. Resp. Dis.* *108*:1205–1207.

Green, M. H. L., Muriel, W. J., and Bridges, B. A., 1976, Use of a simplified fluctuation test to detect low levels of mutagens, *Mutat. Res.* **38**:33–42.

Greenwood, M. R., Clarkson, T. W., and Magos, L., 1972, Transfer of metallic mercury into the fetus, *Experientia* **28**:1455–1456.

Gruber, J. E., and Jenette, K. W., 1978, Metabolism of the carcinogenic chromate in rat-liver chromsomes, *Biochem. Biophys. Res. Commun.* **822**:700–706.

Gruenwald, P., 1958, Malformations caused by necrosis in the embryo, illustrated by the effect of selenium compounds on the chick embryo, *Am. J. Pathol.* **34**:77–95.

Gruenwedel, D. W., and Friend, D., 1980, Long-term effects of methylmercury (II) on the viability of Hela S3 cells, *Bull. Environ. Contam. Toxicol.* **25**:441–447.

Gunn, S., Gould, T., and Anderson, W., 1964, Effect of zinc on cancerogenesis by cadmium, *Proc. Exp. Biol. Med.* **115**:653–657.

Hadjimarkos, D. M., Bonhorst, C. W., and Mattice, J. J., 1959, The selenium concentration in placental tissue and fetal cord blood, *J. Pediatr.* **54**:296–298.

Hall, A., 1905, Increasing use of leads as an abortifacient, *Br. Med. J.* **1**:584–587.

Hall, B. K., 1972, Thallium-induced achondroplasia in the embryonic chick, *Develop. Biol.* **28**:47–60.

Hanlon, D. P., and Ferm, V. H., 1977, Placental permeability of arsenate ion during early embryogenesis in the hamster, *Experientia* **33**:1221–1222.

Happle, R., and Hoehn, H., 1973, Cytogenetic studies on cultured fibroblast-like cells derived from basal cell carcinoma tissue, *Clin. Genet.* **4**:17–24.

Harada, M., 1978, Congenital Minamata disease: Intrauterine methylmercury poisoning, *Teratology* **18**:285–288.

Harris, P., and Holley, M. R., 1972, Lead levels in cord blood, *Pediatrics* **49**:606–608.

Harris, S. B., Wilson, J. G., and Printz, R. H., 1972, Embryotoxicity of methylmercuric chloride in golden hamsters, *Teratology* **6**:139–142.

Hasan, F. M., and Kazemi, H., 1974, Chronic beryllium disease: A continuing epidemiologic hazard, *Chest* **65**:289–293.

Hecker, R. J., Bilgen, T., Bhatnagar, P. S., and Smith, G. A., 1972, Test for chemical induction of male sterility in sugarbeet, *Can. J. Plant Sci.* **52**:927–940.

Heath, J. C., Freeman, M. A. R., and Swanson, S. A. V., 1971, Carcinogenic properties of wear particles from prostheses made in cobalt-chromium alloy, *Lancet* **1**:564–566.

Heddle, J. A., and Bruce, W. R., 1977, Comparison of tests for mutagenicity and carcinogenicity using assays for sperm abnormalities, formation of micronuclei and mutations in *Salmonella*, in *Origins of Human Cancer*, (edited by H. H. Hiatt, J. D. Watson and J. A. Winsten), Cold Spring Harbor Laboratory Press, New York, Vol. 4, pp. 1549–1557.

Hedenstedt, A., Rannug, U., Ramel, C., and Wachtmeister, C., 1979, Mutagenicity and metabolism studies on 12 thiouram and dithiocarbamate compounds used as accelerators in the Swedish rubber industry, *Mutat. Res.* **68**:313–325.

Henke, G., Sachs, H. W., and Bohn, G., 1970, Cadmiumbestimmungen in Leber und Nieren von Kindern und Jugendlichen durch Neutronenaktivierungsanalyse, *Arch. Toxicol.* **26**:8.

Hessler, A., 1974, Effect of lead on algae, I. Effect of Pb on viability of *Platymonas subcordiformis* (Chlorophyta *volvocales*), *Water Air Soil Pollut.* **3**:371–385.

Hessler, A., 1975, The effect of lead on algae, II. Mutagenesis experiments on *Platymonas subcordiformis*, *Mutat. Res.* **31**:43–47.

Hill, A. B., and Faning, E. L., 1948, Studies on the incidence of cancer in a factory handling inorganic compounds of arsenic. I. Mortality experience in the factory, *Br. J. Ind. Med.* **5**:1–6.

Hirano, A., and Kochen, J. A., 1973, Neurotoxic effects of lead in the chick embryo, *Lab. Invest.* **29**:659–668.

Hoagland, M. B., Grier, R. S., and Hood, M. B., 1950, Beryllium and growth. I. Beryllium-induced osteogenic sarcomata, *Cancer Res.* **10**:629–635.

Holmberg, R. E., and Ferm, V. H., 1969, Interrelationship of selenium, cadmium and arsenic in mammalian teratogenesis, *Arch. Environ. Health* **18**:873–877.

Hood, R. D., 1972, Effects of sodium arsenite on fetal development, *Bull. Environ. Contam. Toxicol.* **7**:216.

Hood, R. D., and Bishop, S. L., 1972, Teratogenic effects of sodium arsenate in mice, *Arch. Environ. Health* **24**:62–65.

Hood, R. D., and Piken, C. T., 1972, BAL alleviation of arsenate-induced teratogenesis in mice, *Teratology* **6**:235–238.

Hopkins, L. L., 1965, Distribution in the rat of physiological amounts of injected $Cr^{51}$ (IV) with time, *Am. J. Physiol.* **209**:731–735.

Hubermont, G., Buchet, J. P., Roels, H., and Lauwerys, R., 1978, Placental transfer of lead, mercury and cadmium in women living in a rural area, *Int. Arch. Occup. Environ. Health* **41**:117–124.

Hueper, W. C., 1958, Experimental studies in metal cancerigenesis. X. Cancerigenic effects of chromite ore roast deposited in muscle tissue and pleural cavity of rats, *AMA. Arch. Ind. Health.* **18**:284–291.

Hueper, W. C., and Payne, W. W., 1959, Experimental cancers in rats produced by chromium compounds and their significance in industry and public health, *Am. Indust. Hyg. Assoc. J.* **20**:272–280.

Hurley, L. S., 1981, Teratogenic aspects of manganese, zinc, and copper nutrition, *Physiol. Rev.* **61**:249–295.

IARC (1976), Monographs on the evaluation of the carcinogenic risk of chemicals to humans: Cadmium, nickel, some epoxydes, miscellaneous industrial chemical and general considerations on volatile anaesthetics, International Agency for Research on Cancer, Lyon, Vol II, pp. 39–74.

IARC (1980), Monographs on the evaluation of the carcinogenic risk of chemicals to humans. Some metal and metal compounds, International Agency for Research on Cancer, Lyon, vol. 23. pp. 39–74.

Iijima, S., Matsumoto, N., Lu, C. C., and Katsunuma, H., 1975, Placental transfer of CrCl3 and its effects on foetal growth and development in mice, *Teratology* **12**:198.

Inoue, J., and Watanabe, T., 1978, Toxicity and mutagenicity of cadmium and furylfuramide in *Drosophila melanogaster, Jpn. J. Genet.* **53**:183–190.

Inouye, M., Hoshimo, K., and Murukami, U., 1972, Effects of methylmercuric chloride on embryonic and fetal development in rats and mice, *Annu. Rep. Res. Inst. Environ. Med. Nagoya Univ.* **19**:69–74.

Ishizu, S., Minami, M., Suzuki, A., Yamada, M., Sato, M., and Yamamura, K., 1973, An experimental study on teratogenic effects of cadmium, *Indust. Health* **11**:127–139.

Jacobson, K. B., and Turner, J. E., 1980, The interaction of cadmium and certain other metal ions with proteins and nucleic acids, *Toxicology* **16**:1–37.

Jacobsen, N., Alfheim, I., and Jonsen, J., 1978, Nickel and strontium distribution in some mouse tissues: Passage through placenta and mammary glands, *Res. Commun. Chem. Pathol. Pharmacol.* **20**:571–584.

Jacquet, P., 1976, Effects du plomb administré durant la gestation à des souris C57Bl, *C. R. Soc. Biol.* **170**:1319–1322.

Jacquet, P., 1977, Early embryonic development in lead intoxicated mice, *Arch. Pathol. Lab. Med.* **101**:1641–1643.

Jacquet, P., and Gerber, G. B., 1979, Teratogenic effects of lead in the mouse, *Biomedicine* **30**:223–229.

Jacquet, P., and Tachon, P., 1981, Effects of long-term lead exposure on monkey leucocyte chromosomes, *Toxicology* **8**:165–169.

Jacquet, P., Léonard, A., and Gerber, G. B., 1975, Embryonic death in mouse due to lead exposure, *Experientia* **31**:1312–1313.

Jacquet, P., Léonard, A., and Gerber, G. B., 1976, Action of lead on the early divisions of the mouse embryo, *Toxicology* **6**:129–132.

Jacquet, P., Gerber, G. B., Léonard, A., and Maes, J., 1977a, Plasma hormone levels in normal and lead treated pregnant mice, *Experientia* **33**:1375–1376.

Jacquet, P., Gerber, G. B., and Maes, J., 1977b. Biochemical studies in embryos after exposure of pregnant mice to dietary lead, *Bull. Environ. Contam. Toxicol.* **18**:271–277.

Jacquet, P., Léonard, A., and Gerber, G. B., 1977c, Cytogenetic investigations on mice treated with lead, *J. Toxicol. Environ. Health* **2**:619–624.

Jagiello, G., and Lin, J. S., 1973, An assessment of the effects of mercury on the meiosis of mouse ova, *Mutat. Res.* **17**:93–99.

James, L. F., Lazar, V. A., and Binns, W., 1966, Effects of sublethal doses of certain metals on pregnant ewes and fetal development, *Am. J. Vet. Res.* **27**:132–135.

Jarric, L. F. Bishun, N. P., Bleiweiss, H., Kato, T., and Moralishvilli, E., 1971, Chromosome examinations in patients on lithium carbonate, *Arch. Gen. Psychiatry* **24**:166–168.

Jones, J. M., Higgins, G. M., and Herrick, J. F., 1954, Beryllium-induced osteogenic sarcoma in rabbits, *J. Bone J. Surg.* **36B**:543–552.

Jung, E. G., 1971, Molekularbiologische Untersuchungen zur chronischen Arsenvergiftung, *Z. Haut-Geschl. Kr.* **46:**35–36.

Jung, E. G., and Trachsel, B., 1970, Molekularbiologische Untersuchungen zur Arsencarcinogenese, *Arch. Klin. Exp. Dermatol.* **237:**819–826.

Kalinina, L., and Polukhina, G., 1977, Mutagenic efect of heavy metal salts on Salmonella in activation systems *in vivo* and *in vitro*, *Mutat. Res.* **46:**223–224.

Kalinina, L., Polukhina, G., and Lukasheva, L., 1977, *Salmomella typhimurium* test-system for indication of mutagenic activity of environmental hazards. I. Detection of mutagenic effect of heavy metal salts using *in vivo* and *in vitro* assays without metabolic activation, *Genetica (Moscow)* **13:**1089–1092.

Kanematsu, K., and Kada, T., 1978, Mutagenicity of metal compounds, *Mutat. Res.* **53:**207–208.

Kanematsu, K., Hara, M., and Kada, T., 1980, Rec-assay and mutagenicity studies on metal compounds, *Mutat. Res.* **77:**109–116.

Kasirsky, G., Gautieri, R. F., and Mann, D. E., 1967, Inhibition of cortisone-induced cleft palate in mice by cobaltous chloride, *J. Pharm. Sci.* **56:**1330–1332.

Kasuya, M., 1972, Effects of inorganic aryl, alkyl and other mercury compounds on the outgrowth of cells and fibers from dorsal root ganglia in tissue culture, *Toxicol. Appl. Pharmacol.* **23:**136–146.

Kasuya, M., 1975, The effect of vitamin E on the toxicology of alkyl mercurials in nervous tissue in culture, *Toxicol. Appl. Pharmacol.* **32:**347–354.

Kato, R., 1976, Chromosome breakage associated with organic mercury in Chinese hamster cells in vitro, *Mutat. Res.* **38:**340–341.

Kato, R., Nakamura, A., and Sawai, T., 1976, Chromosome breakage associated with organic mercury in human leucocytes *in vitro* and *in vivo*, *Jpn. J. Hum. Genet.* **20:**256–257.

Kazantzis, G., and Lilly, L. J., 1979, Mutagenic and carcinogenic effects of metals, in *Handbook on the Toxicology of Metals*, (edited by L. Friberg, G. F. Nordberg, and V. B. Vouk) Elsevier, North Holland Biomedical Press, Amsterdam, pp. 237–272.

Keino, H. and Yamamura, H., 1974, Effects of cadmium salts administered to pregnant mice on postnatal development of the offspring, *Teratology* **10:**87.

Keino, H., Watanabe, K., Totsuka, T., and Sato, H., 1975a, Incorporation of intraperitoneally administered cadmium ion in the kidneys and embryos of pregnant mice, *Igaku to Seibutsugaku* **91:**197–200.

Keino, H., Watanabe, K., Totsuka, T., and Sato, H., 1975b, Relation between cadmium concentration in maternal blood and the rate of congenital anomalies in ICR-JCL mice, *Igaku to Seibutsugaku* **91:**201–205.

Kelly, P. J., Jones, T. M., and Peterson, L. F. A., 1961, The effect of beryllium on bone, *J. Bone J. Surg.* **43A:**829–844.

Kelman, B. J., Steinmetz, S. E., Walter, B. K., and Sasser, L. B., 1980, Absorption of methylmercury by the fetal guinea pig during mid to late gestation, *Teratology*, **21:**161–165.

Kennedy, G. L., and Arnold, D. W., 1971, Absence of mutagenic effects after treatment of mice with lead compounds, *E. M. S. News Letter* **5:**37.

Khera, K. S., 1973, Teratogenic effects of methylmercury in the cat: Note on the use of this species as a model for teratogenicity studies, *Teratology* **8:**293–304.

Khera, K. S., and Tabacova, S. A., 1973, Effects of methylmercuric chloride on the progeny of mice and rats treated before or during gestation, *Food Cosmet. Toxicol.* **11:**245–254.

Kihlman, B. A., 1975, Root tips of *Vicia faba* for the study of the induction of chromosomal aberrations, *Mutat. Res.* **31:**401–412.

Kilian, D. J., and Picciano, D., 1976, Cytogenetic surveillance of industrial populations, in *Chemical Mutagens: Principle and Methods for Their Detection* (edited by A. Hollaender) Plenum Press, New York, vol. 4, pp. 321–334.

Kimmel, C. A., Grant, L. D., and Sloan, C. D., 1976, Chronic lead exposure: assessment of developmental toxicity, *Teratology* **13**:23A–28A.

King, H., and Lunford, R. J., 1950, The relation between the constitution of arsenicals and their action on cell division, *J. Chem. Soc.* **8**:2086–2088.

King, R. B., Robkin, M. A., and Shepard, T. H., 1976, Distribution of [203]Hg in pregnant and fetal rats, *Teratology* **13**:275–280.

Kipling, M., and Waterhouse, J., 1967, Cadmium and prostatic carcinoma, *Lancet* **1**:730–731.

Kitamura, S., 1968, Minamata disease, Study group of Minamata disease, Kumamoto University, Japan, pp. 257–266.

Kjellstroem, T., Friberg, L., and Rahnster, B., 1979, Mortality and cancer morbidity among cadmium-exposed workers, *Environ. Health Perspect.* **28**:199–204.

Komczynnski, L., Nowak H., and Reyniak, L., 1963, Effect of cobalt, nickel and iron on mitosis in the roots of the broad bean (*Vicia faba*), *Nature (London)* **198**:1016–1017.

Koos, B. J., and Longo, L. D., 1976, Mercury toxicity in the pregnant woman, fetus and newborn infant, *Am. J. Obstet. Gynecol.* **126**:390–409.

Kopp, J. F., and Kroner, R. C., 1967, A five year study of trace metals in waters of the United States, Fed. Water Pollut. Control, U.S. Dept. Inter., Cincinnati, Ohio.

Kostoff, D., 1939, Effect of the fungicide "Granosan" on a typical growth and chromosome doubling in plants, *Nature (London)* **144**:334.

Kostoff, D., 1940, Atypical growth, abnormal mitosis and polyploidy induced by ethyl-mercury chloride, *Phytopathol. Z.* **23**:90.

Kretzschmar, J. G., Delespaul, I., de Ryck, Th., 1980, Heavy metals in Belgium: A five year survey. *Sci. Total Environ.* **14**:85–87.

Kubinski, H., Morin, N. R., and Zeldin, P. E., 1976, Increased attachment of nucleic acids to eukaryotic and prokaryotic cells induced by chemical and physical carcinogens and mutagens, *Cancer Res.* **6**:3025–3033.

Kumaraswamy, K., and Sekarasetty, M., 1977, Preliminary studies on the effects of cadmium chloride on the meiotic chromosomes, *Curr. Sci.* **46**:475–478.

Kuratsune, M. S., Tokudome, S., Shirakusa, T., Yoshida, M., Tokuitsu, Y., Hayano, T., and Seita, M., 1975, Occupational lung cancer among copper smelters, *Int. J. Cancer* **13**:552–558.

Kury, G., Rev-Kury, L. H., and Crosby, R. J., 1967, The effect of selenous acid on the hematopoietic system of chicken embryos, *Toxicol. Appl. Pharmacol.* **11**:449–458.

Kuschner, M., and Laskfin, S., 1971, Experimental models in environmental carcinogenesis, *Am. J. Pathol.* **64**:183–191.

Kuwahara, S., 1970, Toxicity of mercurials, especially methyl mercury compound in chick embryo, *J. Kumamoto Med. Soc.* **44**:81–89.

Lafontaine, A., Aerts, J., Bruaux, P., Claeys-Thoreau, F., Impens, R., Mahy, P., Roels, H., Van Bruwaene, R., 1977, Le plomb dans l'environnement en Belgique, *Arch. Belg. Med. Soc. Hy. Med.* **1–2**:127.

Lancranjan, T., Popescu, H., Gavanescu, O., Klepsch, J., and Serbanescu, M., 1975, Reproductive ability of workmen occupationally exposed to lead, *Arch. Environ. Health* **300**:396–401.

Lander, J. J., Stanely, R. J., Sumner, H. D., Boswell, D. W., and Aach, R. D., 1975, Angiosarcoma of the liver associated with Fowler's solution (potassium arsenite), *Gastroenterology* **68**:1582–1586.

Laskin, S., Kuschner, M., and Drew, R. T., 1970, Studies in pulmonary carcinogenesis, in *Inhalation carcinogenesis*, (edited by M. G. Hanna, P. Netteshein and J. R. Gilbert), U.S. Atomic Energy Commission, Division Techn. Information, pp. 321–351.

Lauwerys, R., (Rapporteur), 1978, Criteria for dose-effect relationships for cadmium, Comm. Europ. Commun. Luxemburg Pergamon, Oxford.

Lauwerys, R., Buchet, J. P., Roels, H., and Hubermont, G., 1978, Placental transfer of lead, mercury, cadmium and monoxide in women. I. Comparison of the frequency distribution of the biological indices in maternal and umbilical cord blood, *Environ. Res.* **15**:278-289.

Layton, W. M. Jr, and Ferm, V. H., 1980, Protection against cadmium-induced limb malformations by pretreatment with cadmium or mercury, *Teratology* **21**:357-360.

Lecointe, P., Macquet, J. P. and Butour, J. L., 1979, Correlation between the toxicity of platinum drugs to L 1210 leukemia cells and their mutagenic properties, *Biochem. Biophys. Res. Commun.* **90**:209-213.

Lee, A. M., and Froumeni, J. F., 1969, Arsenic and respiratory cancer in man: An occupational study, *J. Natl. Cancer Inst.* **42**:1045-1052.

Lee, I. P., and Dixon, R. L., 1973, Effects of mercury on mouse spermatogenesis studied by cell separation and serial muting, *Toxicol. Appl. Pharmacol.* **25**:464.

Lemen, R. A., Lee, J. S., Wagoner, J. K., and Bleyer, H. P., 1976, Cancer mortality among cadmium production workers, *Ann. N.Y. Acad. Sci.* **271**:273-279.

Lemontt, J. F., Dudney, C. S., Meeks, C. K., and McDougall, K. J., 1981, Heavy metal cytotoxicity and mutagenicity in yeast: Isolation of mutants with altered response to cadmium ion, 12th EMS Annual Meeting, San Diego Cal., March 5-8, Abstr. p. 72.

Léonard, A., 1978, Carcinogenic and mutagenic effects of metals (As, Cd, Cr, Hg, Ni). Present state of knowledge and needs for further studies, in Trace Metals: Exposure and health effects, (edited by E. Di Ferrante) Pergamon, pp. 199-216.

Léonard, A., and Lauwerys, R. R., 1980a, Carcinogenicity and mutagenicity of chromium, *Mutat. Res.* **76**:227-239.

Léonard, A., and Lauwerys, R. R., 1980b, Carcinogenicity, teratogenicity and mutagenicity of arsenic, *Mutat. Res.* **75**:49-62.

Léonard, A., Linden, B., Gerber, G. B., 1972, Etude chez la souris des effets genetiques et cytogenetiques d'une contamination par le plomb, *Proc. Internat. Symp. Environmental Health Aspects of Lead*, Amsterdam, pp. 303-309.

Léonard, A., Deknudt, Gh., and Gilliavod, N., 1975, Genetic and cytogenetic hazards of heavy metals in mammals, *Mutat. Res.* **29**:280-281.

Léonard, A., Gerber, G. B., and Jacquet, P., 1983, Carcinogenicity, teratogenicity and mutagenicity of nickel, *Mutat. Res.* **87**:1-15.

Léonard, A., Lauwerys, R. R., and Jacquet, P., 1981b, Carcinogenicity, teratogenicity and mutagenicity of mercury, *Mutat. Res.* **114**:1-18.

Levan, A., 1945, Cytological reactions induced by inorganic salt solutions, *Nature (London)* **156**:751.

Levan, A., 1971, Cytogenetic effects of hexyl mercury bromide in the Allium test, *J. Indian Bot. Soc.* **50A**:340-349.

Levander, O. A., and Argrett, L. C. 1969, Effects of arsenic mercury, thallium, and lead on selenium metabolism in rats, *Toxicol. Appl. Pharmacol.* **14**:308-314.

Levander, O. A., and Bauman, C. A., 1966, Selenium metabolism. VI. Effect of arsenic on the excretion of selenium in the bile, *Toxicol. Appl. Pharmacol.* **9**:106-115.

Levy, L. S., and Clarck, J., 1975, Further studies on the effect of cadmium on the prostate gland, I. *Ann. Occup. Hyg.* **17**:205-211.

Levy, L. S., Roe, F. J. C., Malcolm, D., Kazantzis, G., Clack, J., and Platt, H. S., 1973, Absence of prostatic changes in rats exposed to cadmium, *Ann. Occup. Hyg.* **16**:111-118.

Levy, L. S., Clack, J., and Roe, F. J. C., 1975, Further studies on the effect of cadmium on the prostate gland, II., *Ann. Occup. Hyg.* **17**:213-220.

Loefroth, G., and Ames, B. N., 1978, Mutagenicity of inorganic compounds in *Salmonella typhimurium*: Arsenic, chromium and selenium, *Mutat. Res.* **53**:65-66.

Loevy, H. T., 1973, Lithium ion in cleft palate teratogenesis in CDl mice, *Proc. Soc. Exp. Biol. Med.* **144**:644–646.

Lower, W. R., 1975, Gene frequencies differences in *Drosophila melanogaster* associated with lead smelting operations, *Mutat. Res.* **31**:315.

Lower, W. R., Rose, P. S., and Drobney, V. K., 1978, *In situ* mutagenic and other toxic effects associated with lead smelting, *Mutat. Res.* **54**:83–93.

Lu, C. C., Matsumoto, N., and Iijima, S., 1976, Placental transfer of $NiCl_2$ to fetuses in mice, *Teratology* **14**:245.

Lu, C. C., Matsumoto, N., and Iijima, S., 1979, Teratogenic effects of nickel chloride on embryonic mice and its transfer to embryonic mice, *Teratology* **19**:137–142.

Luckey, T. D., and Venugopal, B., 1977, Metal toxicity in mammals. Physiologic and chemical basis for metal toxicity, Vol. 2, Plenum Press, New York.

Lugo, G., Cassady, G., and Palmisano, P., 1969, Acute maternal arsenic intoxication with neonatal death, *Am. J. Dis. Child.* **117**:328–330.

Macfarlane, E. W. E., 1950, Somatic mutations produced by organic mercurials in flowering plants, *Genetics* **35**:122–123.

Macfarlane, E. W. E., 1951, Effects of water source on toxicity of mercurial poisons. II. Reactions of Allium root tip cells as indicators of penetration, *Growth* **15**:241–246.

MacRae, W. D., Whiting, R. F., and Stich, H. F., 1979, Sister chromatid exchanges induced in cultured mammalian cells by chromate, *Chem. Biol. Interact.* **26**:281–286.

Majone, F., and Rensi, D., 1979, Mitotic alterations, chromosome alterations and sister chromatid exchanges induced by hexavalent and trivalent chromium on mammalian cells in vitro, *Caryologia* **32**:379–392.

Mancuso, T. F., 1970, Relation of duration of employment and prior respiratory illness to respiratory cancer among beryllium workers, *Environ. Res.* **3**:251–275.

Mandel, L., and Ryser, H. J. P., 1981, The mutagenic effect of cadmium in bacteria and its synergism with alkylating agents, *12th EMS Annual Meeting*, San Diego Ca. March 5–8, Abstr. 89.

Mansour, M. M., Dyer, N. C., Hoffman, L. H., Davies, J., and Brill, A. B., 1975, Placental transfer of mercuric nitrate and methylmercury in the rat, *Am. J. Obstet. Gynecol.* **119**:557–562.

Marsh, D. O. Meyers, G., Clarkson, L., Amin-zaki, I., and Tikritio, S. T., 1977, Fetal methylmercury poisoning: New data on clinical and toxicological aspects, *Trans. Am. Neurol. Assoc.* **102**:69–71.

Mathews, C., and Al-Doori, Z., 1976, The mutagenic effect of the mercury fungicide ceresan M in *Drosophila melanogaster*, *Mutat. Res.* **40**:31–36.

Mathur, A. K., Drikshith, T. S. S., Lal, M. M. and Tandon, S. K., 1978, Distribution of nickel and cytogenetic changes in poisoned rats, *Toxicology* **10**:105–113.

Matsumoto, H., Suzuki, A., and Morita, C., 1967, Preventive effect of penicillamine on the brain defect of fetal rat poisoned transplacentally with methylmercury, *Life Sci.* **6**:2321–2326.

Maxild, J., Andersen, N., Kiel, P., and Stern, R. M., 1978, Mutagenicity of fume particles from metal arc welding on stain steel in the *Salmonella* microsome test, *Mutat. Res.* **56**:235–243.

McClain, R. M., and Becker, B. A., 1970, Placental transport and teratogenicity of lead in rats and mice, *Fed. Proc.* **29**:347.

McClain, R. M., and Becker, B. A., 1975, Teratogenicity, fetal toxicity and placental transfer of lead nitrate in rats, *Toxicol. Appl. Pharmacol.* **31**:72–82.

McLellan, J. S., Vonsmolinski, A. W., Bederka, J. P., and Boulos, B. M., 1974, Development toxicology of lead in the mouse, *Fed. Proc. Fed. Am. Soc. Exp. Biol.* **33**:288.

McNeely, M. D., Sunderman, F. W. Jr, Nechay, M. W., and Levine, H., 1971, Abnormal concentrations of nickel in serum in cases of myocardial infarction, stroke, burns, hepatic cirrhosis, and uremia, *Clin. Chem.* **17**:1123–1128.

Mehra, M., and Kanwar, K. C., 1980, Absorption, distribution and excretion of methylmercury in mice, *Bull. Environ. Contam. Toxicol.* **24**:627–633.

Mertz, W., 1969, Chromium occurence and function in biological systems, *Physiol. Rev.* **49**:163–239.

Mertz, W., Roginski, E. E., Feldmnan, F. J. and Thurman, D. E., 1969, Dependence of chromium transfer into the rat embryo on the chemical form, *J. Nutr.* **99**:363.

Michalowsky, I., 1926, Die experimentelle Erzeugung einer teratoiden Neubildung der Hoden beim Hahn, *Zentrbl. Allg. Path. Anat.* **38**:585–587.

Milham, S., and Strong, T., 1974, Human arsenic exposure in relation to a copper smelter, *Environ. Res.* **7**:176–182.

Ministery of Agriculture, Fisheries and Food, 1979, Survey of lead in food-Working party of the monitoring of food stuffs for heavy metals, HRSO, London.

Minkowitz, S., 1964, Multiple carcinomata following ingestion of medicinal arsenic, *Ann. Int. Med.* **61**:296–299.

Miyaki, M., Murata, I., Osabe, M., and Ono, T., 1977, Effect of metal cations on misincorporation by *E. coli* DNA polymerases, *Biochem. Biophys. Res. Commun.* **77**:854–860.

Moreau, P., and Devoret, R., 1977, Potential carcinogens tested by induction and mutagenesis of prophage in *Escherichia coli* K12, in *Origin of Human Cancer* (edited by H. H. Hratt, J. D. Watson, and J. A. Winston) Cold Spring Harbor, N. Y., Cold Spring Harbor Lab., pp. 1451–1472.

Morgan, J., 1970, Cadmium and zinc abnormalities in bronchogenic carcinoma, *Cancer* **25**:1394–1398.

Morikawa, N., 1961, Pathological studies in organic mercury poisoning, *Kumamoto Med. J.* **14**:87–93.

Morris, H. P., Lang, E. P., Morris, H. J., and Grant R. L., 1938, The growth and reproduction of rats fed diets containing lead acetate and arsenic trioxide, *J. Pharmacol. Exp. Ther.* **64**:420–445.

Mottet, N. K., 1974, Effects of chronic low-dose exposure of rat fetuses to methylmercury hydroxide, *Teratology* **10**:173–190.

Moutschen, J., Moutschen-Dahmen, M., and Degraeve, N., 1965, Modified effects of ethyl methane sulfonate (EMS) at the chromosome level, Sympos. Mechanisms of Mutation and Inducing Factors, Prague, pp. 397–400.

Moxon, A. L., and Dubois, K. P., 1939, The influence of arsenic and other elements on the toxicity of seleniferous grains, *J. Nutr.* **18**:447–457.

Mulvihill, J., Gramm, S., and Ferm, V., 1970, Facial formations in normal and cadmium treated golden hamsters, *J. Embryol. Exp. Morphol.* **24**:393–403.

Murakami, U., Kameyama, Y., and Kato, T., 1956, Effects of a vaginally applied contraceptive with phenylmercuric acetate upon developing embryos and their mother animals, *Ann. Rep. Res. Inst. Environ. Med. Nagoya Univ.*, pp. 88–99.

Muro, L. A., and Goyer, R. A., 1969, Chromosome damage in experimental lead poisoning, *Arch. Pathol.* **87**:660–663.

Nadenko, V. G., Lenchenko, V. G., Arkhipenko, T. A., Saichenko, S. P., and Petrova, N. N., 1979, Embryotoxic effect of nickel ingested with drinking water, *Gig. Sanit.* **6**:86–88.

Nakamuro, K., and Sayato, Y., 1981, Comparative studies of chromosomal aberrations induced by trivalent and pentavalent arsenic, *Mutat. Res.* **88**:73–90.

Nakamuro, K., Yoshikawa, K., Sayato, Y., Kurata, H., Tomomura, and Tomomura A., 1976,

Studies on selenium-related compounds. V. Genetic effects and reactivity with DNA, *Mutat. Res.* **40**:177–183.

Nakamuro, K., Yoshikawa, K., Sayato, Y., and Kurata, H., 1978, Comparative studies of chromosomal aberrations and mutagenicity of trivalent and hexavalent chromium, *Mutat. Res.* **58**:175–181.

National Academy of Science–National Research Council, 1974, Medical and biological effects of environmental polluants: Chromium, Washington, D.C.

National Academy of Science–National Research Council, 1975, Medical and biological effects of environmental polluants: Nickel, Washington, D.C.

National Academy of Science–National Research Council, 1977, Medical and biological effects of environmental polluants: Arsenic, Washington, D.C.

Nestmann, E. R., Matula, T. I., Douglas, G. R., Boza, K. C., and Kowbel, D. J., 1979, Detection of the mutagenic activity of lead chromate using a battery of microbial tests, *Mutat. Res.* **66**:357–365.

Nettesheim, P., and Hammons, A. S., 1971, Induction of squamous cell carcinoma in the respiratory tract of mice, *J. Natl. Cancer Inst.* **47**:697–791.

Neubauer, O., 1946, Arsenical cancer: A review, *Br. J. Cancer* **1**:192–196.

Newbold, R. F., Amos, J., and Connell, J. R., 1979, The cytotoxic, mutagenic and clastogenic effects of chromium containing compounds on mammalian cells in culture, *Mutat. Res.* **67**:55–63.

Newborne, P. M., Glaser, O., Friedman, L., and Stillings, B. R., 1972, Chronic exposure of rats to methylmercury in fish proteins, *Nature (London)* **237**:40–41.

Nielsen, F. H., 1977, Nickel toxicity, in *Advances in Modern Toxicology*, (edited by R. A. Goyer and M. A. Mehlman) Hemisphere Publ. Corp., Washington, vol. 2, pp. 129–146.

Nii Lo Piccolo, G. M., 1972, M. A. Thesis, Western Michigan Univcrisity, Kalamazoo Mi.

Nikiforov, Yu. L., Sakharova, M. N., Beknazaryants, M. M., and Rapoport, I. A., 1970, Specific effects of chromium on puff formation in *Drosophila melanogaster*, *Dokl. Biol. Sci. (Engl. Transl.)* **194**:520–523.

Nishimura, M., and Umeda, M., 1978, Mutagenic effect of some metal compounds on cultured mammalian cells, *Mutat. Res.* **54**:246–247.

Nishimura, M., and Umeda, M., 1979, Induction of chromosomal aberrations in cultured mammalian cells by nickel compounds, *Mutat. Res.* **68**:337–349.

Nishioka, H., 1974, Mutagenesis of metal compounds in bacteria, *Mutat. Res.* **26**:437–438.

Nishioka, H., 1975, Mutagenic activities of metal compounds in bacteria, *Mutat. Res.* **31**:185–189.

Noguki, K., 1958, On the action of lead on the body of refinery workers, particularly on the conception, pregnancy and parturition in the case of females and on the vitality of the new-born. *Excerpta Med.* **17**:515–516.

Nogami, H., and Terashima, Y., 1973, Thallium-induced achondroplasia in the rat, *Teratology* **8**:101–102.

Nolen, G. A. Buehler, E. V., Geil, R. G., and Goldenthal, E. I., 1972, Effects of trisodium nitrilotriacetate on cadmium and methylmercury toxicity and teratogenicity in rats, *Toxicol. Appl. Pharmacol.* **23**:222–237.

Nonaka, I., 1969, An electron microscopical study on the experimental congenital Minamata disease in rat, *Kumamoto Med. J.* **22**:27–40.

Nordenson, I., Beckmann, G., Beckman, L., and Nordstroem, S., 1978, Occupational and environmental risk in and around a smelter in northern Sweden. II. Chromosomal aberrations in workers exposed to arsenic, *Hereditas* **88**:47–50.

Nordenson, I., Beckman, G., Beckman, L., and Nordstroem, S., 1978c, Occupational and environmental risk in and around a smelter in northern Sweden. IV. Chromosomal aberrations in workers exposed to lead, *Hereditas* **88**:263–268.

Norseth, T., 1977, Industrial viewpoints on cancer caused by metals as occupational disease, in *Origins of Human Cancer*, Cold Spring Harbor Laboratory, Cold Spring Harbor.

Norseth, T., and M. Piscator, M., 1979, Nickel, in *Handbook on the Toxicology of Metals*, (edited by L. Friberg, G. F. Nordberg, and V. B. Vouk) Elsevier/North Holland Biomedical Press, Amsterdam, pp. 541–553.

Novey, H. S., and Martel, S. H. 1969, Asthma, arsenic and cancer, *J. Allergy* **44**:315–319.

Nriagu, J. D., 1978, The Biogeochemistry of Lead in the Environment, Vol. 2, Elsevier, Amsterdam.

Null, D. H., Gartside, P. S., and Wei, E., 1973, Methylmercury accumulation in brains of pregnant, nonpregnant and fetal rats, *Life Sci.* **12**:65–72.

Nygren, A., 1949, Cytological studies of the effects of 2,4-D, MCPA and 2,4,5-T on *Allium cepa*, *Ann. R. Agr. Coll. Sweden* **16**:723–728.

Obe, G., Beek, B., and Dudin, G., 1975, Some experiments on the action of lead acetate on human leucocytes *in vitro*, *Mutat. Res.* **29**:283.

Ochi, H., and Tonomura, A., 1975, The low-dose effect of two organic mercury compounds on cultured human fibroblastic cells, *Mutat. Res.* **31**:268.

Oehlkers, F., 1953: Chromosome breaks influenced by chemicals, *Heredity* **6 Suppl**:95–105.

Okada, M., and Oharazawa, H., 1967, Diagnosis of mercury poisoning. Influence of ethyl-mercuric phosphate on pregnant mice and their fetuses, in Report on the cases of mercury poisoning in Niigata, Ministery of Health and Welfare, Tokyo, Stencils 63.

Oliver, T., 1911, Lead poisoning and the race, in *Lead Poisoning*, Lewis, London, p. 192.

Olsen, I., and Jonsen, J., 1979, Whole body autoradiography of $^{63}$Ni in mice throughout gestation, *Toxicology* **12**:165–172.

Olson, F. C., and Massaro, E. J., 1977, Effects of methylmercury on murine fetal amino acid uptake, protein synthesis and palate closure, *Teratology* **16**:187–194.

Oppenheim, J. P., and Fishbein, W. N., 1965, Induction of chromosome breaks in normal cultured human leucocytes by potassium arsenite, hydroxyurea and related compounds, *Cancer Res.* **25**:980–985.

Orgel, A., and Orgel, L. E., 1965, Induction of mutations in bacteriophage T4 with divalent manganese, *J. Mol. Biol.* **14**:453–457.

O'Riordan, M. L., and Evans, H. J., 1974, Absence of significant chromosome damage in males occupationally exposed to lead, *Nature (London)* **274**:50–53.

O'Riordan, M. L., Hughes, E., and Evans, H., 1978, Chromosome studies on blood lymphocytes of men occupationally exposed to cadmium, *Mutat. Res.* **58**:305–311.

Osburn, H. S., 1969, lung cancer in a mining district in Rhodesia, *S. Afr. Med. J.* **43**:1307–1312.

Oswald, H., and Goerttler, K., 1971, Arsenic-induced leucosis in mice after diaplacental and postnatal application, *Verh, Deutsch. Ges. Pathol.* **55**:289–293.

Ott, M. G., Holder, B. B., and Gordon H. L., 1974, Respiratory cancer and occupational exposure to arsenicals, *Arch. Environ. Health* **29**:250–255.

Palmisano, P. A., Sneed, R. C., and Cassady, G., 1969, Untaxed whiskey and fetal lead exposure, *J. Pediatr.* **75**:869–872.

Parizek, J., 1963, Vascular changes at sites of oestrogen biosynthesis produced by parenteral injection of cadmium salts: the destruction of placenta by cadmium salts, *J. Reprod. Fertil.* **7**:263–265.

Parzyk, D., Shaw, S., Kessler, W., Vetter, R., Vansickle, D., and Mayes, R., 1978, Fetal effects of cadmium in pregnant rats on normal and zinc deficient diets, *Bull. Environm. Contam. Toxicol.* **19**:206–214.

Paton, G. R., and Allison, A. C., 1972, Chromosome damage in human cell cultures induced by metal salts, *Mutat. Res.* **16**:332–336.

Paul, C., 1860, Etude sur l'intoxication lente par des préparations de plomb; de son influence sur le produit de la conception, *Arch. Gén. Med.* **15**:513–533.

Payne, W. W., 1960, Production of cancers in mice and rats by chromium compounds, *AMA. Arch Ind. Health* **21**:530–535.

Petres, J., 1972, Zum Einfluss inorganischen Arsens auf die DNA Synthese menschlicher Lymphozyten *in vitro, Hautarzt* **23**:464.

Petres, J., and Berger, A., 1972, Zum Einfluss anorganischen Arsenics auf die DNS-Synthese menschlicher Lymphocyten *in vitro, Arch. Dermatol. Forsch.* **242**:343–352.

Petres, J., Schmid-Ulrich, K., and Wolf, V., 1970, Chromosomenaberrationen an menschlichen Lymphozyten bei chronischen Arsenschaeden, *Dtsch. Med. Wochenschr.* **2**:79–80.

Petres, J., Baron, D., and Kunick, I., 1974, Untersuchungen ueber arsenbedingte Veraenderungen der Nukleinsaeuresynthese *in vitro, Dermatol. Monatsschr.* **160**:724–729.

Petrilli, F. L., and De Flora, S., 1977, Toxicity and mutagenicity of hexavalent chromium in *Salmonella typhimurium, Appl. Environ. Microbiol.* **33**:805–809.

Petrilli, F. L., and De Flora, S., 1978a, Metabolic deactivation of hexavalent chromium mutagenicity, *Mutat. Res.* **54**:139–147.

Petrilli, F. L., and De Flora, S., 1978b, Oxidation of inactive trivalent chromium to the mutagenic hexavalent form, *Mutat. Res.* **58**:167–173.

Petzow, G., Zorn, H., 1974, Toxicology of beryllium-containing materials, *Chemiker-Ztg.* **98**:236–241.

Piechoka, J., 1968, Chemical and toxicological studies of the fungicide phenylmercuric acetate. 1. Studies on the effect of food contaminated with fungitox OR, on rats, *Roczn. Panst. Zakl. Hig.* **19**:385.

Pierro, L. J., and Haynes, J. S., 1976, Cd-induced exencephaly and eye defects in the mouse, *Teratology* **13**:33A

Pilinskaya, M. A., 1970, Chromosome aberrations in the persons contaminated with Ziram, *Genetika (Moscow)* **6**:157–163.

Pilinskaya, M. A., 1971, Cytogenetic effects of the fungicide Ziram in the culture of human lymphocytes *in vitro, Genetika (Moscow)* **7**:138–143.

Pilinskaya, M. A., 1974, Results of cytogenetic examination of persons occupationally contacting with the fungicide Ziram, *Genetika (Moscow)* **10**:140–146.

Pinto, S. S., Enterline, P. E., Henderson, V., and Varner, M. O., 1977, Mortality experience in relation to a measured arsenic trioxide exposure, *Environ. Health Perspect.* **19**:127–130.

Piscator, M., 1971, Transport, distribution, and excretion of cadmium in animals, in *Cadmium in the Environment* (edited by Friberg, L., Piscator, M., and Nordberg, G.), The Chemical Rubber Company, Cleveland, Ohio, p. 33.

Pitkin, R. M., Bahns, J. A., Filer, L. J., and Reynolds, W. A., 1976, Mercury in human maternal and cord blood, placenta and milk, *Proc. Soc. Exp. Biol. Med.* **151**:565–567.

Polukhina, G., Kalinina, L., and Lukasheva, L., 1977, *Salmonella typhimurium* assay test-system for indication of mutagenic effect of environmental hazard. II. Detection of heavy metals salts using *in vitro* assay with metabolic activation, *Genetika* **13**:1492–1494.

Poma, K., Kirsch-Volders, M., and Susanne, C., 1981, Mutagenicity studies on mice given mercuric chloride, *J. Appl. Toxicol.* **1**:314–316.

Popescu, H. I., Negru, L., and Lancranjan, I., 1979, Chromosome aberrations induced by occupational exposure to mercury, *Arch. Environ. Health* **34**:461–463.

Potts, C. L., 1965, Cadmium proteinuria. The health of battery workers exposed to cadmium oxide dust, *Ann. Occup. Hyg.* **8**:55–61.

Powell, J. B., and Taylorson, R. B., 1967, Induced sterility and associated effects of dimethylarsenic acid treatment on pearl millet, *Crop Sci.* **7**:670–672.

Prazmo, W., Ballin, E., Baranowska, H., Ejjchart, A., and Putrament, A., 1975, Manganese mutagenesis in yeast II. Conditions of induction and characteristics of respiratory deficient Saccharomyces cerevisiae mutants induced with manganese and cobalt, *Genet. Res.* **26**:21–29.

Putrament, A., Baranowska, H., Ejchart, A., and Jachymczyk, W., 1977, Manganese mutagenesis in yeast. VI. $Mn^{2+}$ uptake, mitDNA replication and $E^R$ induction. Comparison with other diavalent cations, *Mol. Gen. Genet.* **151**:69–76.

Ramel, C., 1967, Genetic effects of organic mercury compounds, *Hereditas* **57**:445–447.

Ramel, C., 1969, Genetic effects of organic mercury compounds. I. Cytological investigations on Allium roots, *Hereditas* **61**:208–233.

Ramel, C., 1970, Tests of chromosome segregation in *Drosophila*, *Abstr, Ist. Ann. Meet. Env. Mutag. Soc.*, p. 22.

Ramel, C., 1972, Genetic effects, in *Mercury in the Environment* (edited by L. Friberg and D. Vostal) CRC Press, pp. 169–181.

Ramel, C., 1973, The effect of metal compounds on chromosome segregation, *Mutat. Res.* **21**:45–46.

Ramel, C., and Friberg, K., 1974, in *Cadmium in the Environment*, (edited by L. Friberg, M. Piscator, and G. Nordberg) 2nd edition, CRC Press, p. 133.

Ramel, C., and Magnusson, J., 1969, Genetic effects of organic mercury compounds. II. Chromosome segregation in *Drosophila melanogaster*, *Hereditas* **61**:231–254.

Reddy, T. P., and Vaidyanath, K., 1978a, Mutagenic, potentiating and antimutagenic activity of certain metallic ions in the rice genetic system, *Curr. Sci.* **47**:513–515.

Reddy, T. P., and Vaidyanath, K., 1978b, Synergistic interaction of gamma rays and some metallic salts in the induction of chlorophyll mutants in rice, *Mutat. Res.* **52**:361–365.

Reeves, A. L., 1979, Beryllium, in *Handbook on the Toxicology of Metals*, (edited by L. Friberg, G. F. Nordberg, and V. B. Vouk) Elsevier/ North Holland Biomedical Press, Amsterdam, pp. 329–343.

Reeves, A. L., and Vorwald, A. J., 1967, Beryllium carcinogenesis II. Pulmonary deposition and clearance of inhaled beryllium, *Cancer Res.* **27**:446–451.

Reeves, A. L., Deitch, D., and Vorwald, A. J., 1967, Beryllium carcinogenesis. I. Inhalation exposure of rats to beryllium, *Cancer Res.* **27**:439–445.

Regelson, W., Kim, U., Ospina, J., and Holland, J. F., 1968, Hemangioendothelial sarcoma of liver from chronic arsenic intoxication by Fowler's solution, *Cancer* **12**:514–522.

Reynolds, W. A., and Pitkin, R. M., 1975, Transplacental passage of methylmercury and its uptake by Primate fetal tissues, *Proc. Soc. Exp. Biol. Med.* **148**:523–526.

Ribas, B., and Schmidt, W., 1973, Der Einfluss von Cadmium auf die Entwicklung von Huehnerembryos, *Morphol. Jahrb.* **119**:358–366.

Ridgway, L. P., and Karnofsky, D. A., 1952, The effects of metals on the chick embryo: toxicity and production of abnormalities in development, *Ann. N.Y. Acad. Sci.* **55**:203–215.

Rivedahl, E., and Sanner, T., 1980, Synergistic effect on morphological transformation of hamster embryo cells by nickel sulfate and benz(a) pyrene, *Cancer Lett.* **8**:203–208.

Robertson, D. S. F., 1970, Selenium, a possible teratogen, *Lancet* **1**:518–519.

Robson, A. O., and Jelliffe, A. J., 1963, Medical arsenic poisoning and lung cancer, *Br. J. Med.* **2**:207–209.

Roe, F. J. C., 1967, On the potential carcinogenicity of the iron macromolecular complexes, in *Potential Carcinogenic Hazards From Drugs*, (edited by R. Truhaut) Springer Verlag, Berlin, pp. 105–118.

Roe, F. J. C., and Carter, R. L., 1969, Chromium carcinogenesis: calcium chromate as a potent carcinogen for the subcutaneous tissues of the rat, *Br. J. Cancer* **23**:172–176.

Roels, H., Hubermont, G., Buchet, J. P., and Lauwerys, R., 1978, Placental transfer of lead, mercury, cadmium, and carbon monoxide in women. III. Factors influencing the accumulation of heavy metals in the placenta and the relationship between metal concentration in the placenta and in maternal and cord blood, *Environ. Res.* **16**:236–247.

Rohr, G., and Bauchinger, M., 1976, Chromosome analyses in cell cultures of the Chinese hamster after application of cadmium sulfate, *Mutat. Res.* **40**:125–130.

Rondia, D., 1979, Sources, modes and levels of human exposure to nickel and chromium, in *Trace Metals, Exposure and Health Effects*, (edited by E. Di Ferrante) Pergamon Press, Oxford, pp. 117–134.

Rosenfeld, I., and Beath, O. A., 1954, Effect of selenium on reproduction in rats, *Proc. Soc. Exp. Biol. Med.* **87**:295–298.

Rosenthal, E., and Sparber, S. B., 1972, Methylmercury dicyandiamide: Retardation of detour learning in chicks hatched from injected eggs, *Life Sci.* **11**:883–892.

Rossman, T. G., Meyn, M. S., and Troll, W., 1975, Effects of sodium arsenite on the survival of UV-irradiated *Escherichia coli:* Inhibition of a recA-dependent function, *Mutat. Res.* **30**:157–162.

Rossman, T. G., Meyn, M. S., and Troll, W., 1977, Effects of arsenite on DNA repair in *Escherichia coli, Environ. Health Perspect.* **19**:229 233.

Rossman, T. G., Stone, D., Molina, M., and Troll, W., 1980, Absence of arsenite mutagenicity in *E. coli* and Chinese hamster cells, *Environ. Mutagen.* **2**:371–379.

Roth, F., 1958, Bronchial cancer in vintners exposed to arsenic, *Virchow Arch. Pathol. Anat.* **221**:119–137.

Ruposhev, A., 1976a, Cytogenic effect of heavy metal ions on Crepis capillaris L. seeds, *Genetika (Moscow)* **12**:37–43.

Ruposhev, A., 1976b, Modification of the mutagenic effect of ethyleneimine in *Crepis capillaris* L., *Tsitol. Genet.* **10**:111–113.

Ruposhev, A., and Garina, K., 1976, Mutagenic effect of cadmium salts, *Tsitol. Genet.* **10**:437–439.

Ruposhev, A., and Garina, K., 1977, Modification of mutagenic effects of ethyleneimine in *Crepis capillaris* L. Genetika *(Moscow)* **13**:32–36.

Samarawickrama, G., and Webb, M., 1979, Acute effects of cadmium on the pregnant rat and embryo-fetal development, *Environ. Health. Perspect.* **28**:245–250.

Satterlee, H. S., 1960, The arsenic poisoning epidemic of 1900: Its relation to lung cancer in 1960. An exercise in retrospective epidemiology. *N. Engl. J. Med.* **263**:676–684.

Scharpf, L. G. Jr., Hill, I. D., Wright, P. L., Plank, J. G., Keplinger, M. L., and Calandra, J. C., 1972, Effect of sodium nitrilotriacetate on toxicity, teratogenicity, and tissue distribution of cadmium, *Nature (London)* **239**:231–233.

Scharpf, L. G. Jr., Hill, I. D., Wright, P. L., and Keplinger, M. L., 1973, Teratology studies on methylmercury hydroxide and nitrilotriacetate, *Nature (London)* **241**:461–463.

Schmid, E., Bauchinger, M., Pietruck, S., and Hall, G., 1972, Die cytogenetische Wirkung von Blei in menschlichen peripheren Lymphocyten *in vitro* und *in vivo, Mutat. Res.* **16**:401–406.

Schroeder, H. A., and Mitchener, M., 1971a, The teratogenic profile of sodium arsenate in the golden hamster, *Arch. Environ. Health* **22**:557–560.

Schroeder, H. A., and Mitchener, M., 1971b, Toxic effects of trace elements on the reproduction of mice and rats, *Arch. Environ. Health* **23**:102–106.

Schroeder, H. A., Balassa, J. J., and Vinton, W. H. Jr., 1964, Chromium, lead, cadmium, nickel and titanium in mice: Effect on mortality, tumors and tissue levels, *J. Nutr.* **83**:239–250.

Schwanitz, G., Lehnert, G., and Gebhart, E., 1970, Chromosomenschaeden bei beruflicher Bleibelastung, *Dtsch. Med Wochenschr.* **95**:1636–1641.

Schwanitz, G., Gebhart, E., Rott, H. D., Schaller, J. K., Essing, G., Lauer, O., and Prestele, H., 1975, Chromosomenuntersuchungen bei Personen mit beruflicher Bleiexposition, *Dtsch. Med. Wochenschr.* **100**:1007–1011.

Semba, R., Ohta, K., and Yamamura, H., 1974, Low dose preadministration of cadmium prevents cadmium-induced exencephalia, *Teratology* **10**:96A.

Semba, R., Ohta, K., Yamamura, H., and Murakami, Y., 1977, Effect of cadmium pretreatment and fetolethality of cadmium, *Okajimas Folia Anat. Jpn.* **54**:283–288.

Shamberger, R. J., 1971, Is selenium a teratogen? *Lancet* **2**:1137.

Shamberger, R. J., 1979, Beneficial effects of trace elements, in *Toxicity of Heavy Metals in the Environment* (edited by F. W. Oehme) part 2, Marcel Dekker Inc., New York, pp. 689–796.

Shimada, T., Watanabe, T., and Endo, A., 1976, Potential mutagenicity of cadmium in mammalian oocytes, *Mutat. Res.* **40**:389–396.

Shiraishi, Y., and Yosida, T., 1972, Chromosal abnormalities in cultured leucocyte cells from Itai-itai disease patients, *Proc. Jpn. Acad.* **48**:248–25.

Shiraishi, Y., Kurahashi, H., and Yosida, T., 1972, Chromosomal abnormalities in cultured human leucocytes induced by cadmium sulfide, *Proc. Jpn. Acad.* **48**:133–137.

Shirasu, Y., Moriya, M., Kato, K., Furuhashi, A., and Kado, T., 1976, Mutagenicity screening of pesticides in the microbial system, *Mutat. Res.* **40**:19–30.

Shou, M., and Amdisen, A., 1971, Lithium teratogenicity, *Lancet* **1**:1132.

Sirover, M. A., and Loeb, L. A., 1976, Infidelity of DNA synthesis *in vitro*, screening for potential metal mutagens or carcinogens, *Science* **194**:1434–1436.

Sissons, H. A., 1950, Bone sarcomas produced experimentally in the rabbit using compounds of beryllium, *Acta Unio Contra Cancrum* **7**:171.

Skerfving, S., 1974, Methyl mercury exposure, mercury levels in blood and hair and health status in Swedes consuming contaminated fish, *Toxicology* **22**:3–23.

Skerfving, S., Hansson, K., and Lindsten, J., 1970, Chromosome breakage in humans exposed to methylmercury through fish consumption, *Arch. Environ. Health* **21**:133–139.

Skervfing, S., Hansson, K., Mangs, C., Lindsten, J., and Ryman, N., 1974, Methylmercury-induced chromosome damage in man, *Environ. Res.* **7**:83–98.

Smith, R. J., 1981, Beryllium report disputed by listed authors, *Science* **211**:556–557.

Sorsa, M., and Pfeifer, S., 1973, Effects of cadmium on development time and prepupal puffing pattern of Drosophila melanogaster, *Hereditas* **75**:273–277.

Spann, J. W., Heath, R. G., Kreitzer, J. F., and Lock, L. N., 1972, Ethylmercury p-toluene sulfonanilide: lethal and reproductive effects on pheasants, *Science* **175**:328–331.

Sperling, K., Weiss, G., Muenzer, M., and Obe, G., 1970, Chromosomenuntersuchungen an Blei exponierten Arbeitern, "Arbeitsgruppe Blei" der Kommission fuer Umweltgefahren des Bundesgesundheitsamtes, Berlin.

Spyker, J. M., and Chang, L. W., 1974, Delayed effects of prenatal exposure to methylmercury on brain ultrastructure and behavior, *Teratology* **9**:17–37.

Spyker, J. M., and Smithberg, J., 1972, Effects of methylmercury on prenatal development in mice, *Teratology* **5**:181–190.

Sram, R. J., and Beneko, V., 1974, A contribution to the evaluation of the genetic risk of exposure to arsenic, *Cesk. Hyg.* **19**:308–315.

Stack, M. V., Burkett, A. J., and Nickless, G., 1976, Trace metals in teeth at birth, *Bull. Environ. Contam. Toxicol.* **16**:764–766.

Stella, M., Rossi, R., Martinucci, G. B., Rossi, G., and Bonfante, A., 1979, BUDR as a tracer of the possible mutagenic activity of $Pb^{++}$ in human lymphocyte cultures, *Biochem. Exp. Biol.* **14**:221–231.

Stich, H. F., and Kuhnlein, U., 1979, Chromosome breaking activity of human feces and its enhancement by transition metals, *Int. J. Cancer* **24**:284–287.

Stich, H. F., Wei, L., and Whiting, R. F., 1979, Enhancement of the chromosome-damaging action of ascorbate by transition metals, *Cancer Res.* **39**:4145–4151.

Stone, O. J., 1969, The effect of arsenic on inflammation, infection and carcinogenic, *Tex. State J. Med.* **65**:40–43.

Storeng, R., and Jonsen, J., 1980a, Nickel toxicity in early mammalian embryogenesis, *Toxicology Lett.*, Spec. Issue 2nd. Int. Congr. Toxicology, Brussels, p. 110.

Storeng, R., and Jonsen, J., 1980b, Effect of nickel chloride and cadmium acetate on the development of preimplantation mouse embryos *in vitro*, *Toxicology* **17**:183–187.

Storeng, R., and Jonsen, J., 1981, Nickel toxicity in early embryogenesis in mice, *Toxicology* **20**:45–51.

Streffer, C., van Beuningen, D., Molls, M., Schulz, A. P., and Zamboglou, N., 1979, The *in vitro* culture of preimplanted mouse embryos. A model for studying combined effects, in *Late Biological Effects of Ionizing Radiation*, II, STI/PUB/489, IAEA, Vienna.

Su, M. Q., and Okita, G. T., 1976a, Embryocidal and teratogenic effects of methylmercury in mice, *Toxicol. Appl. Pharmacol.* **38**:207–216.

Su, M. Q., and Okita, G. T., 1976b, Behavioral effects on the progeny of mice treated with methylmercury, *Toxicol. Appl. Pharmacol.* **38**:195–205.

Sullivan, R. J., 1969, Preliminary air pollution survey of arsenic and its components, U.S. Dept. of Health, Education, and Welfare, Raleigh, N.C., APTD-69-26.

Sunderman, F. W., Jr., 1971, Metal carcinogenesis in experimental animals, *Food Cosmet. Toxicol.* **9**:105–120.

Sunderman, F. W., Jr., 1976a, A review of the carcinogenicities of nickel, chromium, and arsenic compounds in man and animals, *Prev. Med.* **5**:279–294.

Sunderman, F. W., Jr., 1976b, A review of the carcinogenicities of nickel, chromium and arsenic compounds in man and animals, *Prev. Med.* **5**:279–294.

Sunderman, F. W., Jr., 1977a, Metal carcinogenesis, in *Advances in Modern Toxicology*, (edited by R. A. Goyer and M. A. Mehlman) Hemisphere Publ. Corp., Washington, Vol. 2, pp. 257–295.

Sunderman, F. W., Jr., 1977b, A review of the metabolism and toxicology of nickel, *Ann. Clin. Lab. Sci.* **7**:377–398.

Sunderman, F. W., Jr., 1979, Mechanisms of metal carcinogenesis, *Biol. Trace Element Res.* **1**:63–86.

Sunderman, F. W., and Sunderman, F. W., Jr., 1961, Nickel poisoning XI. Implication of nickel as a pulmonary carcinogen in tobacco smoke, *Am. J. Clin. Pathol.* **35**:203–209.

Sunderman, F. W., Jr., Shen, S. K., Mitchell, J. M., Allpass, P. R., and Damjanov, I., 1978, Embryotoxicity and fetal toxicity of nickel in rats, *Toxicol. Appl. Pharmacol.* **43**:381–390.

Sunderman, F. W., Jr., Allpass, P. R., Mitchell, J. M., Baselt, R. C., and Albert, D. M., 1979, Eye malformations in rats: Induction by prenatal exposure to nickel carbonyl, *Science* **203**:550–553.

Sunderman, F. W., Jr., Shen, S. K., Reid, M. C., and Allpass, P. R., 1980, Teratogenicity and embryotoxicity of nickel carbonyl in Syrian hamsters, in 3. Spurenelementsymposium Nickel, (edited by M. Anke, H. J. Schneide, and C. Brueckner), Karl Marx Universitaet Leipzig, Friedrich Schiller Universitaet Jena, pp. 301–307.

Suraikina, T. I., Zakharova, I. A., Mashkovsky, Yu. Sh., and Fonshtein, L. H., 1979, Study of the mutagenic action of platinum and palladium compounds on bacteria, *Toxicol. Genet.* **13f**:486–491.

Sussman, V. K., Lieben, J., and Cleland, J. G., 1959, An air pollution study of a community surrounding a beryllium plant, *Am. Ind. Hyg. Assoc. J.* **20**:504–510.

Sutou, S., Yamamoto, K., Sendota, H., and Sugiyama, M., 1980, Toxicity, fertility, teratogenicity, and dominant lethal tests in rats administered cadmium subchronically. II. Fertility, teratogenicity and dominant lethal tests, *Ecotoxicol. Environ. Safety* **4**:51–56.

Swieringa, S. H. H., and Basrur, P. K., 1968, Effect of nickel on cultured rat embryo muscle cells, *Lab. Invest.* **19**:663–674.

Takeuchi, I. K., 1972, Environmental mercury contamination, in *Ann Arbor Science*, (edited by R. Hartung and B. Dinman), Ann Arbor, Mich., p. 302.

Takeuchi, I. K., 1979, Embryotoxicity of arsenic acid: Light and electron microscopy of its effect on neurulation-stage rat embryo, *J. Tox. Sci.* **4**:405–416.

Tamoro, M., Banfi, E., Venturini, S., and Monti-Bragadin, C., 1975, Hexavalent chromium compounds are mutagenic for bacteria, in *XVII Congr. Naz. Soc. Ital. Microbiol.*, Padova, p. 411–415.

Task group on metal accumulation, 1973, Accumulation of toxic metals with special reference to their absorption, excretion and biological half-times, *Environ. Physiol. Biochem.* **3**:65–107.

Taussig, F. G., 1936, Abortions, spontaneous and induced, Mosby, St. Louis

Taylor, R. T., Carver, J. H., Hanna, U. L., and Wandres, D. L., 1979, Platinum-induced mutations to 8-azaguanine resistance in Chinese hamster ovary cells, *Mutat. Res.* **67**:65–80.

Taylor, R. T., Hoppe, J. A., Hanna, U. L., and Wu, R., 1979, Platinum tetrachloride mutagenicity and methylation with methylcobalamine, *Environ. Sci. Health* **14**:87–109.

Tazima, Y., 1974, Attempts to induce non-disjunction by means of irradiation and chemical treatment in the silkworm, *Radiat. Res.* **59**:267–268.

Tepper, L. B., 1972, Beryllium, *Crit. Rev. Toxicol.* **1**:235–256.

Terada, H., Katsuta, K., Sasakawa, T., Saito, H., Shrota, H., Fukuchi, K., Sekiya, E., Yokohama, Y., Hirokawa, S., Watanabe, G., Hasegawa, K., Oshina, T., and Sekiguchi, E., 1960, Clinical observations of chronic toxicosis by arsenic, *Nippon Rinsho* **18**:2394–2403.

Timpson, J., and Price, D. J., 1971, Lithium and mitosis, *Lancet* **2**:93.

Tindall, K. R., and Hsie, A. W., 1980, Mutagenic and cytotoxic effects of hexavalent and trivalent chromium in the CHO/HGPRT system, 11th Ann. Meet. Environ. Mutagen Soc., Nashville Tenn. pp. 118–119.

Tindall, K. R., Warren, G. R., and Skaar, P. D., 1978, Metal ion effects in microbial screening systems, *Mutat. Res.* **53**:90–91.

Trepel, F., 1976, Das lymphatische Zellsystem: Struktur, allgemeine Physiologie und allgemeine Pathophysiologie, in *Blut und Blutkrarkheiten, Teil 3, Leuköcytores und retikulöres System* (edited by H. Begemann), Springer-Verlag, Berlin, pp. 1–191.

Tsuda, H., and Kato, K., 1976, Potassium dichromate-induced chromosome aberrations and its control with sodium sulfite in hamster embryonic cells, *Gann* **67**:469–470.

Tsuda, H., and Kato, K., 1977, Chromosomal aberrations and morphological transformation in hamster embryonic cells treated with potassium dichromate *in vitro*, *Mutat. Res.* **46**:87–94.

Umeda, M., and Nishimura, M., 1979, Inducibility of chromosomal aberrations by metal compounds in cultured mammalian cells, *Mutat. Res.* **67**:221–229.

Umeda, M., Saito, K., Hirose, K., and Saito, M., 1969, Cytotoxic effect of inorganic, phenyl and alkyl mercuric compounds on Hela cells, *Jpn. J. Exp. Med.* **39**:47–58.

Van Esch, G. J., and Kroes, R., 1969, The induction of renal tumours by feeding basic lead acetate to mice and hamsters, *Br. J. Cancer* **232**:765–771.

Varma, M. M., Josshi, S. R., and Adeyemi, A. O., 1974, Mutagenicity and infertility following administration of lead subacetate to Swiss male mice, *Experientia* 30:486–487.

Vasudev, V., Krishnamurthy, N., 1979, Dominant lethals induced by cadmium chloride in *Drosophila melanogaster*, *Curr. Sci.* 48:1007–1008.

Venitt, S., and Levy, L. S., 1974, Mutagenicity of chromates in bacteria and its relevance to chromate carcinogenesis, *Nature (London)* 250:493–495.

Venugopal, B., and Luckey, T. D., 1978, *Metal toxicity in mammals 2. Chemical toxicity of metals and metalloids*, Plenum Press, New York.

Verschaeve, L., and Susanne, C., 1978, Genetic hazard of mercury exposure in the dental surgery, Eighth Ann. Meet. Europ. Environ. Mutag. Soc., Dublin, July 1–13, Book of Abstracts p. 93.

Verschaeve, L., Kirsch-Volders, M., Susanne, C., Groettenbriel, C., Haustermans, R., Lecomte, A., and Roossels, D., 1976, Genetic damage induced by occupationally low mercury exposure, *Environ. Res.* 12:306–316.

Verschaeve, L., Kirsch-Volders, M., Hens, L., and Susanne, C., 1978, Chromosome distribution studies in phenylmercury acetate exposed subjects and in age-related controls, *Mutat. Res.* 57:335–347.

Verschaeve, L., Tassignon, J. P., Lefebvre, M., De Stoop, P., and Susanne, C., 1979, Cytogenetic investigation on leucocytes of workers exposed to metallic mercury, *Environ, Mutagen.* 1:259–268.

Vilkina, G., Pomerantzeva, M., and Ramoya, L., 1978, Lack of mutagenic effect of cadmium and zinc salts in somatic and germ mouse cells, *Genetika (Moscow)* 14:2212–2214.

Visek, W. J., Whitney, I. B., Kuhn, U. S. G., and Comar, C. L., 1953, Metabolism of $Cr^{51}$ by animals as influenced by chemical state, *Proc. Soc. Exp. Biol. Med.* 84:610–614.

Van Rosen, G., 1953, Radiomimetic activity and the periodical system of elements, *Bot. Notis.* 140–141.

Van Rosen, G., 1954a, Breaking of chromosomes by the action of elements of the periodical system and some other principles, *Hereditas* 40:258–263.

Van Rosen, G., 1954b, Radiomimetic reactivity arising after treatment employing elements of the periodical system, *Socker* 8:157–273.

Voroshilin, S., Plotko, E., Fink, T., and Nikriforova, V., 1978, Cytogenic effect of inorganic and acetate compounds of tungsten, zinc, cadmium, and cobalt on animal and human somatic cells, *Tsitol. Genet.* 12:241–243.

Vorwald, A. J., Reeves, A. L., and Urban, E. J. C., 1966, Experimental beryllium toxicology, in *Beryllium: Its industrial Hygiene Aspects*, (edited by H. E. Stockinger) Academic Press, New York, pp. 201–234.

Wagoner, J., Infante, P., and Bayliss, D., 1980, Beryllium: An ethiologic agent in the induction of lung cancers, nonneoplastic respiratory disease and heart disease among industrially exposed workers, *Environ. Res.* 21:15–34.

Wahlstrom, R. C., and Olson, O. E., 1959, The effect of selenium on reproduction in swine, *J. Anim. Sci.* 18:141–145.

Waksvik, H., Boyseen, M., Broegger, A., Saxholm, H., and Reith, A., 1980, *In vivo* and *in vitro* studies of mutagenicity and carcinogenicity of nickel compounds in man, Tenth Ann. Meeting Eur. Environ. Mutagen Soc., Athens, Poster 32.

Walker, G. W. R., and Bradley, A. M., 1969, Interacting effects of sodium monohydroarsenate and selenocystin on crossing over in *Drosophila melanogaster*, *Can. J. Genet. Cytol.* 11:677–688.

Wannag, A., 1976, The importance of organ blood mercury when comparing foetal and maternal rat organ distribution of mercury after methylmercury exposure, *Acta Pharmacol. Toxicol.* 38:289–298.

Wannag, A., and Skjaerasen, A., 1975, Mercury in the placenta and foetal membranes as an indication of low mercury exposure, in Proc. Int. Symp. "Recent Advances in the

Assessment of the Health Effects of Environmental Pollution", Paris, June 1974, Commission of the European Community, Luxembourg, Vol. 3, pp. 1233–1238.

Ware, R. A., Chang, L. W., and Burkholder, P. M., 1974, Ultrastructural evidence for fetal liver injury induced by *in utero* exposure to small doses of methylmercury, *Nature (London)* **251**:236–237.

Webb, J. L., 1966, Enzyme and metabolic inhibitors, Academic Press, New York.

Weiss, B., and Doherty, R. A., 1975, Methylmercury poisoning, *Teratology* **12**:311–313.

Weller, V. C., 1975, The blastophoric effects of chronic lead poisoning, *J. Med. Res.* **33**:271–293.

Westfall, B. B., Stohlman, E. F., and Smith, M. I., 1938, The placental transmission of selenium, *J. Pharmacol. Exp. Ther.* **64**:55–57.

WHO, 1976, Environmental health criteria 1. Mercury, World Health Organization, Geneva.

WHO, 1977, Lead, Environmental Health Criteria, World Health Organization, Geneva.

Wide, M., and Nilsson, O., 1977, Differential susceptibility of the embryo to inorganic lead during implantation in the mouse, *Teratology* **16**:273–276.

Wild, D., 1978, Cytogenetic effects in the mouse of 17 chemical mutagens and carcinogens evaluated by the micronucleus test, *Mutat. Res.* **56**:319–327.

Wu, S. H., Oldfield, J. E., and Whanger, P. D., 1971, Effect of selenium, chromium and vitamin E on spermatogenesis, *J. Anim. Sci.* **33**:273.

Wulf, H. C., 1980, Sister chromatid exchanges in human lymphocytes exposed to nickel and lead, *Dan. Med. Bull.* **27**:40–42.

Wyrobek, A. J., and Bruce, W. R., 1978, The induction of sperm cell abnormalities in mice and humans, in *Chemical Mutagens, Principles and Methods for their Detection*, (edited by A. Hollaender) Plenum, New York, Vol. 5, pp. 257–285.

Yamaguchi, S., and Nunotani, H., 1974, Transplacental transport of mercurials in rats at the subclinical dose levels, *Environ. Physiol. Biochem.* **4**:7–15.

Yang, M. G., Krawford, K. S., Garcia, J. D., Wang, J. H. C., and Lei, K. Y., 1972, Deposition of mercury in fetal and maternal brain, *Proc. Soc. Exp. Biol. Med.* **141**:1004–1007.

Yang, M. G., Wang, J. H. C., Garcia, J. D., Post, E. P., and Lei, K. Y., 1973, Mammary transfer of [203]Hg from mother to brains of nursing rats, *Proc. Soc. Exp. Biol. Med.* **142**:723–727.

Yoshikawa, T., Utsumi, J., Okada, T., Moriuchi, M. M., Ozawa, K., and Kaneko, Y., 1960, Concerning the mass outbreak of chronic arsenic toxicosis in Niigata prefecture, *Chiryo* **42**:1739–1749.

Zachariae, H., 1972, Arsenik og cancerrisiko, Ugeskr. Laeg. **134**:2720–2721.

Zanzoni, F., and Jung, E. G., 1980, Arsenic elevates the sister chromatid exchange (SCE) rate in human lymphocytes *in vitro*, *Arch. Dermatol. Res.* **267**:91–95.

Zasukhina, G., and Sinelschikova, T., 1976, Mechanism of the action of certain mutagens on the DNA of human cells, *Dokl. Acad. Nauk SSSR* **230**:719–721.

Zasukhina, G., Shalunova, N., Shvetsova, T., and Lomanova, G., 1975, Increase of virus mutagenic potential in presence of cadmium salts, *Dokl. Acad. Nauk SSSR* **224**:1189–1191.

Zasukhina, G., Sinelschikova, T., Lvova, G., and Kirkova, Z., 1977, Moleculargenetic effects of cadmium chloride, *Mutat. Res.* **454**:169–174.

Zawirska, B., and Medras, K., 1972, Role of the kidneys in disorders of peripheric metabolism of porphyrin during carcinogenesis induced with lead acetate, *Arch. Immunol. Ther. Exp.* (Warsz) **20**:257–272.

Zollinger, W. X., 1953, Kidney adenomas and carcinomas in rats caused by chronic lead poisoning and their relationship to corresponding human neoplasms, *Virchows Arch. Pathol. Anat. Physiol.* **323**:694–710.

# Mutagenicity, Carcinogenicity, and Teratogenicity of Insecticides

## J. and M. Moutschen-Dahmen and N. Degraeve

## 1. INTRODUCTION

The origin of insecticides is rooted in antiquity. Plinius the Elder recommended arsenic to kill insects as early as 70 A.D. Arsenic sulfide is reported to have been used by the Chinese in the 16th century, and salts of various metals were utilized as insecticides in the 19th century.

The use of natural substances extracted from plants also became widespread centuries ago. Pyrethrum is said to have been introduced in Europe from the far east by Marco Polo. Root extracts of Derris, which gave rise to the modern insecticide rotenone, were first used for killing insects in 1848, almost at the same time as tobacco extracts were used. We should also mention that, during the last decades of the 19th century, the introduction of hydrogen cyanide and dinitrophenol as insecticides and, in the beginning of the 20th century, of methylbromide, naphthalene and paradichlorobenzene took place.

Just before World War II, the shortage of so-called natural insecticides, principally nicotine and pyrethrin, forced several countries to synthesize replacement substances. This substitution was the origin of chlorinated insecticides. Historically speaking, the chlorinated compound hexachlorocyclohexane, the commercial formulation of which is Lindane or Gammexan, was the first synthesized organochlorine (as early as 1825). However, its insecticidal properties were not recognized before 1935, and it was produced industrially at the same time as other chlorinated compounds.

The insecticidal properties of DDT were first mentioned in 1939 by

**J. and M. Moutschen-Dahmen and N. Degraeve** • University of Liège, Genetics Department, 15 rue Forgeur, B-4000 Liège, Belgium.

Müller, who was looking for a substance which could combine liposolubility and toxic properties. The substance called Eulan BL, known as a stomach poison for insects and used as acaricide, served as the framework for a series of syntheses which led to the contact poison DDT. In 1943 its industrial production started, and it was released on several markets by 1944. The success obtained with DDT stimulated several researchers to synthesize new chlorinated derivatives. Thus, Methoxychlor and DDD, two DDT analogues, were produced in 1946.

Compounds which are chemically more readily dehydrochlorinated have a much higher insecticidal activity than DDT. This observation led to the discovery of new insecticides, among which were the wide class of cyclodienes synthesized from completely different frameworks than that of DDT.

Scientists were rewarded by pursuing the somewhat naive idea that chemical dehydrochlorination liberates hydrogen chloride, which is toxic at the site of action, into the tissues of insects. In fact, from 1940 to 1950, within no more than a decade, almost all the chlorinated insecticides used to date had been synthesized.

The history of organophosphorus insecticides is somewhat different. The incidental discovery of this group of compounds arose from the desire to find nerve poisons with military potential. Thus was the situation which led, at the beginning of World War II, to the synthesis of the so-called G gases, which were organophosphorus derivatives with high anticholinesterase properties. As by-products of this search for anticholinesterase molecules, three organophosphorus insecticides, TEPP, Schradan, and Parathion, were synthesized; the latter is still used. They were, along with other insecticides, produced commercially after the war.

The history of carbamate insecticides can be traced back to the Calabar bean, a seed from the legume *Physostigma venenosum*, a tree known to have been used in West Africa for a long period of time. In the middle of the 19th century, the Calabar bean was sent to Scotland, and some European laboratories succeeded in extracting from it two powerful alkaloids: Eserine and Physostigmine, which are still used today in medicine. The formulas of these two alkaloids were established in the first part of this century, and their toxic properties thoroughly investigated. The medical importance of these drugs incited chemists to synthesize new molecules, all characterized by the presence of the carbamate moiety. In fact, the discovery of the anticholinesterase activity of these drugs suggested toxicity for insects. They did not, however, show any insecticidal properties, due to the presence of a quaternary amino group in the molecule which prevented their penetration of the insect cuticle. It was therefore necessary to synthesize unchanged lipid-soluble molecules on the model of Physostigmine.

One had to wait until 1940 for Dimetan, the first carbamate that exhibited insecticidal properties against the house fly. In 1953, a new carbamate was synthesized which appeared to be one of the most promising insecticides; it was first called Sevin, then Carbaryl. The synthesis of this compound was published in the literature in 1957, and it was then released on the market. Thus, for every group of insecticides, a long period of time generally elapses between the discovery of the synthesis procedure, the recognition of insecticidal activity, the investigation of toxic properties, and the clearance for marketing.

Among the thousands of methylcarbamates synthesized during the last two decades, only a dozen could be released on the market as commercial insecticides. After the discovery, between 1940 and 1950, of the great classes of synthetic insecticides, commercial production increased.

In the United States, the production of DDT increased after 1960 to a peak in 1964 (of 200,000 to 250,000 tons). One quarter to one fifth of this production was used to control human disease vectors, especially malaria eradication. In 1966, DDT, Aldrin, and Toxaphene represented more than half of the production of insecticides in the U.S.A., i.e., between 50–75% of the world's production. A slight decrease between 1964 and 1966 was compensated for by an increase in the production of organophosphorus insecticides. In 1969, some American states restricted the use of DDT and its analogues. They were banned in 1972, along with 15 other pesticides that were formulated into hundreds of products. The decision arose from the long persistence of chlorinated insecticides in the environment (see below), the possibility of adverse long-term effects, and the increasing resistance of insects to pesticides. Today 400 species of insects and mites are resistant to pesticides, more than twice as many as in 1965. In several countries, however, the production of the main classes of insecticides remains high, as in Belgium (see Table I).

The environmental hazards created by insecticides differ very much from one class to another. Organophosphorus insecticides, being readily degraded or metabolized, do not persist for a long time in the environment except occasionally, as cyclic side chains. However, the risk of acute accidents in manufacturing plants or injury to agricultural workers, as revealed by occupational studies, is higher than with other classes of insecticides. It should also be recalled that one compound (Trichlorfon or Metrifonate) is not only used as an insecticide, but also as a pharmaceutical drug in the treatment of *Schistosomiasis*, at doses far higher than those which stem from exposure to insecticides.

Chlorinated insecticide residues, on the other hand, are most persistent. They can be found on pulverized foods, e.g., fruits and vegetables. In fruits they have an affinity for peels, so that peeling followed by boiling removes

Table I
Production of Insecticides Sold in Belgium
During the Years 1979–1980
(expressed as kg of active compound)[a]

| Type of insecticide | Year | |
|---|---|---|
| | 1979 | 1980 |
| Chlorinated | 112, 141 | 139, 509 |
| Organophosphorus | 166, 418 | 173, 225 |
| Carbamates | 124, 522 | 118, 849 |
| Pyrethroids | 40 | 1262 |
| From plant origin other than pyrethroids | 604 | 369 |
| Synergistic (piperonyl butoxide) | 985 | 948 |

[a]Data from the Ministère de l'Agriculture (Belgium).

almost all organochlorine residues. The problem of dairy milk is more important. Chlorinated insecticides can accumulate in fat, especially via the waste products incorporated in animal food. Chlorinated insecticides were detected in human adipose tissues: Dieldrin was found to be 0.2 ppm in the United Kingdom and 0.2–0.3 ppm in the U.S.A.; DDT was up to 3 ppm in the United Kingdom and northern Europe, and 6–12 ppm in southern and eastern Europe. Chlorinated insecticides are said to concentrate in the trophic chain. They can be detected in an aquatic environment, but at seemingly the same concentration as in other environments. Due to the great variety of organisms and environments involved, it is presently very difficult to generalize on the behavior of chlorinated insecticides.

Birds, especially predators, can accumulate chlorinated insecticides more readily than mammals, even leading to death (5 to 10% of predators). DDT has been found in eggs (6 ppm in heron eggs).

Carbamates can enter the animal body fluid when applied directly to animals for insect control, or indirectly after eating contaminated foods. In the latter case, the degradation products should be accounted for. However, feeding cows with a contaminated food containing 50–450 ppm Carbaryl for two weeks did not result in detectable amounts in their milk or in modification of the organoleptic properties. In meat, residues can be found but do not persist for a long time. After spraying chickens abundantly, 1 ppm could be detected in muscle and 2 ppm in fat. Carbaryl only appeared in eggs after high oral doses.

Since Carbamates are not used as soil insecticides, there are few works published, on this subject, but there is reason to believe that they are rapidly decomposed, being well metabolized by microorganisms. The introduction of carbamates to water is only incidental. As to their presence in air, a few experimental data are available. Dissipation curves of the residues have been carefully investigated, especially in fruits and vegetables.

According to these observations, it does not seem that carbamate insecticides accumulate in the trophic chain. However, it should be determined whether some metabolic products could create risks under certain conditions. A comprehensive review of the persistence of pesticides in the environment has recently been done by Edwards (1973).

## 2. CHEMICAL AND BIOCHEMICAL PROPERTIES

### 2.1. Chlorinated Insecticides

#### 2.1.1. Chemical Properties

The chlorinated cyclic hydrocarbons that are used for their high insecticidal properties belong to different classes of molecules.

First are the diphenyl derivatives, the best known of which is DDT. One analogue, DDD, which is a metabolite of DDT, has insecticidal properties of its own. Commercial DDTs are generally mixtures of similar compounds, one of which is DDD. Such molecules are resistant to light and oxidation. This exceptional stability accounts for the difficulty of removing residues from soil, water, and foodstuffs.

Another widely used, commercially prepared compound is Methoxychlor, an analogue of DDT. Still another class of cyclic chlorinated compounds is that of cyclodienes, which have a chlorine-substituted endomethylene bridge. These are of four types:

1. Aldrin (or its isomer Isodrin) and its oxidation product Dieldrin (or its isomer Endrin);
2. Telodrin;
3. Chlordane, Heptachlor, or its oxidation product heptachlor-epoxide;
4. Endosulfan, which contains a sulfur atom in the cycle.

Kepone and Mirex are chlorinated derivatives from cyclobutapentalene. Lindane (gammexane or BHC) is a mixture of eight well described stereoisomers, the gamma stereoisomer being the effective insecticide. Paradichlorobenzene has chemical properties similar to those of Lindane. The last of these chlorinated compounds is the camphene named Toxaphene. These compounds are almost insoluble in water, but highly soluble in fats, which explains their accumulation in fat deposits.

Commercial products are generally mixtures of several compounds. They are also frequently mixed with insecticides of other groups, e.g., carbamates or organophosphates in a great variety of solvents, which sometimes makes it difficult to assess the risks for man.

The formulas of the compounds mentioned above are listed in Table II. These compounds have been investigated for their mutagenic, carcinogenic, or teratogenic properties.

## 2.1.2. Biochemical Properties

All vertebrates have evolved protective mechanisms against the toxic action of organochlorine insecticides.

Injected organochlorine compounds are almost entirely absorbed from the gastrointestinal tract and transported to the liver through the portal vein, before being spread among other organs. Fecal excretion seems to be predominant. These compounds can, however, persist for a long time in fluids and tissues before being eliminated.

In mammals, DDT biotransformations involve two separate reductive dehydrochlorination pathways. The metabolite of DDT, DDE [(bis-para-chlorophenyl) 2,2-dichloro-1, 1-ethylene)] is the major storage product found in fats, especially in the liver, along with nonmetabolized molecules. This metabolite is as toxic as DDT for mammals, but loses its insecticidal property, which explains the resistance of various insects to DDE. In a further step, DDE is transformed into DDA (para-dichlorodiphenyl-acetic acid), which is principally excreted as a labile glucuronide conjugate.

In general, cyclodienes are first transformed into stable epoxides by a liver enzymatic system equivalent to the mono-oxygenase of the microsomal fraction which requires $NADPH_2$ and $O_2$. Epoxide derivatives stored in the adipose tissues may then undergo further metabolic transformations involving hydroxylation, dechlorination, oxidation, and conjugation, and are eventually converted into hydrophilic compounds excreted mainly by the fecal route.

In this respect, Aldrin and Heptachlor are initially epoxidized respectively into Dieldrin and Heptachlor epoxide, which are stored as such in fat deposits. They may undergo further transformations in mammals, e.g., dechlorination, hydroxilation, oxidation, or conjugation. The hydrophylic metabolic products are excreted via the fecal route. Toxaphene is partly dechlorinized, giving rise to free chloride for excretion. The metabolites of Toxaphene are water-soluble, and for this reason, this insecticide does not accumulate as much in adipose tissues. For Lindane, dehalogenation followed by a thiol conjugation (with Glutathion) is predominant. Because this insecticide is a mixture of several isomers, the metabolic pathways strongly depend on the composition of the mixture. Some isomers can be degraded not only by the liver microsomes, but also by cytosol and even mitochondria. This degradation can also occur in extrahepatic tissues. For paradichlorobenzene, monohydroxylation is the main metabolic route.

## Table II

| a. - Chlorinated insecticides of the DDT group | b. - Insecticides of the Diene-organochlorine group |
|---|---|

a. - Chlorinated insecticides of the DDT group

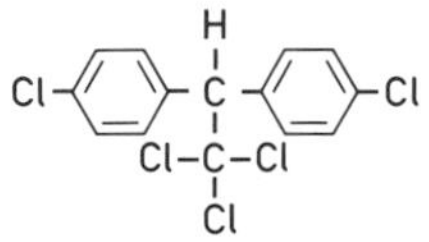

DDT

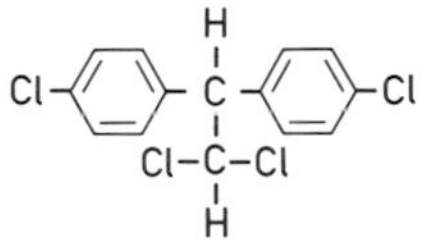

DDD

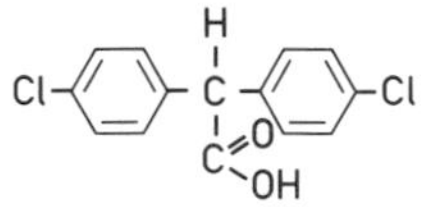

DDA

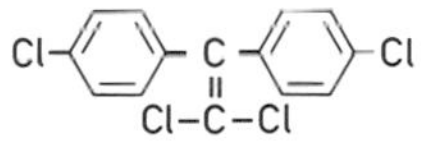

DDE

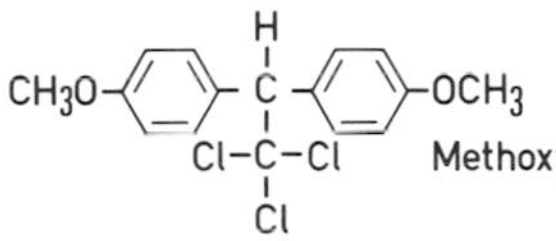

Methoxychlor

c. - Gamma-1,2,3,4,5,6-hexachlorocyclohexane

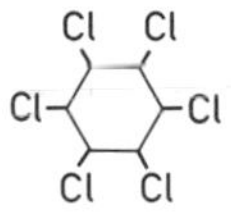

Lindane

d. - Polychloroterpene

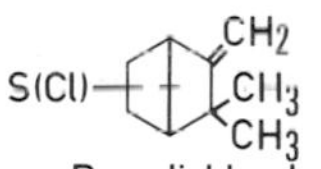

Toxaphene

e. - Paradichlorobenzene

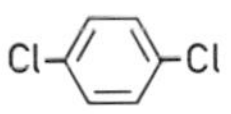

b. - Insecticides of the Diene-organochlorine group

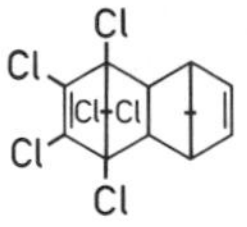

Aldrin

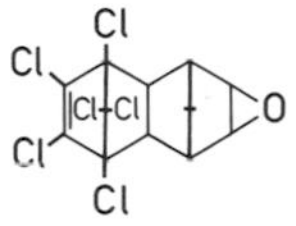

Dieldrin
Endrin

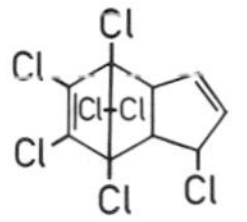

Heptachlor

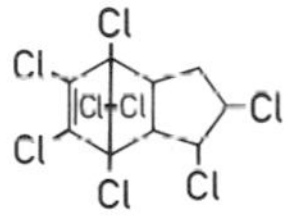

Chlordane

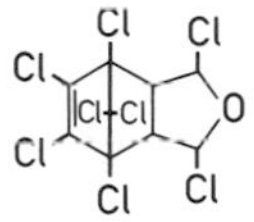

Isobenzan
(Telodrin®)

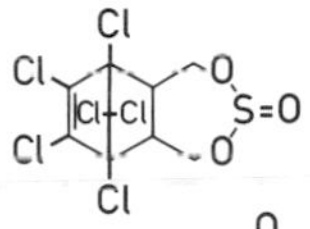

Endosulfan

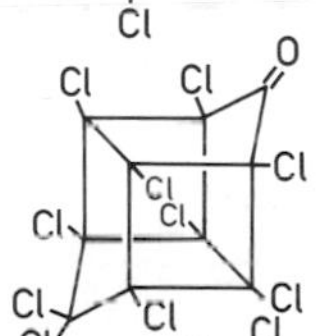

Chlordecone

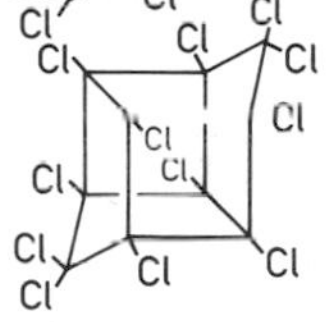

Mirex

All metabolic pathways of chlorinated insecticides have been recently reviewed in detail (Brooks, 1974). Chlorinated insecticides are large spectrum insecticides. They easily cross the chitinous framework of sensitive insects, and paralyze principally the peripheral nerves. The mechanism of action at the molecular level is far from understood, and is probably not exactly the same for each class of chlorinated compound. Chlorinated compounds are known to act by a mechanism quite different from a simple enzyme inhibition, as is the case for organophosphates and carbamates. DDT and analogues, whose mechanism of action was well investigated, have insecticidal properties that depend on two chlorobenzenes. The reaction with the receptor site is governed by steric effects. Holan (1969) suggested that DDT and its analogues may interact with the molecular layers of a unit membrane, mainly of the sensory nerves, so that the aromatic rings form a complex with the outer protein layer. The capacity of several insect species to dehydrochlorinate DDT to DDE, which developed in some house fly strains and is under genetic control, partly explains their DDT resistance. (For a review, see Brown, 1969).

## 2.2. Organophosphorus Insecticides

### 2.2.1. Chemical Properties

Under this name are several compounds, the general structure of which is:

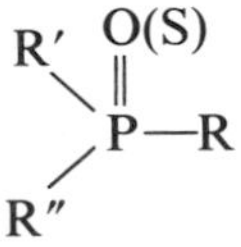

$$\begin{array}{c} R' \\ \diagdown \\ \diagup \\ R'' \end{array} \overset{O(S)}{\underset{\|}{P}}-R$$

Most of these compounds are derived from phosphoric acid, but a few are derived from phosphonic acid (e.g., Trichlorfon). In the structure above, O is replaced by S in the group of thiophosphates. The R' and R'' radicals are generally alkyl groups (especially methyl or ethyl), but can also be alkoxy, phenoxy amino, or substituted amino groups. The R group comprises a large variety of radicals, some aliphatic, some cyclic, all with a labile P—R bond.

The preferential attack at the phosphorus atom followed by the cleavage of the P—O bond leads to *phosphorylation*, whereas the preferential attack at the carbon atom (in radicals R' and R'') leads to *alkylation*. In some cases, the attack occurs at the electrophilic sites.

Hydrolysis of organophosphorus insecticides occurs in water, which leads to diesters of phosphoric acid, alcohols, thiols, and phenols. Further hydrolysis to monoester and eventually to phosphate can also occur. These properties help to explain the relative lack of persistence of organophosphates in the environment, as compared to organochlorine insecticides.

Due to their great biological importance, the alkylating properties of organophosphorus insecticides have been extensively investigated by the Preussman's reaction with 4-(4-nitrobenzyl) pyridine. However, by this method, firm conclusions on the extent of the reaction with DNA *in vivo* can scarcely be drawn. The alkylation of DNA *in vitro* was mostly investigated with Dichlorvos (see Section 3.2). Principal formulas investigated for alterogenic properties are summarized in Table III.

## Table III

**A. - PHOSPHATES AND RELATED COMPOUNDS.**

$(CH_3O)_2 \overset{O}{\underset{\|}{P}}\_OCH=CCl_2$ — Dichlorvos

$(C_2H_5O)_2 \overset{O}{\underset{\|}{P}}\_O\_C$ ... Cl — Chlorfenvinphos

$(CH_3O)_2 \overset{O}{\underset{\|}{P}}\_O\_C$ ... Cl — Tetrachlorvinphos

$(CH_3O)_2 \overset{O}{\underset{\|}{P}}\_O\_C=\overset{H}{C}\_\overset{O}{\underset{\|}{C}}\_O\_CH$ ... Crotoxyphos
with $CH_3$ and $CH_3$

$(CH_3O)_2 \overset{O}{\underset{\|}{P}}\_O\_\overset{CH_3}{C}=\overset{H}{C}\_\overset{O}{\underset{\|}{C}}\_O\_CH_3$ — Mevinphos

$(CH_3O)_2 \overset{O}{\underset{\|}{P}}\_O\_C=\overset{Cl}{C}\_\overset{O}{\underset{\|}{C}}\_N\overset{C_2H_5}{\underset{C_2H_5}{}}$ — Phosphamidon
with $CH_3$

$(CH_3O)_2 \overset{O}{\underset{\|}{P}}\_O\_C=\overset{H}{C}\_\overset{O}{\underset{\|}{C}}\_NHCH_3$ — Monocrotophos
with $CH_3$

$(CH_3O)_2 \overset{O}{\underset{\|}{P}}\_O\_C=\overset{H}{C}\_\overset{O}{\underset{\|}{C}}\_N\overset{CH_3}{\underset{CH_3}{}}$ — Dicrotophos
with $CH_3$

**C. - PHOSPHOROTHIOLOTHIONATES.**

$(CH_3O)_2 \overset{S}{\underset{\|}{P}}\_S\_CH\_\overset{O}{\underset{\|}{C}}\_OC_2H_5$ — Malathion
$CH_2\_C\_OC_2H_5$ with O

$(C_2H_5O)_2 \overset{S}{\underset{\|}{P}}\_S\_CH_2\_S\_\overset{S}{\underset{\|}{P}}(OC_2H_5)_2$ — Ethion

$(CH_3O)_2 \overset{S}{\underset{\|}{P}}\_S\_CH_2\_N$ ... — Phosmet

$(RO)_2 \overset{S}{\underset{\|}{P}}\_S\_CH_2\_N$ ... — $R=CH_3$ Azinphos-methyl, $R=C_2H_5$ Azinphos-ethyl

$(CH_3O)_2 \overset{S}{\underset{\|}{P}}\_S\_CH_2\_N$ ... $N=C\_OCH_3$ — Methidathion

$(CH_3O)_2 \overset{S}{\underset{\|}{P}}\_S\_CH_2\_\overset{O}{\underset{\|}{C}}\_NHCH_3$ — Dimethoate

$(CH_3O)_2 \overset{S}{\underset{\|}{P}}\_S\_CH_2\_CH_2\_NH\overset{O}{\underset{\|}{C}}\_CH_3$ — Amiphos

$(CH_3O)_2 \overset{S}{\underset{\|}{P}}\_S\_CH_2\_\overset{O}{\underset{\|}{C}}\_N\overset{CH_3}{\underset{CHO}{}}$ — Formothion

**B. - PHOSPHOROTHIONATES.**

$(RO)_2 \overset{S}{\underset{\|}{P}}\_O$ ... $NO_2$ — $R=CH_3$ Parathion-methyl, $R=C_2H_5$ Parathion-ethyl

$(CH_3O)_2 \overset{S}{\underset{\|}{P}}\_O$ ... $NO_2$ with $CH_3$ — Fenitrothion

$(RO)_2 \overset{S}{\underset{\|}{P}}\_O$ ... Cl, Br, Cl — $R=CH_3$ Bromophos-methyl, $R=C_2H_5$ Bromophos-ethyl

$(CH_3O)_2 \overset{S}{\underset{\|}{P}}\_O$ ... Cl, I — Iodofenphos

$(CH_3O)_2 \overset{S}{\underset{\|}{P}}\_O$ ... $SCH_3$ with $CH_3$ — Fenthion

$(CH_3O)_2 \overset{S}{\underset{\|}{P}}\_O$ ... CN — Cyanophos

$(CH_3O)_2 \overset{S}{\underset{\|}{P}}\_O$ ... $S$ ... $O\_\overset{S}{\underset{\|}{P}}(OCH_3)_2$ — Abate

$(RO)_2 \overset{S}{\underset{\|}{P}}\_O$ ... $N(CH_3)_2$ with $CH_3$ — $R=CH_3$ Pirimiphos-methyl, $R=C_2H_5$ Pirimiphos-ethyl

$(C_2H_5O)_2 \overset{S}{\underset{\|}{P}}\_O$ ... $CH(CH_3)_2$ with $CH_3$ — Diazinon

$(C_2H_5O)_2 \overset{S}{\underset{\|}{P}}\_O$ ... Cl, Cl, Cl — Chlorpyrifos

**D. - PHOSPHOROTHIOLATES.**

$(C_2H_5O)_2 \overset{O}{\underset{\|}{P}}\_S\_CH_2$ ... — Kitazin

$(CH_3O)_2 \overset{O}{\underset{\|}{P}}\_S\_CH_2\_CH_2\_S\_\overset{CH_3}{CH}\_\overset{O}{\underset{\|}{C}}NHCH_3$ — Vamidothion

$(CH_3O)_2 \overset{O}{\underset{\|}{P}}\_S\_CH_2\_CH_2\_\overset{O}{\underset{\|}{S}}\_C_2H_5$ — Oxydemeton-methyl

**E. - PHOSPHORAMIDATE.**

$\overset{CH_3O}{\underset{CH_3NH}{}}>\overset{O}{\underset{\|}{P}}\_O$ ... $C(CH_3)_3$ with Cl — Crufomate(Ruelene)

**F. - PHOSPHONATE.**

$(CH_3O)_2 \overset{O}{\underset{\|}{P}}\_CH\_CCl_3$ with OH — Trichlorfon

## 2.2.2. Biochemical Properties

The insecticidal properties of organophosphates depend on the presence of the organic phosphate radical (Section 2.2.1), through which they can inactivate cholinesterases by phosphorylation and extend their main toxic effects to sensitive organisms.

The reaction with the enzyme occurs by the covalent attachment of the inhibitor through the electrophilic P atom to the esteratic site of the enzyme's active center, which is apparently a serine hydroxyl group. In spite of their wide structural diversity, organophosphate compounds react with a great uniformity.

A large proportion of organophosphates require metabolic trans-formations *in vivo* to inhibit cholinesterases. This is the case with thiophosphates, which are first oxidated to phosphates, leading to enhancement of the phosphorylating capacity. This activation is effected by the microsomal mixed-function oxidase. Dehalogenation is also considered a process of activation rather than detoxication.

There are a great variety of detoxicating reactions in animals, depending of the nature of R, R' and R" (Section 2.2.1). Among the most important of these reactions are the hydrolysis of carboxyester or carboxy amide groups, hydrolysis of the phosphoric ester linkage, O-dealkylation, reduction of the nitro-group, dechlorination, and conjugation.

The rate of degradation of most organophosphates is generally rapid in mammalian tissues. For Dichlorvos, the half-life has been reported to be 13.5 min. in rat kidneys (Blair *et al.*, 1975). The insecticidal properties of organophosphorus insecticides are evidently linked to the inhibition of cholinesterases at the endings of the nerves. In insects, acetylcholine acts as transmitter in the synapses of the central nervous system, but not the peripheral nerves. Also, it has been shown that in the fly brain, acetyl-cholinesterase is somewhat different from the mammalian enzyme.

Strong organophosphates used as insect chemosterilants, e.g., Hempa, will not be considered in the present chapter, since they are not, strictly speaking, insecticides. They show obvious alterogenic properties even at low doses. Chemical and biochemical properties of organophosphates have been recently reviewed (Eto, 1974).

## 2.3. Carbamate Insecticides

### 2.3.1. Chemical Properties

The backbone of all carbamates is carbamic acid:

$$\underset{\text{HO}-\text{C}-\text{NH}_2}{\overset{\overset{\displaystyle O}{\parallel}}{}}$$

It does not exist freely, but can be stabilized by adding an alkyl group. The ethyl ester, well known as urethane, is carcinogenic for mammals.

The structure and properties of carbamate insecticides discussed in this chapter are quite different from urethane. The general formula is

$$R-O-\overset{\overset{\displaystyle O}{\|}}{C}-N\overset{\displaystyle R'}{\underset{\displaystyle R''}{<}}$$

in which R' and R" are usually methyl groups or hydrogen atoms. R comprises various radicals, among which are aromatic, heterocyclic, and pyrazolyl structures.

Carbaryl and Carbofuran are the most widely used carbamate insecticides. They are aryl carbamate esters, respectively prepared from 1-naphthol and 2.3-dihydro-2.2-dimethyl-7-hydroxybenzofuran. New insecticides of this class have recently been synthesized from enols and dimethylcarbamic acid, but so far Carbaryl is almost the only carbamate insecticide which has been tested for alterogenic properties.

Carbamates can be obtained as pure crystalline solids, which facilitate chemical and biological investigations. They are slightly soluble in water, but can be dissolved in a large variety of solvents. Most of them are susceptible to light, heat, and air oxidation, so they do not create many environmental hazards (Section 1). The formulas of specific carbamate insecticides are given in Table IV. The chemistry, biochemistry, and toxicology of carbamates have been recently reviewed (Kuhr and Dorough, 1976).

## 2.3.2. Biochemical Properties

Carbamate insecticides show a low toxicity for mammals. Metabolic processes operate at a high rate. The primary biotransformation is usually oxidative involving the mixed-function-oxidase system. For most methyl carbamates, aromatic hydroxylation is the major attack to which the molecule is submitted in both living animals and *in vitro* microsomal systems. The hydroxy-metabolites are excreted mainly as sulfate or $\beta$-glucuronide conjugates.

In mammals, Carbaryl is principally metabolized in the liver, leading to 1-naphthyl *N*-hydroxymethylcarbamate, 4-hydroxy-1-naphthyl *N*-methylcarbamate, and 5-hydroxyl-1-naphthyl *N*-methylcarbamate, and then conjugated with these hydroxylated molecules (mainly glucuronide conjugation).

The metabolic pathways seem to be the same in rat and human livers, but differ in insects where they are metabolized through non-hydrolitic pathways. Methyl carbamates are converted to water-soluble molecules, but keep intact

Table IV

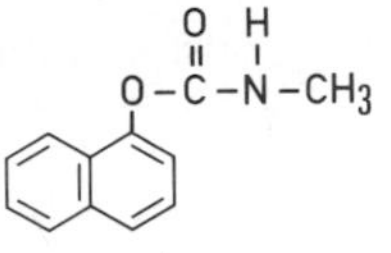

Carbaryl

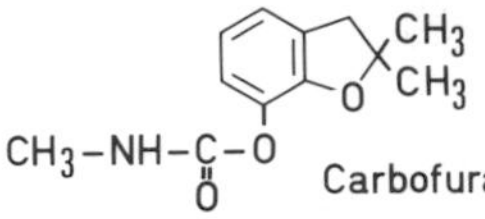

Carbofuran

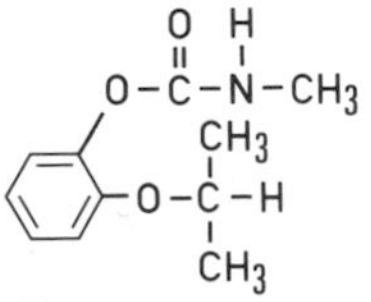

Propoxur

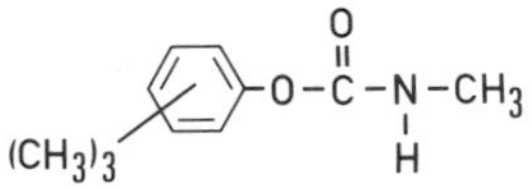

Landrin

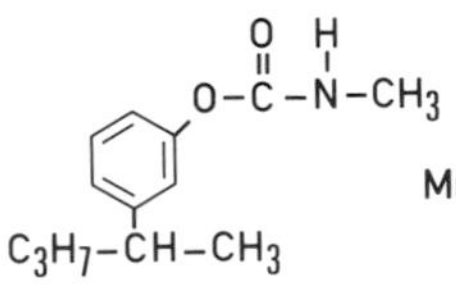

Mixture of

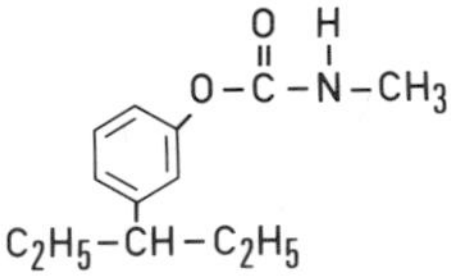

Bux-Ten®

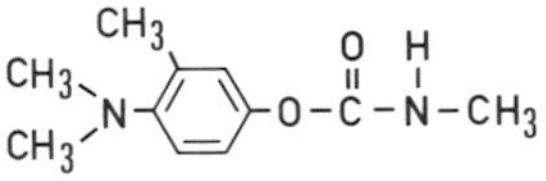

Aminocarb

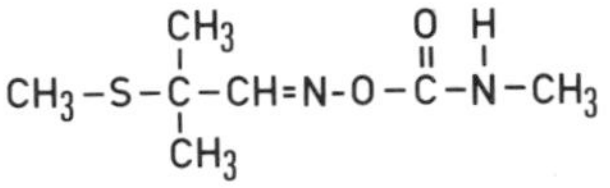

Aldicarb

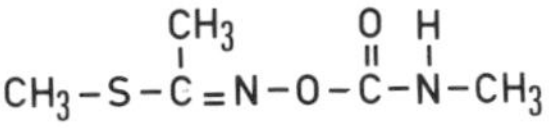

Methomyl

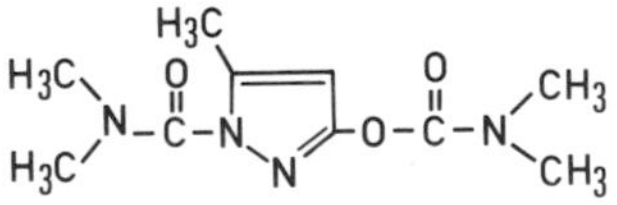

Dimetilan

the carbamate moiety. In resistant or more tolerant insect species, there is less absorption, more excretion, and a faster metabolism, generally due to a higher level of NADPH-dependent oxidative enzymes.

There is a great similarity between the mode of action of organophosphorus compounds and carbamates in all kinds of animals. The toxicity is due to the inhibition of acetylcholinesterase in the central nervous system, leading to paralysis. A difference from organophosphorus insecticides is that carbamates do not require metabolic conversion to exhibit toxic effects. Moreover, the inhibition can be reversible, and the active enzyme is sometimes quickly regenerated. The kinetics of inhibition were carefully

investigated, and involve carbamoylation of the enzyme (binding covalently
of the electrophilic carbamoyl groups) to esteratic sites of the enzymes.
Carbamates transfer an acidic group to this site yielding an acetylated enzyme
complex. In spite of this knowledge, the actual cause of death of treated
insects is not fully elucidated.

## 2.4. Miscellaneous Insecticides

### 2.4.1. Chemical Properties

Before World War II, lead arsenate was one of the leading insecticides
(for the toxicological hazards of this substance, see Chapter 2). It is still
occasionally used. Naphthalene has been in favor for a long time as an
insecticide. Like chlorinated compounds, it is almost insoluble in water, but
soluble in lipids and in several organic solvents.

Apart from the synthetic compounds, this class of insecticides includes
three types of naturally occurring molecules: nicotinoid-like, rotenoid-like,
and pyrethroid-like.

Nicotinoid-like compounds include nicotine, particularly the water
soluble type used in the U.S.A. as a 40% solution of nicotine sulfate called
Black Leaf 40. Solutions of the free base are also used as fumigants. As a
contact poison, nicotine is utilized more efficiently as a soap in the form of
naphthalenate, laurate, or oleate.

Rotenoid compounds, including rotenone, are practically insoluble in
water. They decompose upon exposure to light and air, and they oxidize in
organic solvents. They may eventually deposit crystals of dehydrorotenone
and rotenone, and both derivatives are highly toxic for insects.

Among the pyrethroid-like compounds, the natural products comprise
Pyrethrins I and II, which differ by a side chain. These substances are
insoluble in water and should be dissolved in solvents for spraying.

There are also a number of synthetic analogues, such as Allethrin,
Fenothrin, Furamethrin, Propathrin, Resmethrin, Permethrin, and Tetramethrin. Some of these have been tested for toxic properties. The formulas of
these substances are given in Table V. It should also be mentioned that the
compound piperonyl butoxide, which is not by itself an insecticide, is used for
synergistic effects with several classes of insecticides in aerosols or liquid-
soluble powders.

### 2.4.2. Biochemical Properties

In mammals, nicotine is extensively metabolized; minor quantities are
eliminated unchanged in urine. Other metabolites appear, e.g., cotinine,
hydroxycotinine, nicotynine, 3-pyridylacetic acid, and $\gamma$(3-pyridyl)
$\beta$-oxo-N-methylbutyramide.

## Table V

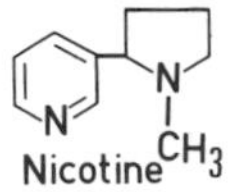

Nicotine

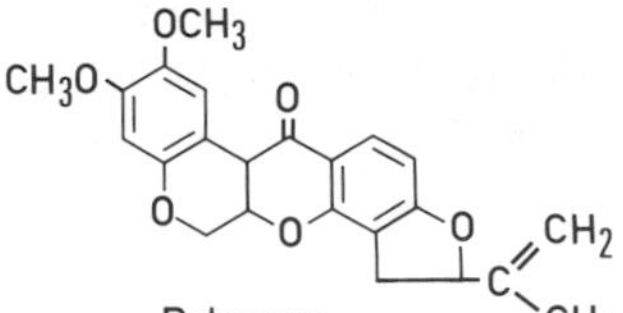

Rotenone

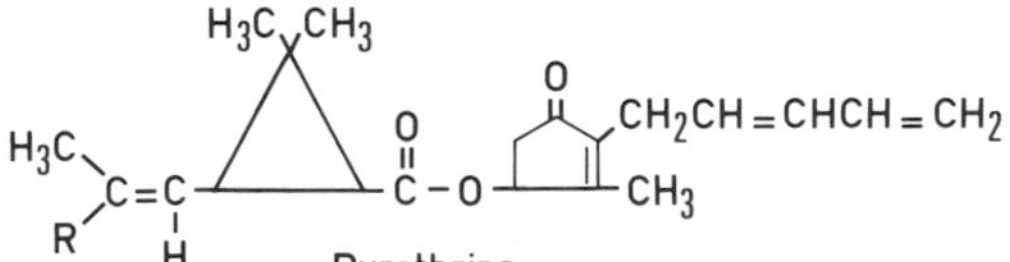

Pyrethrins

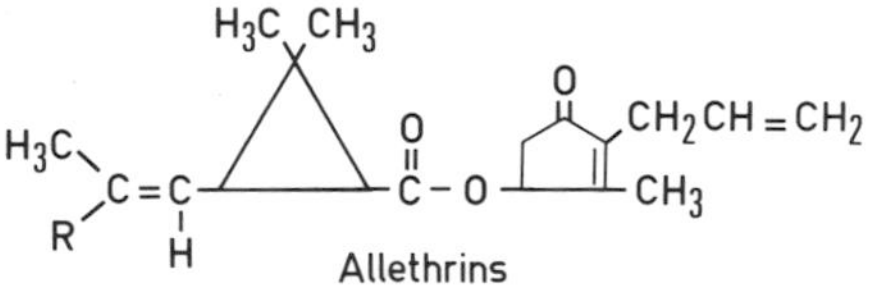

Allethrins

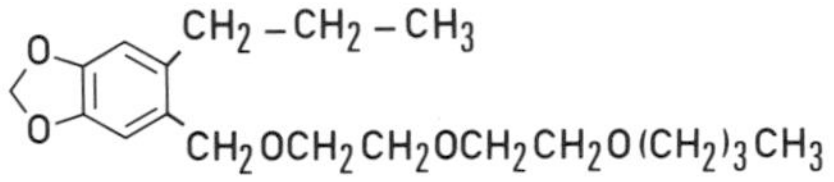

Piperonyl butoxide

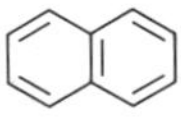

Naphthalin

There are three successive sequences of modifications of the molecule. First is hydroxylation, followed by scission and reclosure of the pyrrolidine ring, which yields cotinine. Further reaction consists in $N$-methylation of the pyridine ring, yielding methylnicotine. The last reaction is demethylation of $N$-pyrrolidine, synthesizing nornicotine, converted by oxidation into desmethylnicotine.

In insects, the cationized nitrogen of the pyrrolidine moiety of the nicotine binds to the anionic site of the postsynaptic membrane of the central nervous system of sensitive insects. No inhibiting action of cholinesterases could be demonstrated, however.

In mammals, rotenoid compounds are metabolized in the mixed-function oxidase system by hydroxylation, forming rotenolone at $C_7$, then at the terminal methyl group $C_{24}$, and then by epoxidation of the isopropenyl double bond. Rotenone epoxide is finally converted into the dihydroxy derivatives.

In insects, rotenoid compounds block the respiration of NADH-linked substrates of isolated mitochondria. It seems that the *prima facie* is the inhibition of glutamic dehydrogenase which results in an inhibition of the respiratory metabolism, first in the nerve and then in the muscle.

For pyrethroid compounds, the isobutenyl side chain is generally transformed into a carboxylic group sometimes involving successive oxidations in the liver mixed-function oxidase. There is low toxicity of these molecules for mammals due to the facility of hydrolytic attack by esterases.

In insects, pyrethroid compounds do not inhibit cholinesterases. They act by inducing a neurotoxin which is not a pyrethroid metabolite, and is then released in the hemolymph. The nature of this neurotoxin is not clear. An aromatic amine which contains an ester group has been suggested.

The mode of action of the three classes of substances has been reviewd by Yamamoto (1970). More specifically, synthetic pyrethroids have been investigated by Miyamoto (1976).

Naphthalene has several metabolic pathways. In mammals, it undergoes hydroxylation and mercapturic acid synthesis. However, hydroxylation is the main pathway, leading to mono- and dihydroxylated active metabolites.

## 3. MUTAGENICITY

### 3.1. Chlorinated Insecticides

The chlorinated insecticides can be classified into different groups according to their chemical structures.

### 3.1.1. DDT and Related Compounds

The mutagenicity of DDT was extensively studied in both prokaryotes and eukaryotes.

In bacteria, negative results were reported in *E. coli* (Ashwood-Smith *et al.*, 1972; Fahrig, 1974), *S. typhimurium* (Shirasu *et al.*, 1975; Marshall *et al.*, 1976; Bartsch *et al.*, 1980), *B. subtilis* (Shirasu *et al.*, 1976), and *S. marcescens* (Fahrig, 1974), as well as in host-mediated assays with *S. typhimurium* and *S. marcescens* as indicators (Buselmaier *et al.*, 1973) (see Table VI).

No increase in the frequency of mitotic gene conversions was observed in *S. cerevisiae* (Fahrig, 1974), and the number of mutants was not significantly enhanced in *Neurospora* after direct treatment, or in a host-mediated assay in mice (Clark, 1974). Saturated water solutions of DDT were observed to have a weak C-mitotic effect in higher plants (Vaarama, 1947).

In testing the sex-linked recessive mutations in *Drosophila melanogaster*, Vogel (1972) considered DDT to be a very weak mutagen, but DDA, the

**Table VI**

**Effects of Chlorinated Insecticides on Prokaryotes**

| Tested substance | Organism | Strain | Effect | With S9 added | References |
|---|---|---|---|---|---|
| DDT | S. typhimurium | TA1535, TA1536, TA1537, TA1538 | − | Yes | Marshall et al., 1976 |
| | | 4 TA strains | − | Yes | Shirasu et al., 1975 |
| | | G46, TA98, TA100, TA1530, TA1535, TA1538 | − | Yes | Bartsch et al., 1980 |
| | E. coli | Gal R$^s$ | − | | Fahrig, 1974 |
| | | WP2 Try$^-$ | − | | Ashwood-Smith et al., 1972 |
| | B. subtilis | H17 rec$^-$, M45 rec$^-$ | − | | Shirasu et al., 1976 |
| Methoxychlor | E. coli | WP2 Try$^-$ | − | | Ashwood-Smith et al., 1972 |
| | | WP2 uvr A | − | | Brusick et al., 1980 |
| | S. typhimurium | TA98, TA1535, TA1537, TA1538 | − | Yes | Grant et al., 1976 |
| | | TA98, TA1535, TA1538 | − | | Quinto et al., 1981 |
| Aldrin | E. coli | Gal R$^s$ | − | | Fahrig, 1974 |
| | | WP2 Try$^-$ | − | | Ashwood-Smith et al., 1972 |
| | S. typhimurium | 4 TA strains | − | Yes | Shirasu et al., 1975 |
| | | TA98, TA100, TA1535, TA1537, TA1538 | − | Yes | Simmon et al., 1977 |
| | | TA98, TA100, TA1537, TA1538 | − | Yes | Simmon and Kaukanen, 1978a |

| Compound | Organism | Strain/genotype | | | Reference |
|---|---|---|---|---|---|
| Dieldrin | B. subtilis | H17 rec⁻, M45 rec⁻ | — | | Shirasu et al., 1976 |
| | E. coli | Gal Rˢ | — | | Fahrig, 1974 |
| | S. typhimurium | WP2 Try⁻ | — | Yes | Ashwood-Smith et al., 1972 |
| | | TA1535, TA1536, TA1537, TA1538 | — | Yes | Marshall et al., 1976 |
| | | TA98, TA100, TA1535, TA1537, TA1538 | — | Yes | Mc Cann et al., 1975 |
| | | Nonindicated | — | Yes | Bidwell et al., 1975 |
| | | TA98, TA100, TA1535, TA1538 | — | Yes | Anderson and Styles, 1978 |
| | | TA98, TA100, TA1537, TA1538 | — | Yes | Simmon and Kaukanen, 1978b |
| | | TA98, TA100 | — | Yes | Wade et al., 1979 |
| Endrin | B. subtilis | H17 rec⁻, M45 rec⁻ | — | | Shirasu et al., 1976 |
| | E. coli | Gal Rˢ | — | | Fahrig, 1974 |
| | S. typhimurium | WP2 uvr A | — | | Brusick et al., 1980 |
| Heptachlor | S. typhimurium | TA1535, TA1536, TA1537, TA1538 | — | Yes | Marshall et al., 1976 |
| | B. subtilis | H17 rec⁻, M45 rec⁻ | — | | Shirasu et al., 1976 |
| Chlordane | E. coli | WP2 Try⁻ | — | | Ashwood-Smith et al., 1972 |
| Kepone | S. typhimurium | TA98, TA100, TA1535, TA1537 | — | Yes | Schoeny et al., 1979 |
| Mirex | S. typhimurium | TA98, TA100, TA1535, TA1537 | — | Yes | Schoeny et al., 1979 |
| Lindane | E. coli | WP2 Try⁻ | — | | Ashwood-Smith et al., 1972 |
| | | Gal Rˢ | — | | Fahrig, 1974 |
| Endosulfan | S. typhimurium | TA98, TA1535, TA1538 | — | | Quinto et al., 1981 |

principal urinary excretion product of DDT in mammals, was found to induce recessive lethals. In the same species, Clark (1974) obtained an increase of dominant lethal mutations in early spermatid and spermatocyte stages, and a high frequency of nondisjunction of the X and Y chromosomes at the spermatocyte stage. However, treatment of a population of the Canton S strain for 8 months did not cause any increase in the frequency of second chromosome recessive lethal mutations (Clark, 1974). No evidence of mutagenic activity was noted in *Bracon hebetor* (Grosch and Valcovic, 1967).

No breakage of colicinogenic plasmid E1 and no unscheduled DNA synthesis in human fibroblast cultures were found after *in vitro* treatment (Griffin and Hill, 1978; Ahmed *et al.*, 1977). Both chromosome breaks and exchanges were observed in kangaroo rat cells treated *in vitro* with $p, p'$-DDT (10 $\mu$g/ml/24 hr) (Palmer *et al.*, 1972).

In the V79 Chinese hamster cell line, DDT (30 and 35 $\mu$g/ml/24 hr) was ineffective for the induction of chromosome aberrations and 8-azaguanine forward mutations. Its metabolite DDE gave positive results in both tests (Kelly-Garvert and Legator, 1973). Mahr and Miltenburger (1976), using another cell line, obtained chromosome breaks with an 81 ppm/4 hr dose. Lower doses (49 ppm/4 hr or 8 ppm/3 months) were inactive.

No significant increase in the incidence of chromosome aberrations was found in human and rabbit blood cultures submitted to DDT (Hart *et al.*, 1972; Lessa *et al.*, 1976).

Chromosome breakage was obtained in bone marrow metaphases of Balb/c mice treated with DDT (200 to 400 mg/kg i.p.). Lower doses (100 and 150 mg/kg i.p.) were ineffective (Johnson and Jalal, 1973). A significant increase of chromosome deletions was observed by Larsen and Jalal (1974) at 50 mg/kg i.p. and higher doses (100 to 250 mg/kg i.p.). In contrast, in another mouse strain the micronucleus test was negative even at doses as high as 300 mg/kg (Jenssen and Ramel, 1980). Diakinesis analyzed 36 hr after a 2 × 150 mg/kg treatment showed an enhanced frequency of breaks and univalents, but not of gaps and exchanges (Clark, 1974).

There was no evidence of a greater incidence of recessive "invisible" mutations (6 biochemical loci) in mice fed DDT (250 ppm) during 5 generations (Wallace *et al.*, 1976), and no sperm anomalies were induced by DDT (5 × 10 or 30 mg/kg i.p.) in mice (Wyrobek and Bruce, 1975).

Several authors have tested the mutagenic activity of DDT in the dominant lethal mutation test in mice (Table VII). Negative results were obtained by Epstein and Shafner (1968) with a 105 mg/kg dose and by Epstein *et al.*, (1972) under different experimental conditions. These data were confirmed by Buselmaier *et al.* (1973).

However, after acute (2 × 150 mg/kg) and chronic (2 × 100 mg/kg/week for 10 weeks) treatments, Clark (1974) observed a decreased number of

Table VII
Dominant Lethal Mutation Studies in Mice with Chlorinated Insecticides

| Tested substance | Dose range | Route | Effect | Reference |
|---|---|---|---|---|
| DDT | 105 mg/kg | i.p. | − | Epstein and Shafner, 1968 |
| | 105–130 mg/kg | i.p. | − | Epstein et al., 1972 |
| | 15–30 mg/kg | 5 × per os | − | Epstein et al., 1972 |
| | 10–100 mg/kg | 48 × per os | − | Epstein et al., 1972 |
| | 150 mg/kg | 2 × | + | Clark, 1974 |
| | 100 mg/kg | Twice a week over 10 week. | + | Clark, 1974 |
| Aldrin | 8–40 mg/kg | i.p. | − | Epstein et al., 1972 |
| | 0.5–1.0 mg/kg | 5 × per os | − | Epstein et al., 1972 |
| Endrin | 3.8 mg/kg | i.p. | − | Epstein et al., 1972 |
| | 0.1–0.25 mg/kg | 5 × per os | − | Epstein et al., 1972 |
| Dieldrin | 5.2–26 mg/kg | i.p. | − | Epstein et al., 1972 |
| | 2–3 mg/kg | 5 × per os | − | Epstein et al., 1972 |
| | 0.08–8.0 mg/kg | per os | − | Bidwell et al., 1975 |
| | 12.5–25 mg/kg | per os | − | Dean et al., 1975 |
| Heptachlor | 4.8–24 mg/kg | i.p. | − | Epstein et al., 1972 |
| | 5–10 mg/kg | 5 × per os | − | Epstein et al., 1972 |
| Chlordane | 48–240 mg/kg | i.p. | − | Epstein et al., 1972 |
| | 50 mg/kg | 5 × per os | − | Epstein et al., 1972 |
| Toxaphene | 36–180 mg/kg | i.p. | − | Epstein et al., 1972 |
| | 40–80 mg/kg | 5 × per os | − | Epstein et al., 1972 |

implants and an increased frequency of dead embryos. A 3-week dominant lethal mutation test was also performed on rats. Single oral doses (25 to 100 mg/kg) and intraperitoneal multiple doses (5 × 20, 40 or 80 mg/kg) did not modify the percentage of pre- and post-implantation losses (Palmer et al., 1973).

No significant difference in the frequency of cells with chromosomal aberrations was observed when workers from three insecticide plants who had direct contact with DDT were compared with controls from the same plants who did not have direct contact with DDT (Rabello et al., 1975).

Methoxychlor (methoxy DDT) was tested in bacteria. Negative results were obtained in E. coli (Ashwood-Smith et al., 1972; Brusick et al., 1980) and in S. typhimurium (Grant et al., 1976; Probst et al., 1981; Quinto et al., 1981).

No mutagenic activity was obtained in the Muller-5 test in Drosophila (Benes and Sram, 1969).

### 3.1.2. Cyclodienes: Aldrin and Dieldrin

The genetic effects of these compounds have recently been reviewed by Ashwood-Smith (1981).

Aldrin, together with such related compounds as Dieldrin and its isomer Endrin, failed to induce mutations in prokaryotes (Table VI). Aldrin was ineffective in *E. coli* (Ashwood-Smith *et al.*, 1972; Fahrig, 1974), *S. typhimurium* (Shirasu *et al.*, 1975; Simmon *et al.*, 1977; Simmon and Kauhanen, 1978a), *B. subtilis* (Shirasu *et al.*, 1976), and *S. marcescens* (Fahrig, 1974). Negative results were also obtained with Endrin in *E. coli* (Fahrig, 1974; Brusick *et al.*, 1980), and *S. marcescens* (Fahrig, 1974), and with Dieldrin in *E. coli* (Ashwood-Smith *et al.*, 1972; Fahrig, 1974), *B. subtilis* (Shirasu *et al.*, 1975), and *S. marcescens* (Fahrig, 1974). No increased frequency of mutations was observed in *S. typhimurium* in a direct bacterial test with and without rat liver homogenate, in host-mediated assay, and in blood or urine tests for active metabolites (Bidwell *et al.*, 1975; McCann *et al.*, 1975; Marshall *et al.*, 1976; Anderson and Styles, 1978; Simmon and Kauhanen, 1978b; Wade *et al.*, 1979).

In the yeast *Saccharomyces cerevisiae*, back mutations were observed by Guerzoni *et al.*, (1976) after treatment with Aldrin, but negative data were obtained for mitotic gene conversion with Aldrin, Endrin, and Dieldrin (Fahrig, 1974), and in a host-mediated assay in mice treated with Aldrin (5 and 10 mg/kg *per os*) (Dean *et al.*, 1975).

*Hordeum vulgare* root tip cells treated with Endrin (500 to 1500 ppm) showed chromosome aberrations in both metaphases and anaphases (Wuu and Grant, 1966). Seed treatments and plant sprays induced only a low frequency of anomalies in meiosis (Wuu and Grant, 1967).

No increase in the frequency of recessive lethals was induced by Aldrin, Dieldrin and Endrin in the Muller-5 test in *Drosophila* (Benes and Sram, 1969). Dieldrin showed no mutagenic activity in *Bracon hebetor* (Grosch and Valcovic, 1967).

*In vitro*, Aldrin and Dieldrin produced unscheduled DNA synthesis in human fibroblast cultures (Ahmed *et al.*, 1977), but not in primary rat hepatocytes (Probst *et al.*, 1981), and no breakage of colicinogenic plasmid E1 (Griffin and Hill, 1978). Chromosome aberrations were obtained in cultured human lymphocytes after Aldrin treatments (Georgian, 1975), in cultured human embryonic lung cells (Majumdar *et al.*, 1976), and in a human lymphoblastoid cell line (Trepanier *et al.*, 1977) after Dieldrin treatments.

Nevertheless, all but one result obtained for mammals treated *in vivo* were negative (Table VII). The micronucleus test was negative for Swiss albino mice receiving Aldrin (13 mg/kg *per os*) (Usha Rani *et al.*, 1980). Higher i.p. doses (19 and 38 mg/kg) produced chromosome aberrations in bone marrow cells of AKR mice and Wistar rats (Georgian, 1975). In an eight-week dominant lethal mutation test in mice, 8 mg/kg i.p. doses gave normal data. A number of early deaths, higher than control values, were obtained at 40 mg/kg i.p. (5th week after the treatment), 5 × 0.5 mg/kg *per os*

(8th week), and $5 \times 1$ mg/kg *per os* (2nd week) dose levels, but these were reported as being not statistically significant (Epstein *et al.*, 1972).

In the same test, Endrin (0.76 and 3.8 mg/kg i.p. or $5 \times 0.1$ and 0.25 mg/kg *per os*) gave only negative results (Epstein *et al.*, 1972).

Dieldrin (5.2 and 26 mg/kg i.p. or $5 \times 2$ and 3 mg/kg *per os*) produced fetal deaths and pre-implantation losses within control limits (Epstein *et al.*, 1972). Doses ranging from 0.08 to 8 mg/kg *per os* were ineffective in the micronucleus test, the metaphase analysis, the dominant lethal mutation test, and the heritable translocation test in mice (Bidwell *et al*, 1975). These data were confirmed for the dominant lethal mutation test in mice (12.5 and 25 mg/kg *per os*) and in cytogenetic studies in Chinese hamsters (30 and 60 mg/kg oral) (Dean *et al.*, 1975).

Chromosome analysis was performed on lymphocyte cultures *in vitro* from Dieldrin plant workers. No increase, as compared to a control population, was pointed out (Dean *et al.*, 1975).

### 3.1.3. Cyclodienes: Heptachlor and Chlordane

Heptachlor gave negative results in the Rec-assay in *Bacillus subtilis* (Shirasu *et al.*, 1976), and did not induce revertants in *Salmonella typhimurium* (Marshall *et al.*, 1976; Probst *et al.*, 1981; Shirasu *et al.*, 1982).

Heptachlor and Heptachlor-epoxide showed no mutagenic activity in the Muller-5 test in *Drosophila* (Benes and Sram, 1969). No *in vitro* breakage of colicinogenic plasmid E1 was observed (Griffin and Hill, 1978). Unscheduled DNA synthesis in human fibroblast culture was demonstrated only in the presence of S9 microsomal fraction (Ahmed *et al.*, 1977).

The testicular DNA synthesis was normal in mice after oral treatment (40 mg/kg) (Seiler, 1977a).

In the dominant lethal mutation test in mice, Heptachlor (4.8 and 24 mg/kg i.p. or $5 \times 5$ and 10 mg/kg *per os*) and Heptachlor-epoxide (6 and 30 mg/kg i.p. or $5 \times 8$ mg/kg *per os*) gave pre- and post-implantation losses within control limits (Epstein *et al.*, 1972). This result was confirmed for the 7.5 and 15 mg/kg doses (Arnold *et al.*, 1977).

In contrast, male rats receiving Heptachlor (1 and 5 ppm) in their diet during three generations showed an increased number of abnormal metaphases in bone marrow cells, and produced an increased number of resorbed fetuses in the dominant lethal mutation test (Cerey *et al.*, 1973).

Chlordane was ineffective in *E. coli* (Ashwood-Smith *et al.*, 1972), in *Salmonella typhimurium* (Probst *et al.*, 1981; Gentile *et al.*, 1982) and for the *in vitro* breakage of colicinogenic plasmid E1 (Griffin and Hill, 1978). It induced unscheduled DNA synthesis in human fibroblast cultures, but this effect disappeared when S9 microsomal fraction was present during the treatment (Ahmed *et al.*, 1977).

Negative results were obtained in the dominant lethal mutation test in mice receiving 48 or 240 mg/kg i.p. (Epstein *et al.*, 1972). A small but not significant increase of early deaths was observed when males receiving 5 × 50 mg/kg *per os* were mated 5 weeks after the treatment (Epstein *et al.*, 1972). In this test α-chlordane (42 and 290 mg/kg i.p. or 5 × 75 mg/kg *per os*) and δ-chlordane (5 × 50 mg/kg *per os*) gave negative results (Epstein *et al.*, 1972).

No increase in the frequency of dominant lethal mutations was obtained with male mice receiving 50 and 100 mg/kg of technical Chlordane *per os* or i.p. (Arnold *et al.*, 1977).

### 3.1.4. Chlordecone and Mirex

Chlordecone is better known under its trade name Kepone®. Kepone and Mirex gave negative results in the *Salmonella* Ames test (Schoeny *et al.*, 1979; Probst *et al.*, 1981).

In a dominant lethal mutation test in rats, Mirex (1.5, 3, and 6 mg/kg) revealed no significant difference from the control group (Khera *et al.*, 1976).

### 3.1.5. Lindane and Paradichlorobenzene

Lindane had no mutagenic activity in *E. coli* (Ashwood-Smith *et al.*, 1972; Fahrig, 1974), *S. marcescens* (Fahrig, 1974), and *S. cerevisiae* (Fahrig, 1974; Guerzoni *et al.*, 1976). In higher plants, C-mitotic effects with an increased number of polyploid cells and induction of chromosome breaks were reported by Nybom and Knutsson (1947), Poussel (1948), Kostoff (1948), D'Amato (1949, 1950), and Zeller and Haüser (1974).

Negative results were obtained in the Muller-5 test in *Drosophila* (Benes and Sram, 1969). No unscheduled DNA synthesis was demonstrated in human fibroblast cultures (Ahmed *et al.*, 1977).

A 75 mg/kg i.p. dose was ineffective in the micronucleus test in mice (Jenssen and Ramel, 1980). No appreciable increase of chromatid- and chromosome-type aberrations was found in lymphocytes of Lindane-producing workers (Kiraly *et al.*, 1979).

Paradichlorobenzene was exclusively tested on plants. It has long been recommended as a prefixing agent at low doses due to its ability to induce C-mitoses (Derman and Scott, 1940; Meyer, 1945; Sharma an Mookerjea, 1955; Darlington and La Cour, 1969).

At high doses, e.g., saturated solutions, it induces chromosome fragments and bridges, and polyploid cells in several species, especially *Allium* and *Lens esculenta* (Carey and McDonough, 1943; Oehlkers, 1952; Sharma and Bhattacharya, 1956; Srivastava, 1966; Sarbhoy, 1971; Naithani and Sarbhoy, 1973; Jain and Goswami, 1977; Sarbhoy, 1980). Paradichlorobenzene has even been recommended as a polyploidizing agent (Carey and McDonough, 1943).

### 3.1.6. Toxaphene

Toxaphene did not induce *in vitro* breakage of colicinogenic plasmid E1 (Griffin and Hill, 1978). Intraperitoneal injections (36 and 180 mg/kg) and oral treatments (5 × 40 and 80 mg/kg) caused early fetal deaths and pre-implantation losses within control limits in a dominant lethal mutation test in mice (Epstein *et al.*, 1972).

### 3.1.7. Endosulfan

Endosulfan was ineffective in the Ames test (Shirasu *et al.*, 1982), but induced both gene convertants and revertants in *Saccharomyces cerevisiae* (Yadav *et al.*, 1982).

### 3.2. Organophosphorus Insecticides

### 3.2.1. Prokaryotes

Organophosphorus compounds have been tested mainly on various strains of three bacterial species: *E. coli*, *Salmonella typhimurium*, and *Serratia marcescens*, and to a lesser extent on *Klebsiella pneumoniae*, *Streptomyces sp.*, and *Bacillus subtilis*. The majority of the tests were performed *in vitro*, but a few compounds were also tested in host-mediated assays.

Preliminary experiments on *E. coli* Sd4 suggested mutagenicity of Dichlorvos due to DNA alkylation (Löfroth *et al.*, 1969, and Löfroth, 1970). This conclusion was extended to the strain WP2 (Ashwood-Smith, 1972). In further experiments with the same organism, there are some divergences between the tests, since a clear cut dose-effect relationship for induction of streptomycin resistance (Wild, 1973) or 5-methyltryptophan resistance (Mohn, 1973a and b) was found, whereas reversion on an agar plate test was completely negative. An explanation of the negative results in *E. coli* would be that, in most cases, DNA repair genes rec $A^+$ and exr $A^+$ are required for mutagenic activity. The low mutability of these two genes indicates that mutations induced by Dichlorvos and perhaps other organophosphates result from misrepair of lesions by the error-prone rec $A^+$/exr $A^+$ repair system (Bridges *et al.*, 1973).

More recently, 140 organophosphorus compounds were tested in *E. coli* WP2 and the results were compared with those obtained in *Salmonella typhimurium* and with the activity in *Drosophila* (*vide infra*) (Dyer and Hanna, 1973; Hanna and Dyer 1975). It was concluded that 20% of the compounds tested yielded positive mutagenic responses by producing base substitutions rather than frameshift mutations (Hanna and Dyer, 1975). Dichlorvos also gave positive results in a reverse mutation assay with *E. coli* WP2 and WP2 uvr A (Brusick *et al.*, 1980). Mutagenicity screening was performed with 88 insecticides in *S. typhimurium* and *E. coli* WP2 hcr, with and without metabolic activation (Shirasu *et al.*, 1982). Twenty-five insecticides gave positive effects. Among 36 organophosphorus compounds, 15 induced a significant level of mutations. Dichlorvos was also found to enhance the mutation rate of other bacterial species such as *Klebsiella pneumoniae* or *S. typhimurium* (Voogd *et al.*, 1972), and to induce reversions in the agar plate test (Dean, 1972a). Dichlorvos had positive effects in *Bacillus subtilis* (Shirasu *et al.*, 1976). It was retested in *Salmonella* and *Streptomyces*, where it also had positive effects (Carere *et al.*, 1978). On the other hand, the National Cancer Institute (1977) did not report any effects in *Salmonella typhimurium* and concluded that there is no evidence for mutagenicity with or without mice S9 liver microsomal fraction.

A few tests were performed with bacteria *in vivo* with the host-mediated assay. A subcutaneous injection of mice (25 mg/kg) did not increase the revertant frequency of histidine-requiring *Salmonella typhimurium* strain G46 and *Serratia marcescens* strain a21 at 75 mg/kg (Buselmaier *et al.*, 1972).

The effects of organophosphorus insecticides, other than Dichlorvos, are summarized in Table VIII. It can be seen that there is generally good agreement among the results of different researchers. However, for Malathion and Dimethoate there are some discrepancies. For Dimethoate and Phosphamidon, Usha *et al.* (1980) found positive effects in the host-mediated assay using Swiss albino mice as host and *S. typhimurium* G46 as marker, but at fairly high doses (two oral doses separated by a 24 hr interval, respectively, 51.7 mg/kg for Dimethoate and 5 mg/kg for Phosphamidon).

Three compounds—Dichlorvos, Malathion and Methylparathion—also induced breakage in plasmid DNA (Griffin and Hill, 1978).

In all these works, researchers attempted to correlate structure and mutagenicity of the compounds, and concluded that all methyl esters tested were mutagenic in microorganisms, but only at high concentrations. However, due to the great variations in the response of different species and even of different strains, it would be very difficult to determine a no-effect dose for humans after experiments on bacteria only.

### 3.2.2. Eukaryotes

#### 3.2.2a. Eukaryotic microorganisms. Four lower eukaryotes were tested, including two yeasts, *Saccharomyces cerevisiae* and *Schizosaccharomyces pombe*, and the moulds *Aspergillus nidulans* and *Neurospora crassa*.

In *Aspergillus nidulans*, Dichlorvos was reported to induce somatic recombination in two different tests (Bignami *et al.*, 1977; Aulicino *et al.*, 1976; Morpurgo *et al.*, 1977). No effect could be detected in *Neurospora* at the locus ad-3 after Dichlorvos treatments in gaseous phase, i.e., at concentrations much lower than for other microorganisms (Michalek and Brockmann, 1969).

In *Saccharomyces cerevisiae*, gene conversion was induced by Dichlorvos at doses ranging from 5 to 40 mM (5 hr). This effect was dose-dependent (Dean *et al.*, 1972; Fahrig, 1973). This compound was also tested in host-mediated assays in mice by inhalation or orally. Negative effects were reported, which could be explained by the rapid metabolism of the substance in mammals (Dean *et al.*, 1972). Trichlorfon also induced mitotic recombination in *S. cerevisiae* (Poole *et al.*, 1977).

Other organophosphorus compounds also induce gene conversion in *Saccharomyces cerevisiae*; such compounds include Dimethoate, Bidrin, and Oxydemeton-methyl at concentrations 30–300 mM/5 hr. Methylparathion, Ethylparathion, Malathion, Guthion, and Fenthion were also tested in the same system with and without microsomal fraction S9 from rat liver. Only Guthion yielded positive results (Simmon *et al.*, 1976). However, para-nitrophenol, which is a metabolite of ethyl- or methylparathion, induced gene conversion (Fahrig, 1974). In *Schizosaccharomyces pombe* (ad 6), the detoxication processes by S9 microsomal fraction from mouse liver were investigated for 12 compounds including thiophosphates and trimethyl- and triethylphosphates as controls. There was in general a good correlation between biological and chemical data (alkylating reactions) (Moutschen *et al.*, 1979; Degraeve *et al.*, 1980; Gilot-Delhalle *et al.*, 1983). In this test system, S9 fraction considerably decreases the mutagenic effect.

**3.2.2b. Higher plants.** There are relatively few investigations on the mutagenic effects of organophosphorus compounds in plant systems. It is, however, of interest to define specifically how pulverization induces genetic damage, eventually altering plant populations. This is especially important for crops. All the results obtained so far are reported in Table IX.

Most of the tested compounds are commercial, and sometimes have a low degree of purity. In such experimental conditions, impurities are expected to be responsible for at least a part of the effects observed. This is the case with "Rogor," for which the cytological effects of the pure substance were compared with the effects of the commercial one, and found to be greater in the latter case (Amer and Farah, 1974).

Beside classical chromosome or chromatid damage, multipolar divisions, C-mitosis, abnormal chromosome separation, and in some cases, induction of tetraploid or aneuploid cells were observed.

After exposure to "Rogor," meiosis was investigated under two separate experimental conditions, i.e., after seed soaking and after direct spraying at the seedling and flowering stages. The transmission of chromosome aberrations to the next generations was found to be very low.

**3.2.2c. Insects.** Research papers on the genetic effects of organophosphorus compounds in insects are not numerous, probably because of the high toxicity of these compounds.

## Table VIII
### Effects of Organophosphorus Insecticides on Prokaryotes (for Dichlorvos see text)

| Tested substance | Organism | Strain | Effect | With S9 added | References |
|---|---|---|---|---|---|
| Trichlorfon | *E. coli* | WP2 uvr A | + | | Brusick et al., 1980 |
| | *S. typhimurium* | Not specified | + | | Carere et al., 1978 |
| | *Streptomyces coelicolor* | Not specified | + | | Carere et al., 1978 |
| | *E. coli* | WP2 | + | | Poole et al., 1977 |
| | *S. typhimurium* | TA98, TA100, TA1535, TA1537, TA1538 | TA100 | | Poole et al., 1977 |
| Fenthion | *E. coli* | WP2 uvr A | − | | Brusick et al., 1980 |
| | *E. coli* | WP2 | − | | Shirasu et al., 1976 |
| | *S. typhimurium* | Not specified | − | | Shirasu et al., 1976 |
| | *B. subtilis* | H17 rec⁻, M45 rec⁻ | − | | Shirasu et al., 1976 |
| | *S. typhimurium* | | − | Yes | Simmon et al., 1976 |
| Parathion (ethyl) | *E. coli* | WP2 uvr A | − | | Brusick et al., 1980 |
| | *E. coli* | K12/gal $R^S$ | − | | Mohn, 1973a,b |
| | *S. typhimurium* | | − | Yes | Simmon et al., 1976 |
| | *S. typhimurium* | TA98, TA100 | − | Yes | NIH, 1979[a] |
| Parathion (methyl) | *E. coli* | WP2 uvr A | − | | Brusick et al., 1980 |
| | *S. typhimurium* | Not specified | − | | |
| | *Streptomyces coelicolor* | Not specified | − | | Carere et al., 1978 |
| Malathion | *E. coli* | WP2 | − | | Dean, 1972 |
| | *E. coli* | K12/gal $R^S$ | ? | | Mohn, 1973a,b |
| | *S. typhimurium* | | − | Yes | Simmon et al., 1976 |
| | *E. coli* | WP2 uvr A | − | | Brusick et al., 1980 |
| | *E. coli* | WP2 | − | | Dean, 1972 |
| | *E. coli* | K12/gal $R^S$ | − | | Mohn, 1973a,b |
| | *B. subtilis* | Rec⁻/Exc⁻ | ± | | Shiau et al., 1980 |
| | *S. typhimurium* | | − | Yes | Simmon et al., 1976 |
| Ethion | *E. coli* | WP2 uvr A | − | | Brusick et al., 1980 |
| Vamidothion | *E. coli* | WP2 uvr A | + | | Brusick et al., 1976 |

| Compound | Test organism | Strain | Result | | Reference |
|---|---|---|---|---|---|
| | *E. coli* | WP2 | + | | Brusick *et al.*, 1980 |
| | *E. coli* | WP2 | + | | Shirasu *et al.*, 1976 |
| | *S. typhimurium* | | + | | Shirasu *et al.*, 1976 |
| | *B. subtilis* | | + | | Shirasu *et al.*, 1976 |
| Demeton | *E. coli* | WP2 uvr A | + | | Brusick *et al.*, 1980 |
| Oxydemeton (methyl) | *E. coli* | K12/gal $R^S$ | + | | Mohn, 1973a,b |
| Guthion | *E. coli* | WP2 uvr A | − | | Brusick *et al.*, 1980 |
| | *S. typhimurium* | | − | | Carere *et al.*, 1978 |
| | *Streptomyces coelicor* | | − | | Carere *et al.*, 1976 |
| Diazinon | *S. typhimurium* | | − | Yes | Simmon *et al.*, 1976 |
| | *E. coli* | K12/gal $R^S$ | − | | Mohn, 1973a,b |
| | *S. typhimurium* | WP2 | − | | Shirasu *et al.*, 1976 |
| | *B. subtilis* | H17 Rec$^-$, M45 Rec$^-$ | − | | Shirasu *et al.*, 1976 |
| Dimethoate | *E. coli* | K12/gal $R^S$ | + | | Shirasu *et al.*, 1976 |
| | *E. coli* | WP12 | − | | Mohn, 1973a,b |
| | *S. typhimurium* | | − | | Shirasu *et al.*, 1976 |
| | *B. subtilis* | H17 Rec$^-$, M45 Rec$^-$ | − | | Shirasu *et al.*, 1976 |
| Tetrachlorvinphos | *E. coli* | WP2 | − | | Dean, 1972 |
| | *S. typhimurium* | TA98, TA100 | − | Yes | NIH, 1978[a] |
| Mevinphos | *E. coli* | WP2 | − | | Dean, 1972 |
| Dicrotophos | *E. coli* | WP2 | − | | Dean, 1972 |
| | *Serratia marcescens* | HY/L 13 | − | | Dean, 1972 |
| | *marcescens* | HY/L 21 | − | | Dean, 1972 |
| Crotoxyphos | *E. coli* | WP2 | − | | Dean, 1972 |
| Chlorfenvinphos | *E. coli* | WP2 | − | | Dean, 1972 |
| Monocrotophos (Azodrin) | *E. coli* | WP2 | − | | Dean, 1972 |
| Phosmet (Imidan) | *S. typhimurium* | | − | Yes | Simmon *et al.*, 1976 |
| | *E. coli* | WP2 | − | | Shirasu *et al.*, 1976 |
| | *S. typhimurium* | | − | | Shirasu *et al.*, 1976 |
| | *B. subtilis* | H17 Rec$^-$, M45 Rec$^-$ | − | | Shirasu *et al.*, 1976 |
| Iodofenphos | *S. typhimurium* | TA98, TA100 | − | Yes | NIH, 1978[a] |

[a] National Institute of Health (quoted in Bartsch *et al.*, 1980)

**Table IX**

**Clastogenic Effects of Organophosphorus Insecticides in Plants**

| Tested substance | Dose range | Biological systems | Organ treated | Cytological effects | Reference |
|---|---|---|---|---|---|
| Dimecron 100 | 0.025–0.1 g/ml | *Vicia faba* | Root tips | + | Reddy and Rao, 1969 |
| Rogor 40 | 12–24 hr | *Vicia faba* | Pollen mother cell raised from treated seeds | + | Reddy and Rao, 1969 |
| Folidol (E 605 Bayer) | 0.0001–0.05 g/100 ml 1–24 hr | *Allium cepa* | Root tips | + | Ravindran, 1971 |
| Rogor | 0.0625–0.5 g/100 ml | *Vicia faba* | Seeds and root tips | + | Amer and Farah, 1974 |
| | 0.0313–0.25 g/100 ml | *Gossypium barbadense* | | + | Amer and Farah, 1974 |
| Rogor | 0.1 g/100 ml continuous | *Vicia faba* | Pollen mother cells | + | Amer and Farah, 1976 |
| Dimecron | 0.1 g/100 ml | *Hordeum vulgare* | Presoaked caryopses | + | Singh et al., 1979 |
| Citrobane | | | | + | Singh et al., 1979 |

| Compound | Concentration | Species | Material | Result | Reference |
|---|---|---|---|---|---|
| Thimet | | | | + | Singh et al., 1979 |
| Counter | | | | + | Singh et al., 1979 |
| Disyston | | | | + | Singh et al., 1979 |
| Cythion | | | | + | Singh et al., 1979 |
| Ambithion | | | | + | Singh et al., 1979 |
| Folithion | 0.025–0.1 g/100 ml | Hordeum vulgare | Presoaked caryopses | + | Grover and Tyagi, 1980 |
| Lebaycid | | | | + | Grover and Tyagi, 1980 |
| Kitazin | | | | + | Grover and Tyagi, 1980 |
| Dichlorvos | | Hordeum vulgare | | Clastogen: + Chlorophyll M2: – | Bhan and Kaul, 1975 |
| Trichlorfon | | Hordeum vulgare | Caryopses | + | Panda and Sharma, 1980 |
| Dichlorvos | | | Pollen mother cells | + | Panda and Sharma, 1980 |
| Trichlorfon | | | Caryopses | Chlorophyll M2: + | Panda and Sharma, 1979 |
| Dichlorvos | | | Pollen mother cells | + | Panda and Sharma, 1980 |
| Trichlorfon | | Triticum durum | Caryopses | + | Logvinenko and Morgun, 1978 |
| Phtalophos | | Triticum durum | | + | Logvinenko and Morgun, 1978 |
| Dichlorvos | Air vapor (not precise) | Allium cepa | Seeds | + | Sax and Sax, 1968 |

Sex-linked lethal mutations (in the Muller-5 test) were induced by Trichlorfon, Fenitrothion, and Bromophos after sublethal injections (Benes and Sram, 1969), which makes it difficult to compare the results with mammalian data. Oxydemetonmethyl gave different results according to the insecticide sensitivity of the strain used. In normal sensitive males that were fed the compound, no effect was recorded, whereas the mutagenic level could be reached in a highly resistant strain (Hikone R), although the increase of mutation rate was small (Vogel, 1974).

The chromosome-breaking ability of Dichlorvos was also tested in *Drosophila*, and damage was directly observed in salivary glands (Gupta and Singh, 1974). Hanna and Dyer (1975) compared the activity of seven compounds in bacteria and *Drosophila*. Owing to the high toxicity of the compounds tested, recessive lethal mutations were accumulated by continually exposing populations over an 18-month period for selecting resistant strains. Six of the compounds were mutagenic. In contrast, neither Kramers and Knaap (1975) nor Sobels and Todd (1979) induced sex-linked lethal mutations in *Drosophila* after acute treatments with Dichlorvos. Metrifonate did not increase the frequency of sex-linked and autosomic recessive lethal mutations (Lamb, 1977).

Finally, Bhunya and Dash (1976) investigated the clastogenic effects of Dimethoate in the spermatocytes of the grasshopper *Poecilocerus pictus*. They described an action on the cell spindle, in which some affinity of the compounds for the protein moiety of the chromosomes and for hetero-chromatin was noted. The highest aberration frequency is thought to be significant.

No definite conclusions could be drawn from these genetic studies of insects, but it seems that high or even sublethal doses must be reached to induce slight mutagenic effects.

### 3.2.2d. Mammals

(i) *In vitro*. Cultured mammalian cells, including those of man, are more sensitive to the toxic action of organophosphates than are micro-organisms. The clastogenic effects reported are summarized in Table X. In the large majority of these studies, a cytotoxic effect was observed, but it should be kept in mind that substances like DMSO or ethyl alcohol were utilized as solvents, which are themselves toxic.

Moreover, in protein-rich culture media, organophosphates are more rapidly degraded. This was especially demonstrated for Dichlorvos (Blair *et al.*, 1975), which was found to alkylate the DNA of the HeLa cells (Lawley *et al.*, 1974) and mouse cells (Segerbäck, 1981). In addition to the experiments reported in Table X, V79 Chinese hamster cells were tested for 8-azaguanine-resistant mutations after treatments with Dichlorvos at doses up to 1 mM/2 hr and no effect was found (Wild quoted in Wild, 1975).

In the work of Alam *et al.* (1974) on Chinese hamster cells, it is shown that the distribution of breaks in two chromosomes deviates significantly from a random pattern, from which the authors suggest that Guthion may produce viable mutants.

Of 17 investigated organophosphorus compounds, 8 were found to induce sister chromatid exchanges in Chinese hamster V79 cells cultured *in vivo* (Chen *et al.* 1981; 1982). In the same test system, the same eight compounds were activated by S-9 mix, but to different extent (Chen *et al.*, 1982). Nine organophosphorus insecticides (of 10 tested) were also shown to induce sister chromatid exchanges in Chinese hamster ovary cells (Nishio and Uyeki, 1981). The oxygen-containing compounds induced significantly higher frequenices of sister chromatid exchanges than sulfur-containing compounds. From these data, it was suggested that SCE induction is a common property of organophosphorus insecticides.

(i.i) *In vivo.* Two kinds of *in vivo* tests have been performed on mammals: the investigation of chromosome damage in bone marrow cells or the testes, and the dominant lethal mutation test. Table XI summarizes the clastogenic effects. Only one study produced highly positive effects, and that was on guinea pig spermatogonia after intratesticular injection of Parathion.

In recent investigations (unpublished), we tested the effects of this substance after intraperitoneal injections of 10 mg/kg in mice, which corresponds to 0.33 mg per animal, a dose 6.6 times higher than that for a guinea pig. We obtained no evidence of clastogenicity in bone marrow and testis (spermatogonia and diakinesis). Moreover, it should be pointed out that intratesticular injection is quite an unusual route. This unexpectedly large effect should be interpreted cautiously until an especially high sensitivity of guinea pig chromosomes is demonstrated. In almost all the studies mentioned in Table XI, all the clastogenic effects are recorded, i.e., chromosome and chromatid aberrations, including breaks and exchanges. In the work of Bhunya and Behera (1975), no damage is mentioned except for the centromeric fusions of chromosomes. Under the experimental conditions, this might be interpreted as a direct effect of the commercial product on metaphase chromosomes, possibly leading to stickiness, or alternatively to a C-mitotic effect.

From these studies, it can be concluded that the clastogenic effects of all organophosphorus compounds tested are low and generally not significant.

Most of the results obtained in the dominant lethal mutation test in mice are reported in Table XII. Despite the great variety of treatments, it seems that the methodology of the test is fairly comparable in all these works. Dichlorvos and its possible precursor Trichlorfon are, as for other test systems, the most commonly investigated.

Dichlorvos yielded negative results after both acute and chronic treatments, regardless of doses or routes. The results obtained with Trichlorfon are

**Table X**

**Effects of Organophosphorous Compounds on Mammalian Cells Cultured *in vitro***

| Tested substance | Dose range | Organism | Test system | Effect observed | Reference |
|---|---|---|---|---|---|
| Dichlorvos | Up to 40 µg/ml | Man | Lymphocytes | Only toxic | Dean, 1972b |
| | 2.5–10 µg/ml/48 hr | Man | Lymphocytes | SCE slight increase | Nicholas *et al.*, 1978 |
| | 2.5–10 µg/ml/48 hr | Man | Fetal lung fibroblasts | SCE decrease | Nicholas *et al.*, 1978 |
| | 22–221 µg/ml/16 hr | Chinese hamster | V79 | SCE increased Chr. aber. increased | Tezuka *et al.*, 1980 |
| Trichlorfon | 0.02–20 µg/ml | Man | Lymphocytes | Chr. aber. increased | Kurinniy and Pilinskaia 1977 |
| Malathion | 0.1–10 µg/ml 4–12 hr | Mouse | L cells | Chr. stickiness | Dulout *et al.*, 1978 |
| | 2 × 2, 5–2 × 20 µg/ml | Man | Fetal lung fibroblasts | SCE increased | Nicholas *et al.*, 1979 |
| Azinphosmethyl | 120 µg/ml/18 hr | Chinese hamster | CHO K1 | Chr. breaks and exchanges | Alam and Kasatiya, 1974 |
| | 60–120 µg/ml/18 hr | Chinese hamster | CHO K1 | Chr. breaks and exchanges | Alam *et al.*, 1974 |
| | | Man | WI-38 | Chr. breaks and exchanges | Alam and Kasatiya, 1975 |

| Compound | Dose | Species | Cell line | Effect | Reference |
|---|---|---|---|---|---|
| Diazinon | 0.1 mg/ml | Man | HEp-2 | Chr. breaks and exchanges | Alam and Kasatiya, 1976 |
| | | Chinese hamster | CHL | Tox. without S9 chr. gaps and breaks and exchanges | Matsuoka et al., 1979 |
| Methylparathion | 10, 20, 40 $\mu$g/ml; 28, 34 hr | Chinese hamster | V79 | SCE no chr. aberration | Chen et al., 1981 |
| | 10–40 $\mu$g/ml/72 hr | Man | Burkitt lymphoma cell line B35M | SCE no chr. aberration | Chen et al., 1981 |
| | 10–40 $\mu$g/ml/72 hr | Man | Normal human lymphoid cell line Jeff. | SCE no chr. aberration | Chen et al., 1981 |
| Demeton | 10, 20, 40, 80, 160 $\mu$g/ml; 30 hr | Chinese hamster | V79 | SCE no chr. aberration | Chen et al., 1981 |
| Trichlorfon | 10–80 mg/ml/31 hr | Chinese hamster | V79 | SCE no chr. aberration | Chen et al., 1981 |
| Dimethoate | 10–80 mg/ml/29 hr | Chinese hamster | V79 | SCE no chr. aberration | Chen et al., 1981 |
| Malathion | 10–80 mg/ml/28, 31 hr | Chinese hamster | V79 | SCE no chr. aberration | Chen et al., 1981 |
| Methidathion | 10–80 $\mu$g/ml/30, 29 hr | Chinese hamster | V79 | SCE increased | Chen et al., 1981 |
| Diazinon | 10–80 $\mu$g/ml/29 hr | Chinese hamster | V79 | SCE no effect | Chen et al., 1981 |
| Disyston | 10–80 $\mu$g/ml/28, 29 hr | Chinese hamster | V79 | SCE no effect | Chen et al., 1981 |

## Table XI
### Clastogenic Effects of Organophosphorus Compounds on Mammalian Cells *in vivo*

| Tested substance | Dose range | Route | Organism | Tissue | Effect | Reference |
|---|---|---|---|---|---|---|
| Dichlorvos | 72 μg/liter/16 hr for 21 days | Inhalation | Mouse | Bone marrow | No | Dean and Thorpe, 1972a |
| | | | | Testis | No | Dean and Thorpe, 1972a |
| | 1.15–2/mg/kg | Per *os* | Chinese hamster | Bone marrow | No | Dean and Thorpe, 1972a |
| | 32 μg/liter/16 hr | Inhalation | | Testis | No | Dean and Thorpe, 1972a |
| | [a] | [a] | Mouse | Bone marrow[b] | No | Park and Lee, 1977 |
| | [a] | [a] | Mouse | Bone marrow[b] | No | Molina et al., 1978 |
| | 10 mg/kg | Injection | Mouse | Bone marrow, | No | Moutschen et al., 1981 |
| | 2 ppm/5 days/week/7 weeks | | | Testis | No | Moutschen et al., 1981 |
| Trichlorfon | [a] | [a] | Mouse | Bone marrow[b] | No | Park and Lee, 1977 |
| | 100 mg/kg | i.p. injection | Mouse | Bone marrow, | No | Moutschen et al., 1981 |
| | | | | Testis | No | Moutschen et al., 1981 |
| | 5 × 20 mg/kg | i.p. injection | Mouse | Bone marrow | No | Degraeve et al., 1981 |
| | | | | Testis | No | Degraeve et al., 1981 |
| Parathion | 0.05 mg/animal | Intratesticular injection | Guinea pig | Testis | Highly positive | Dikshith, 1973 |
| Methylparathion | 5–20 mg/kg | i.p. injection | Mouse | Bone marrow | No | Huang, 1972 |
| Fenitrothion | 10–80 ppm | per *os* | Rat | Bone marrow | No | Benes et al., 1973 |
| Dimethoate (Rogor) | 1 ml/100 g | i.p. injection | Mouse | Bone marrow[c] | Positive | Bhunya and Behera, 1975 |

[a] Doses and route not given in abstract.
[b] Micronucleus test only.
[c] Centromeric fusions only.

**Table XII**

**Dominant Lethal Mutation Studies in Mice with Organophosphorus Insecticides**

| Tested substance | Type of treatment | Dose range | Route | Effect | Reference |
|---|---|---|---|---|---|
| Dichlorvos | Acute | 5–10 mg/kg | Oral | – | Epstein et al., 1972 |
| | Acute | 13–16, 5 mg/kg | i.p. | – | Epstein et al., 1972 |
| | Chronic | 30–50 μg/liter/16 hr 4 weeks | Inhalation | – | Dean and Thorpe, 1972b |
| | Chronic | 2.1–5.8 μg/liter/23 hr 4 weeks | Inhalation | – | Dean and Thrope, 1972b |
| | Chronic | 25–50 mg/kg per day/2 weeks | Oral | – | Dean and Blair, 1976 |
| | Chronic | 2–8 μg/liter/5, 10, 15 days | Inhalation[a] | – | Dean and Blair, 1976 |
| | Acute | 10 mg/kg | i.p. | – | Moutschen et al., 1981 |
| | Chronic | 2 ppm/5 days a week/7 weeks | Intubation | – | Moutschen et al., 1981 |
| Trichlorfon | Acute | 405 mg/kg | i.p. | + | Dedek et al., 1975 |
| | Acute | 405 mg/kg | i.p. | + | Schiemann, 1975 |
| | Subacute | 54 mg/kg per day 5 weeks | i.p. | + | Schiemann, 1975 |
| | Acute | 176–405 mg/kg | i.p. | + | Fischer et al., 1977 |
| | Acute | $3–4.5 \times 10^{-2}$ M | i.p. | – | Becker and Schöneich, 1980 |
| | Acute | 100 mg/kg | i.p. | – | Moutschen et al., 1981 |
| | Chronic | 0.5 ppm/5 days a week/7 weeks | Intubation | – | Moutschen et al., 1981 |
| | Subacute | $5 \times 20$ mg/kg each two weeks | i.p. | – | Degraeve et al., 1981 |
| Dimethoate | Acute | Not precise | i.p. | + | Gerstengarbe, 1975 |
| | Chronic | Not precise | i.p. | ± | Gerstengarbe, 1975 |
| Azinphosmethyl (Guthion) | Acute | Not precise | i.p. | – | Arnold, 1971 |
| Parathion | Chronic | 7 weeks | In diet | – | Jorgenson et al., 1976 |
| | Chronic | 7 weeks | In diet | – | Jorgenson et al., 1976 |
| Methylparathion | Chronic | 7 weeks | In diet | – | Jorgenson et al., 1976 |
| Malathion | Chronic | 7 weeks | In diet | – | Jorgenson et al., 1976 |

[a] Only females were exposed.

more difficult to interpret. Positive effects were reported only at doses considerably higher than those used for anthelmintic therapeutics in man which, in turn, overstate considerably the risks of acute or chronic poisoning when the substance is used as an insecticide.

Another explanation for the discrepancy arises from the different degrees of purity of the tested compounds, e.g., technical Dichlorvos contains up to 0.8% Trimethylphosphate, which has been shown to be mutagenic in several systems. The last five compounds for which the effects are reported in Table XII were technical preparations and possibly also Dimethoate. This latter substance was found to be potentially mutagenic, causing damage in all phases of spermatogenesis, with acute treatments being more active than chronic ones. According to Gerstengarbe (1975), treatments induce factors lethal to the X chromosome.

Dimethoate at an acute dose of 10 mg/kg i.p. or chronic treatment (0.6 ppm 5 days a week for 7 weeks) was ineffective in a dominant mutation test and in inducing clastogenic effects in mouse bone marrow (Degraeve and Moutschen, 1983).

The effects of several commercial mixtures containing organophosphorus compounds were also analyzed. Phosan-plus, which contains Malathion and Dimethoate (and also the organochlorine Methoxychlor), induced some chromosome damage in mouse spermatogonia which, however, did not result in abnormal spermatozoids. Tests for clastogenicity in bone marrow cells and dominant lethal mutations were negative (Degraeve et al., 1977). This slight damage could also be interpreted as the effect of impurities. Recently, three commercial mixtures were tested in mice for clastogenicity and dominant lethal mutations (unpublished personal data): Luxan (containing Fenitrothion and Dimethoate), Metadipterex (containing Trichlorfon and Demeton-S-methylsulfoxide), and Dynafos (containing Malathion, Dichlorvos and also Carbaryl, see below). They did not show any clastogenic or mutagenic effects even at rather high doses.

Finally, a few epidemiological studies with organophosphorus compounds should be mentioned. Chromosomes from the blood were investigated after the acute intoxication of patients who had been exposed to several organophosphates: Malathion, Trichlorfon, Methylparathion, Mevinphos, Dimethoate, and Diazinon (Trinh Van Bao et al., 1974). Blood samples were collected for lymphocyte cultures (except for patients who died in the acute period) at three intervals: immediately (3 to 6 days), and then at about 30 and 180 days after the intoxication. A significant but temporary increase of chromatid breaks and stable aberrations of the chromosome type was reported, but only after exposure to Malathion, Trichlorfon, Mevinphos, and Methylparathion, with a maximum for Malathion. For the three latter compounds, the intoxication was too small for reliable evaluation. The level of intoxication remained at a 7-fold increase above normal levels after one month, and decreased almost to control levels after 6 months.

Workers with occupational exposures through insecticide application were investigated after exposures to mixed compounds (Yoder et al., 1973), even in some cases, organochlorines and Carbaryl. Two blood samples were collected—one in the winter time with no recent exposures, and a second in the spraying period. A 6-fold increase of chromosome damage was observed during the spraying season.

Another epidemiological study was conducted by Kiraly et al. (1979), who reported an increased frequency of chromatid aberrations in occupationally exposed workers, as compared to the controls. However, the level of aberrations was not significantly higher than in the unexposed persons working in the same factory. It is clear that definite conclusions could scarcely be drawn from these studies due to the difficulty of selecting adequate controls, of estimating the dose received, and of establishing a causal relationship, especially after exposure to commercial mixtures.

## 3.3. Carbamate Insecticides

### 3.3.1. Carbaryl

The mutagenicity of Carbaryl has been tested on a great variety of organisms. In bacteria, the results were generally negative. It is the case in *Escherichia coli* (Ashwood-Smith et al., 1972; Fahrig, 1974; Brusick et al., 1980), *Salmonella typhimurium* (Mc Cann et al., 1975; Marshall et al., 1976; Blevins et al., 1977b), *Bacillus subtilis* (Shirasu et al., 1976) and *Serratia marcescens* (Fahrig, 1974) (see Table XIII). A host-mediated assay with *S. typhimurium* as indicator was also negative (Usha Rani et al., 1980).

In the yeast *Saccharomyces cerevisiae*, negative results were reported by Fahrig (1974) and by Siebert and Eisenbrand (1974) for the induction of mitotic gene conversion, but Guerzoni et al. (1976) obtained an increase of back mutations.

In *Hordeum vulgare*, Wuu and Grant (1966, 1967) observed an enhanced number of chromosome breaks in mitosis and a slight effect in meiosis. Chromosome abnormalities were also found in *Vicia faba* and *Gossypium barbadense* (Amer et al., 1971). In contrast, after treatment of seeds and root tips of *Nigella damascena*, no effect was observed by Degraeve et al. (1976) and Moutschen-Dahmen et al. (1976).

Intraperitoneal injection of Carbaryl in *Poecilocerus pictus* induced clumping and stickiness of chromosomes, but no structural chromosome aberrations (Reddy et al., 1974).

Human skin cells, both normal and *Xeroderma pigmentosum*, showed no DNA strand breaks (Regan et al., 1976). Breaks, exchanges, and gaps were observed in a Chinese hamster fibroblast cell line (Ishidate and Odashima, 1977), and unscheduled DNA synthesis in human fibroblast cultures *in vitro* was demonstrated by Ahmed et al. (1977).

All the results obtained on mammals *in vivo* were negative. No inhibition of testicular DNA synthesis was observed after treatment of mice (50 mg/kg

**Table XIII**

**Effects of Carbamate Insecticides on Prokaryotes**

| Tested substance | Organism | Strain | Effect | With S9 added | References |
|---|---|---|---|---|---|
| Carbaryl | E. coli | WP2 Try⁻ | — | | Ashwood-Smith et al., 1972 |
| | | WP2 uvr A | — | | Brusick et al., 1980 |
| | | Gal Rˢ | — | | Fahrig, 1974 |
| | S. typhimurium | TA1535, TA1536, TA1537, TA1538 | — | Yes | Marshall et al., 1976 |
| | | TA98, TA100, TA1535, TA1537, TA1538 | — | Yes | Mc Cann et al., 1975 |
| | | TA98, TA100, TA1535, TA1537, TA1538 | — | Yes | Blevins et al., 1977b |
| | B. subtilis | H17 rec⁻, M45 rec⁻ | — | | Shirasu et al., 1976 |
| Baygon | E. coli | WP2 uvr A | — | | Brusick et al., 1980 |
| | S. typhimurium | TA98, TA100, TA1535, TA1537, TA1538 | — | Yes | Blevins et al., 1977b |
| Bux-ten | S. typhimurium | TA98, TA100, TA1535, TA1537, TA1538 | — | Yes | Blevins et al., 1977b |
| Landrin | S. typhimurium | TA98, TA100, TA1535, TA1537, TA1538 | — | Yes | Blevins et al., 1977b |
| Methomyl | S. typhimurium | TA98, TA100, TA1535, TA1537, TA1538 | — | Yes | Blevins et al., 1977b |
| Aminocarb | S. typhimurium | TA98, TA1535, TA1538 | — | | Quinto et al., 1981 |
| Dimetilan | S. typhimurium | TA98, TA1535, TA1538 | — | | Quinto et al., 1981 |

*per os*) (Seiler, 1977a). The micronucleus test gave negative results after oral treatments at doses ranging from 20 to 146 mg/kg (Degraeve *et al*, 1976; Seiler, 1977b; Usha Rani *et al.*, 1980). No chromosome breakage was observed in bone marrow metaphases of treated mice ($1 \times 3$ mg/kg i.p. or $7 \times 3$ mg/kg *per os*) (Degraeve *et al.*, 1976).

In the dominant lethal mutation test in mice, Carbaryl ($5 \times 50$ and 1000 mg/kg *per os*) induced early fetal deaths and preimplantation losses within control limits (Epstein *et al.*, 1972). In the same test, male rats of the second generation treated daily at doses of 25, 100, and 200 mg/kg in their diet or 3.25 and 100 mg/kg per intubation gave negative results (Weil *et al.*, 1973).

### 3.3.2. Other Carbamate Insecticides

Only a few data are available concerning mutagenic effects of the other carbamate insecticides. Propoxur (Baygon) yielded negative results in the *Salmonella* Ames test (Blevins *et al.*, 1977b; Shirasu *et al.*, 1982), and in the *Saccharomyces cerevisiae* mitotic gene conversion assay (Siebert and Eisenbrand, 1974; Siebert and Lemperle, 1974). Propoxur is ineffective in mice in the micronucleus test (25 mg/kg *per os*) and in the dominant lethal mutation test at the same dose (Seiler, 1977b; Tyrkiel, 1977). However, a higher dose (50 mg/kg *per os* during 5 days) induced a considerable increase in the incidence of early embryonic deaths during the two first weeks after treatment. During and after the third week, no such difference was noted between experimental and control groups (Tyrkiel, 1977).

Aminocarb, Bux–ten, Dimetilan, Landrin, and Methomyl gave negative results in the *Salmonella* Ames test (Blevins *et al.*, 1977b; Quinto *et al.*, 1981), and Aminocarb did not induce back mutations in *Saccharomyces cerevisiae* (Guerzoni *et al.*, 1976). No single-strand breaks of human skin cell DNA were observed after treatment with Aldicarb, Carbofuran, Landrin, and Methomyl (Blevins, 1977a). Carbofuran gave contradictory results in *Salmonella* (Gentile *et al.*, 1982; Shirasu *et al.*, 1982) and negative evidence in *Saccharomyces* (Gentile *et al.*, 1982).

In mice, treatment with Carbofuran (10 mg/kg *per os*) did not enhance the frequency of micronucleated polychromatic erythrocytes in bone marrow (Seiler, 1977a).

Even if the majority of the results obtained with carbamate insecticides were negative, their nitroso-derivatives seem to have a mutagenic activity, at least in microorganisms. Such is the case in *E. coli* for Carbaryl (Elespuru *et al.*, 1974), in *S. typhimurium* for Carbaryl (Marshall *et al.*, 1976; Blevins *et al.*, 1977b), Propoxur, Landrin, Methomyl, and Bux-ten (Blevins *et al.*, 1977b), in *H. influenzae* for Carbaryl (Beattie and Kimball, 1974; Beattie, 1975), and in *S. cerevisiae* for Carbaryl and Propoxur (Siebert and Eisenbrand, 1974). Nevertheless, *in vivo* treatments with both carbamates and NaNO$_2$ gave negative results in the micronucleus test for Carbaryl (Degraeve *et al.*, 1976; Seiler, 1977b), Propoxur (Seiler, 1977b), and Carbofuran (Seiler, 1977b).

## 3.4. Miscellaneous Insecticides

The pioneer works of Kostoff (1931) demonstrated the possiblity of inducing with nicotine sulphate fumigations heteroploidy in *Nicotiana tabaccum* and *Solanum melongena*. Since insecticide fumigations with tobacco powder are used rather than nicotine sulphate, the effects could be due to a large variety of compounds. It is in fact well known that in several biological systems, the nicotine from smoke-condensates is not important as a contribution to mutagenic potency, e.g., *Salmonella typhimurium* TA 98 in the presence of S9 Mix (Mizusaki *et al.*, 1977).

In prokaryotes, two tests for mutagenicity screening were performed with pyrethroid compounds (Miyamoto, 1976), i.e., Pyrethrin, Furamethrin, Tetramethrin, Allethrin, Fenothrin, Permethrin, and Resmethrin. (For the last four compounds all isomers were tested). Pyrethroid compounds were first used in a test of reversion of the amino-acid requirement of tryptophan and histidine, respectively, in *E. coli* and *S. typhimurium*, and in a test of the inhibition zone of the DNA-repair-deficient mutants in several strains of *E. coli*, *B. subtilis*, and *S. typhimurium*. These compounds did not induce mutagenic effects at the unique concentration of 10 mg/plate in both tests, even when using DMSO as solvent. In addition, in a host-mediated assay with mice at oral doses of up to the LD50, no mutagenic effect was obtained in *Salmonella typhimurium* G46, recovered 3 hours after treatment with one of the following compounds: Pyrethrin, Allethrin, Permethrin, and Resmethrin (all isomers tested for the three last substances) (Miyamoto, 1976). Permethrin and Decamethrin do not induce revertants in *S. typhimurium* T100 and T98 (Bartsch *et al.*, 1980). In contrast, Allethrin was strongly positive at relatively low doses (0.0019 mg/ml in Chinese hamster cells CHL, but only when it was activated with S9 Mix rat liver (Matsuoka *et al.*, 1979). The results of the experiments on the mutagenic effects of pyrethroid compounds are still too scanty to allow us to draw definite conclusions.

The last natural insecticide investigated for mutagenicity was Rotenone. Negative results were obtained in the Ames test (Probst *et al.*, 1981; Shirasu *et al.*, 1982). It was tested for the induction of unscheduled DNA synthesis in SV40 transformed human cells (VA-4) at concentrations ranging from 1–1000 $\mu$M with and without rat liver microsomal fractions. No adverse effects could be detected in this test system (Ahmed *et al.*., 1977).

Naphthalene has long been known to induce polyploidy in plants. It was active in the *Allium* test at a dilution 1/1000 for long periods (up to 3 days) (Agostini, 1957).

## 4. CARCINOGENICITY

### 4.1. Chlorinated Insecticides

#### 4.1.1. DDT and Related Compounds

The first experiments by Fitzhugh and Nelson (1947) on rats suggested tumorigenic activity by DDT in the liver. Bennison and Mostofi (1950) failed to induce benign or malignant tumors after painting the skin of mice with a 5% DDT solution of kerosene for a 52 week period. Kimbrough *et al.* (1964) observed leukemia in rats that were fed a purified high-fat diet containing DDT. Since leukemia also occurred in the control group receiving the same high-fat diet, they concluded that the promoting factor was not DDT, but some component of the purified diet. Kemèny and Tarján (1966) investigated the effects of chemically administered small amounts of DDT in the diet of mice, and repeated this trial (Tarján and Kemèny, 1969) in a five generation experiment. The diet contained 2.8–3.0 ppm of DDT, but the control level was 0.2–0.4 ppm. They observed leukocytosis as well as a greater incidence of leukemia and malignant tumors in the treated group, especially in the later generations. Pulmonary tumors were most frequent, although tumors of various organs also occurred.

Innes *et al.* (1969) found a significantly increased incidence of tumors in mice at very high dose levels (46.4 mg/kg/day). It should be pointed out that in these experiments, hybrid mice and newborns, which are particularly tumor-susceptible, had been selected for experiments. In the experiments of Tomatis *et al.* (1972), there was only an increased incidence of liver tumors, excluding a variety of other tumors naturally occurring in the mouse strain used (CF₁). The same group of researchers conducted a multigenerational study on the same mouse strain (Turosov *et al.*, 1973). The mice received 2, 10, 50, and 250 ppm DDT in their diet for six generations. Researchers noticed an increased incidence of liver tumors but not of other organs. It should be pointed out that the general incidence of tumors varied greatly from one generation to another. A few brain tumors were reported in the treated groups but not in the control. This observation, if confirmed, might be of significance if we keep in mind the effect of DDT on the nervous system, especially in acute intoxications.

More recently, Rossi *et al.* (1977) performed a long-term experiment on the Wistar rat. Technical DDT was mixed into the diet at 500 ppm for the whole lifespan. Liver cell tumors developed in treated animals of both sexes (45%), but the incidence was much higher in females (56%) than in males (35%). This difference remained unexplained. The incidence of liver tumors also increased with age. It should be pointed out that none of these tumors had metastasized. They consisted in nodular growth which compressed the surrounding parenchyma but did not infiltrate it. The total incidence of tumors was also investigated, but was higher in the control than in the treated animals. There was also a reduction of adrenal tumors in treated rats. Such observations were also made years before by Laws (1971), who stated that he obtained evidence of antitumorigenic effects of DDT. This has also been noted for the analogue DDD which has had some application in the chemotherapy of adrenal tumors (Bergenstal et al., 1960). Syrian golden hamsters given a dose of 125, 250, and 500 ppm in the diet for the whole life span did not show an increase of any kind of tumors (Cabral and Shubik, 1977), so these authors note the absence of evidence of tumorigenic effects in this rodent.

Epidemiological studies with DDT and pesticides in general are not easy to perform due to the difficulty of finding unexposed populations. One has to compare the incidence of tumors in populations with different degrees of exposure to the same substance. Ortelee (1958) investigated a group of men with occupational exposures to DDT, along with an excretion study of metabolites. A similar study was performed by Laws and Biros (1967). If, on the one hand, no ill effects of DDT could be recorded, on the other hand, no correlation with the incidence of tumors could be established. A certain proportion of workers were reexamined by Laws et al. (1973), with an average exposure of 21 years to DDT. No liver disease could be detected. Poland (1970) investigated the same group of workers to detect any effect of long exposures to DDT on phenylbutazone and cortisol metabolism and concluded that this metabolism was not particularly affected.

Attempts were also made to correlate the amount of DDT and its metabolites, especially DDE, in blood and fat with the incidence of tumors. Maier-Bode (1960) did not detect any differences of storage of DDT and DDE in two groups of patients, divided according to those who died of carcinomas or of other diseases. Robinson et al. (1965) and Hofmann et al. (1967) reached the same conclusions using a larger sample. In contrast, Casarett et al. (1968) found a higher level of DDT, of the two metabolites DDD and DDE, and also of other organochlorine insecticides, in patients who died of carcinomas, but these researchers drew attention to the fact that, in people who lost weight or were cachectic, the amount of insecticide could have been artificially enhanced. However, Radomski et al. (1968) reported increased organochlorine contents in patients suffering from cancers, but failed to correlate the fat level with the body weight, as was the case in the observations of Casarett et al. (1968).

Extensive experimental work has been performed with Methoxychlor, a structural analogue of DDT. A review of FDA experiments was recently published on Methoxychlor's carcinogenicity and toxicity (Reuber, 1980). After subcutaneous injection of 0.02-ml of solutions of 0.05% and 5.0% in trioctanoin and also after skin painting (0.1 mg in 0.20 ml of acetone), Hodge *et al.* (1966) failed to detect any neoplasms, and concluded that the oral route was to be preferred for further experiments. Hepatomas were induced in C3H and BALB/c mice that were fed a diet containing 750 ppm of technical Methoxychlor for a two-year period. Carcinomas of the testis were also observed in the BALB/c strain, but not in the C3H strain under the same experimental conditions. BALB/c males were more susceptible than females to the development of carcinomas at all sites for unexplained reasons (Davis, 1969; Reuber, 1979). B6C3F$_1$ mice were given Methoxychlor in the diet at two dose levels, respectively, 750 and 1500 ppm/14 days or 1000 and 2000 ppm/532 days in the female, and 1400 and 2800 ppm/14 days or 1750 and 3500 ppm/532 days in the male (National Cancer Institute, 1978b). Hemangiosarcomas of the vertebrae were found to be strikingly enhanced in females. The incidence of other neoplasms was also increased, although not systematically investigated.

Haag *et al.* (1950) treated albino rats with diet-added Methoxychlor at concentrations ranging from 300–10,000 ppm, but no firm conclusions could be drawn from these experiments on limited numbers of animals. In contrast, the data of Hodge *et al.* (1952) strongly suggest that Methoxychlor is carcinogenic in rats. They treated rats with Methoxychlor, incorporating it into the diet at doses ranging from 25–1600 ppm for two years. Neoplasms of different kinds were especially frequent in females.

Hepatomas also developed in Osborne–Mendel rats fed a diet containing concentrations of Methoxychlor, ranging from 10–2000 ppm for 104 weeks. Carcinomas of the ovary were significantly increased in treated females, as were neoplasms of the pituitary, adrenal, and mammary glands (Nelson, 1951). There is no clear dose–effect relationship, the effects being more marked at high doses.

Miniature swine given food with Methoxychlor (up to 2 g/kg/day for various periods) under several experimental conditions developed chronic interstitial fibrosis of the kidney in both sexes. Treated females also showed hyperplasia of the mammary gland and uterus, suggesting an oestrogen-like effect (Bierbower, 1966).

In castrated mature male swine given Methoxychlor, development of the glandular tissue of the mammary gland was noted (Bierbower, 1967a), whereas immature castrated male swine only had hyperplasia of the ducts of the mammary gland (Bierbower, 1967b). In all these experiments, chronic renal disease occurred (Bierbower, 1966, 1967a and b) but no induction of neoplasms was reported.

The skin of rabbits was painted with Methoxychlor (30% in Dimethylphtalate at concentrations ranging from 0.5 to 4.0 ml/kg/day, 5 days a week for 109 days). In males, this treatment resulted in atrophy of the testis proportional to the dose. There was also renal disease in both sexes (Nelson, 1942).

Radomski *et al.* (1965), after treating Osborne–Mendel rats (80 ppm for two years), concluded that the incidence of tumors was not increased. However, in this particular case, the frequency of tumors was especially high in the control groups, while the dose was low compared with other studies using the same strain.

Deichmann *et al.* (1967) observed an increased incidence of carcinomas in Osborne–Mendel rats fed a diet containing 1000 ppm of recrystallized Methoxychlor for 27 months. The analysis of tumors is however, not complete, so no definite conclusions can be drawn. Results are also inconclusive in experiments with dogs fed diets with Methoxychlor 20-300 mg/kg/day for one year, possibly due to the small sample size (Hodge *et al.*, 1952). The same can be said for the dog study of Nelson (1953) in which 300 mg/kg/day was added to the diet for 3.5 years, although in both studies, dogs of treated groups generally died from Methoxychlor-induced diseases other than neoplasms.

There was also an experiment performed with a mixture of insecticides in rats (Radomski *et al.*, 1965) who were fed 50 ppm of each compound: Methoxychlor, DDT, Aramite, and thiourea. It was concluded that a carcinogenic effect of the mixture on the liver exists. However, a mixture containing 80 ppm of each compound did not increase the incidence of tumors, and as mentioned before, the spontaneous incidence of liver neoplasms in these experiments was unusually high.

Organochlorine insecticides have also been tested for correlating carcinogenicity and mutagenicity in microorganisms (for a review: Bartsch *et al.*, 1980). These types of tests should be considered rather biased as compared with direct evaluation of carcinogenicity by direct experimentation on mammals. DDT and its metabolites DDE and DDD have been tested on *Salmonella typhimurium* strains TA98 and TA100, with and without mouse liver microsomal fractions. Since no mutagenic activity could be detected, there is no correlation between mutagenicity and positive carcinogenicity as reported by IARC (1974). The same organism demonstrated the noncarcinogenicity of Methoxychlor, but apparently on the basis of an incomplete analysis of the available data.

From all the data reported here, it appears difficult to draw generalized conclusions about the carcinogenicity of Methoxychlor. There is a great variety of responses with doses, routes of administration, the mammalian species tested, and particularly the strain selected for investigation. However, since it has been pertinently demonstrated that DDT analogues exert an oestrogenic activity (Bierbower, 1966, 1967a, 1967b; Bitman and Cecil, 1970; and Reuber, 1979), some of the results presented here are particularly relevant. In all cases in which neoplasms of the testis or mammary adenocarcinomas were obviously induced (as in BALB/c mouse strain, Reuber, 1980) on the basis of well organized long-term experiments and accurate histopathological protocols, this oestrogenic property of some organochlorine insecticides should be borne in mind.

### 4.1.2. Cyclodienes: Aldrin and Dieldrin

In early works, Ortega *et al.* (1957) observed an enlargement of liver cells after acute treatments with Dieldrin. This effect, similar to that obtained with DDT, was confirmed by further works (Kimbrough *et al.*, 1971).

After feeding mice with a diet containing 10 ppm Aldrin or Dieldrin, Davis and Fitzhugh (1962) reported a statistically significant increase of hepatomas. However, since these tumors did not result in metastases, especially lung metastases, these researchers considered these compounds to be tumorigenic but not carcinogenic. In further experiments, Fitzhugh *et al.* (1964) tested the two compounds in rats. They found the same increase of tumor incidence as before, but could not establish a dose-effect relationship. Walker *et al.* (1969) fed rats with a diet containing 10 ppm Dieldrin for two years. They did not find any increase of tumor incidence, but reported liver lesions due to the insecticide in female rats. This was confirmed after a revaluation of these data (Stevenson *et al.*, 1976). However, after the same kinds of oral treatments, the same group of researchers reported an increase in the number of liver tumors in mice with, in some cases, lung metastasis (Thorpe and Walker, 1973). Dieldrin given to Syrian golden hamsters (180 ppm/120 weeks) gave completely negative results (endocrine organ tumors and hepatomas) (Cabral *et al.*, 1979).

All these works show a great variability of response to Dieldrin with the animal species selected for experiment; this variability was also evident from the data of Zavon (1970), who failed to demonstrate tumorigenicity in *Rhesus* monkeys. One can even mention some results which lead to opposite conclusions.

Diechmann *et al.* (1970) treated rats with Aldrin and Dieldrin at doses ranging from 20 to 50 ppm (in food) for the whole life span, and showed a decrease in the incidence of all types of tumors which seems to be dose-related. They interpret these data as the possible result of the induction of microsomal enzymes, leading to an increased excretion of steroid hormones, thus resulting in a decrease in the incidence of tumors for which these substances played a role. They also consider alternatively the possibility of reaction via the adrenal glands.

Finally, in a more recent work, the National Cancer Institute performed detailed experiments on mice and rats (Federal Register, 1978). Aldrin was added to the diet (30 or 60 ppm) of Osborne–Mendel rats. Thyroid and adrenal tumors were observed, but the relation to the treatment still seems questionable. In B6C3F$_1$ mice which received 4 and 6 ppm of Aldrin in the diet, a significant number of hepatocarcinomas occurred; these were dose-dependent in males only. Rats (strain Fischer 344) were also treated by

Dieldrin in doses of 2, 10, and 50 ppm. There was no difference in the incidence of tumors between the treated and the control groups. This report concludes that there is a dose-related increase of hepatocarcinomas only in the case of B6C3F₁ mice, but as stated before, the spontaneous occurrence of this type of carcinoma is particularly high in this strain.

Some epidemiological studies with DDT and related compounds (*vide supra*) were at the same time performed with Dieldrin or other organochlorine insecticides. Robinson *et al.* (1965) did not find any difference between highly and weakly exposed workers to Dieldrin. In the study of Casarett *et al.* (1968), the negative effect observed for DDT was confirmed for Dieldrin and Heptachlor epoxide. In a study of workers exposed for a long time to cyclodienes (Aldrin, Dieldrin, Endrin and Telodrin), Jager (1970) did not find a statistically significant difference in the incidence of cancers between experimental and control groups.

In conclusion, there is no evidence of carcinogenicity in man (IARC, 1974; van Raalte, 1977; Sternberg, 1979).

### 4.1.3. Cyclodienes: Chlordane and Heptachlor

There are several unpublished reports concerning the carcinogenic properties of these two compounds. According to Epstein (1976), who surveyed all the available documents from different sources, Chlordane increases the incidence of hepatocarcinomas in rodents. However, an epidemiological study of workers exposed to Heptachlor epoxide concluded there was a negative effect (Casarett *et al.*, 1968).

### 4.1.4. Chlordecone and Mirex

Long-term studies conducted by the National Cancer Institute (reported in Chemical Toxicology, 1976) revealed carcinogenic activity by Chlordecone. In this assay, B6C3F₁ mice and Osborne–Mendel rats were fed a diet containing, respectively, 20, 23, and 40 ppm for mice and 18, 24, and 26 ppm for rats during an 80-week period. A certain proportion of treated animals developed hepatocarcinomas, with mice appearing to be more sensitive than rats. No cancers were found in the controls during the same period. A group of workers from a Kepone manufacturing plant examined over a long period showed liver and testicular damage as well as nervous symptoms. No hepatocarcinomas were reported, however (Huff and Gerstner, 1977; Taylor *et al.*, 1978; Cohn *et al.*, 1978).

Mirex, an analogue of Kepone which can be partly transformed into Kepone, produced similar effects. Its ability to increase the incidence of hepatomas was reported by Innes *et al.* (1969) in mice. This long-term study was repeated in Charles River CD rats (50 and 100 ppm in the diet) by Ulland *et al.* (1977), who confirmed their previous preliminary results.

### 4.1.5. Lindane

Early experiments with rats did not show any evidence of tumor induction with this compound (Fitzhugh *et al.*, 1950; Truhaut, 1954). Further experiments for chronic toxicity were performed. Nagasaki *et al.* (1972a and b) compared the effect in two strains of mice, one with low (dd) and the other with high ($CF_1$), spontaneous liver incidence. Both groups were fed a diet containing 200 ppm of the alpha and 400 ppm of the beta isomer, and the incidence of liver tumors was very significantly increased. These results were confirmed by Thorpe and Walker (1973) who also observed lung metastases, which leaves no doubt as to the malignancy of these tumors. In a more recent long-term feeding study, Weisse and Herbst (1977) did not notice tumorigenic effects in Chbi NMRI (SPF) mice. In this latter experiment, besides the high spontaneous incidence of liver adenomas, the doses used were considerably lower than in previous studies, i.e., 1, 2, 5, 25, and 50 ppm/80 weeks.

In a three-generation feeding study with CD rats given 20, 50, and 100 ppm of Lindane, there was neither a depletion of the reproductive function nor an increase in gross malformations (Palmer *et al.*, 1978b). These researchers only observed enlarged hepatocytes of the type found after exposure to several chlorinated insecticides.

Beagle dogs were fed with diets containing respectively 25, 50, and 100 ppm/104 weeks, and 200 ppm/32 weeks (Rivett *et al.*, 1978). A liver enlargement was observed without histopathological transformations or tumorigenic effects. One factor which can explain some divergences among the results reported above is the simultaneous occurrence of various isomers of Lindane.

### 4.1.6. Toxaphene

In an early study, histopathological changes of the liver were reported in rats (Ortega *et al.*, 1957). In a three generation study of rats and mice that were fed 25 and 100 ppm of Toxaphene added to the diet, no adverse effects were produced (Chernoff and Carver, 1976).

### 4.2. Organophosphorus insecticides

Few organophosphorus compounds have been extensively tested for carcinogenicity.

Metrifonate was mixed in the food of rats and dogs (50–100 ppm) in long-term experiments. No increase in the incidence of tumors was noticed (Lorke and Löser, 1965). In these experiments, however, the daily uptake was not known exactly, so that no comparison with human therapy (where it is used at doses higher than an insecticide) could be established. Pure (98%) Metrifonate was given to rats (30 mg/kg *per os* or subcutaneously for 700–800 days) along with croton oil. Liver steatosis, necrosis, and cirrhosis were observed, and only one carcinoma appeared (Gibel *et al.*, 1971). In another experiment, Metrifonate was given twice weekly (15 mg/kg *per os* or intramuscularly) for the animal's entire lifespan and 11 on 40 treated rats developed tumors, mainly spleen and liver sarcomas (Gibel *et al.*, 1973). Damage to the hematopoietic system was also reported (Gibel *et al.*, 1973; Stieglitz *et al.*, 1974) at lower doses than in previous experiments (Gibel *et al.*, 1971). However, WHO/FAO committees (FAO, 1977, 1979) did not consider the carcinogenic effects of Metrifonate as established.

Dichlorvos was also investigated in long-term feeding studies. After feeding rats at concentrations ranging from 0.1 to 500 ppm, Witherup *et al.* (1971) did not find any effect on the incidence of tumors. In more recent experiments (National Cancer Institute, 1977), both rats and mice were exposed to a low and a high dose of Dichlorvos (daily doses for rats, respectively, 150 and 325 mg/kg, and 318 and 635 mg/kg for mice); No significant increase in tumor incidence was reported. In a two year inhalation study, rats were exposed to an atmosphere containing 0, 0.05, 0.5, and 5 $\mu g/l$ Dichlorvos for 23 hours daily. No dose-related increase in tumors could be established (Blair *et al.*, 1976). It should be pointed out that in these latter experiments, the doses were low and the mortality as well as the spontaneous tumor incidence were high. Recently, carcinogenicity of Dichlorvos was reviewed (Reuber, 1981). From all the studies, it was concluded that Dichlorvos is carcinogenic for rats and mice, but only toxic for dogs and swine.

There are still conflicting results about the carcinogenicity of Metrifonate and especially Dichlorvos, due to the difficulty of evaluating the purity of the drugs.

Recently, an attempt was made to correlate the mutagenicity in two strains of *S. typhimurium* TA100 and TA98 with the carcinogenicity in animals in order to validate short-term assays for detecting carcinogenic substances (see Bartsch *et al.*, 1980). The following compounds were tested with and without microsomal fractions, except for Dichlorvos: Abate (Temephos), Dichlorvos, Gardona (Tetrachlorvinphos), Iodofenphos, and Parathion. There was in fact no correlation. Dichlorvos, which induced mutations in this test system (Section 3.2.), was not considered a carcinogen (NCI, 1977), whereas Gardona which does not induce mutations (Section 4.2.), is considered carcinogenic (NCI, 1978a). Although Parathion was nonmutagenic in several test systems (Section 3.2.), its carcinogenicity is still questionable (NCI, 1979).

### 4.3. Carbamate Insecticides

The reaction of Carbaryl with nitrites and its kinetics were investigated in detail (Eisenbrand *et al.*, 1975; Beraud *et al.*, 1979; see also Section 3.3.).

In 1969, Shimkin *et al.* administered Carbaryl incorported in tricapsylin to mice, and tried to observe the incidence of lung tumors. The results of these experiments could not be interpreted, and only suggested that further work needed to be done. The nitroso-derivative was given by intubation to Sprague–Dawley rats (130 mg/kg in olive oil twice weekly) (Eisenbrand et al., 1976). Carcinomas of the forestomach were observed, but they never occurred in the control group during the observation period. In the same strain, nitroso-Carbaryl, nitroso-N-methylurethane, and nitroso-N-ethylurethane were given, respectively, at 50 and 300 mg, 32 mg, and 29 mg (Lijinsky and Taylor, 1976), inducing the same kind of squamous tumors. Lijinsky and Taylor repeated the experiment, giving to pregnant female rats a dose of 300 mg during a ten-day period with or without adding a solution of 4% nitrite. They concluded that Carbaryl alone does not induce tumors either in dams or offspring. The addition of nitrite did not result in a significant increase in tumors (Lijinsky and Taylor, 1977). On the basis of the experiments available in 1976, an IARC report (1976) concluded that nitroso-Carbaryl had been shown to be carcinogenic in rats. These experiments were extended to other nitroso-derivatives of N-methyl-carbamates in the same strain of rat (Lijinsky and Schmähl, 1978).

In this research, the following derivatives were investigated for carcino-genicity: nitroso-Carbofuran, nitroso-Baygon, nitroso-Landrin, nitroso-Bux-ten, nitroso-Methomyl, and nitroso-Aldicarb in Sprague–Dawley rats given by gavage at a dose of 1.0 ml/kg of a solution in corn oil. All doses were equimolar to a dose of nitroso-Carbaryl of 60 mg/kg, with one treatment given each week for 10 successive weeks, except for nitroso-Carbofuran (16.5 mg/kg, 23 weeks); nitroso-Methomyl and nitroso-Bux-ten were considerably weaker than nitroso-Carbaryl. The survival of the animals was so low after nitroso-methylphenylcarbamate, nitroso-Carbofuran, and nitroso-Aldicarb, that it was not possible to assess the levels of cancer incidence.

In a large scale experiment, the nitroso-methylcarbamates induced fewer tumors, the most effective being nitroso-Baygon, nitroso-Carbofuran, and nitroso-Landrin.

The difficulty of this research lies in evaluating the concentrations of nitroso-Carbaryl or similar compounds actually formed in the stomach (Beraud et al., 1979), and in defining the conditions which could create occupational hazards. No effect of Carbaryl alone or of other carbamate insecticides has been described so far (see above). However, since other carbamate esters which are used as herbicides—including isopropyl-carbamate—have been shown to be carcinogenic (Larsen, 1947; Innes, 1969), further research on this point is recommended.

### 4.4. Miscellaneous Insecticides

Since pure nicotine has never been used as an insecticide, it will not be considered here in detail. There have been reports, however, which show negative evidence (Bartsch et al., 1980).

As stated in Section 3.4., the risk created by fumigations should be investigated in quite different classes of molecules, e.g., polycyclic aromatic hydrocarbons. This risk is probably quite low compared to that of cigarette smoke, since nicotine is infrequently used as an insecticide.

After experimental chronic treatments with mixtures of pyrethroids 380 mg/kg/day, orally for 90 days, only cell necrosis could be observed (Bond and De Feo, 1969). These mixtures were also found to induce liver vacuolisation at 450 mg/kg of a 9% solution in peanut oil (Kimbrough et al., 1968).

The toxicity of pyrethroids was decreased after adding piperonyl butoxide which has synergistic effects as an insecticide (Bond and De Feo, 1969). The following compounds were investigated for chronic effects in long-term studies: Allethrin, Fenothrin, Furamethrin, Permethrin, and Resmethrin (Miyamoto, 1976). Liver abnormalities were observed in rats. Proliferation and cell infiltration of bile ducts were observed after treatments of 12 and 24 weeks of Allethrin and Furamethrin. Proliferation after a 24-week treatment with Allethrin, and some hypertrophy after a 24-week therapy of Permethrin at doses ranging from 100 to 5000 ppm in some experiences and 1000–1500 ppm in others were also observed.

From these experiments, it can be concluded that pyrethroid insecticides do not exert true tumorigenic activity. Piperonyl butoxide, a compound of low toxicity for mammals, was tested in a long-term feeding study using rats (5000 and 10,000 ppm). Liver damage comparable to that obtained with chlorinated insecticides was reported, but there were no true tumors (Lehman, 1948, 1952).

## 5. TERATOGENICITY

### 5.1. Chlorinated Insecticides

Few data have been published on the teratogenic activity of DDT. It was found to be teratogenic for chick and quail embryos (David and Lutz-Ostertag, 1972; Lutz-Ostertag and David, 1973). In contrast, a negative result was obtained in the killifish *Fundulus heteroclitus* (Weis and Weis, 1974). A long-term treatment of BALB/c mice who received during five generations a diet containing 2.8 to 3.0 ppm DDT, corresponding to a daily intake of 0.4 to 0.7 mg/kg, produced no effect on the litter size (Tarján and Kemèny, 1969). In the same way, in BALB/c and CFW strains, 7 ppm in the diet was not embryotoxic (Ware and Good, 1967). The effects of acute, subacute, and chronic treatments have been studied in the AB Jena/Halle strain (Schmidt, 1975). A 300 mg/kg i.p. dose on days 3, 7, 10, or 14 *p.c.* increased the post-implantation mortality and a 2.5 mg/kg/day i.p. dose from the first to 14th day *p.c.* increased both pre- and post-implantation lethality. The same result was obtained after chronic treatment (60 days) *per os* at 2.5 mg/kg/day.

The experiments on rats fed a diet containing 2.4 ppm (Feaster *et al.*, 1972) or 20 and 200 ppm (Ottoboni, 1969) showed no effect on fecundity.

At 50 and 100 mg/kg/day from the 6th to the 15th day *p.c.*, Methoxychlor had no embryotoxic or teratogenic activity in Wistar rats (Khera *et al.*, 1978).

In birds (chick, quail, pheasant), Aldrin induced malformations, especially of the genital tract (Lutz-Ostertag and Lutz, 1969). Mice fed during five generations a diet containing 25 ppm Aldrin alone or combined with DDT (25 ppm), or Chlordane (25 ppm), showed a decreased rate of pregnancy and a reduced number of young per litter (Deichmann and Keplinger, 1966). In the golden hamster, a single oral dose (25 mg/kg) on day 7, 8, or 9 *p.c.* was teratogenic but not embryotoxic. At 50 mg/kg a high incidence of fetal death and congenital anomalies (cleft palate, webbed foot) occurred (Ottolenghi *et al.*, 1974).

A similar result was obtained in golden hamsters with Dieldrin. A single oral dose at 15 mg/kg on day 7, 8, or 9 *p.c.* was teratogenic but not embryotoxic, while 30 mg/kg/day was both embryotoxic and teratogenic (Ottolenghi *et al.*, 1974). Chernoff *et al.* (1975) treated pregnant mice and rats from the 7th to the 16th day *p.c.* with 1.5, 3, and 6 mg/kg/day Dieldrin by intubation. In rats, the results were negative. In mice, at the highest dose an increase in supernumerary ribs and a decrease in ossification centers was noted. Boucard *et al.* (1970) treated the same species from the first to 14th and from the 6th to 14th day of pregnancy with 2 doses of Dieldrin (2.5 µg/kg/day and 3.4 mg/kg/day). Though the authors conclude that Dieldrin is teratogenic, it should be remarked that the percentage of abnormal fetuses was very low and no dose-effect relationship was observed.

Endrin seems to be teratogenic in rodents. In hamsters, a single oral dose (2.5 or 5 mg/kg) on day 7, 8, or 9 *p.c.* caused teratogenic effects (Ottolenghi *et al.*, 1974; Chernoff *et al.*, 1979). Oral treatment (0.75 to 3.5 mg/kg/day) from the 5th to 14th day *p.c.* was fetotoxic, but only slightly teratogenic (Chernoff *et al.*, 1979).

In rats and mice, chronic treatments before mating (0.58 mg/kg/week) had fetotoxic and teratogenic effects. The shorter the time between final administration and mating, the greater the incidence of embryonic mortality (Noda *et al.*, 1972a).

Pregnant rats and mice were treated from the 7th to the 16th day *p.c.* by Kepone (Chernoff and Rogers, 1976). In rats, the 2 and 6 mg/kg/day doses reduced fetal weight. The highest dose (10 mg/kg/day) produced 20% mortality in treated females and fetotoxicity in embryos (reduced fetal weight, reduced degree of ossification, edema, undescended testes). In mice (2, 4, 8, and 12 mg/kg/day), fetotoxicity (increased fetal mortality, club foot) was observed only at the highest dose.

Added to the food of mice, Mirex (5 ppm) produced a slight decrease in litter size (Ware and Good, 1967). Two experiments in rats gave positive results. In the first (intubation from the 6th to 15th day *p.c.*), the lowest doses (1.5 and 3 mg/kg/day) produced no effect, but a 12.5 mg/kg/day dose induced maternal toxicity, pregnancy failure, decreased fetal survival, and increased incidence of visceral anomalies (Khera *et al.*, 1976). In the second experiment, 5 and 7 mg/kg/day doses by intubation from the 7th to 16th day *p.c.* were not fetotoxic or teratogenic, while higher doses (9.5 and 19 mg/kg/day) were both (Chernoff *et al.*, 1979).

Palmer *et al.* (1978a) tested the teratogenic activity of Lindane at 3 dose levels (5, 10, and 15 mg/kg/day) in New Zealand rabbits (from the 6th to 18th day *p.c.*) and CFY rats (from the 6th to 16th day *p.c.*). There was no evidence of any teratogenic effect. No effect on fertility and no major malformations were observed in CD rats treated with Lindane at 20, 50, or 100 ppm in the diet (Palmer *et al.*, 1978b). This result was confirmed in Wistar rats from the 6th to 15th day *p.c.* at 6.25, 12.5, and 25 mg/kg/day doses (Khera *et al.*, 1979).

Endosulfan induced malformations after treatment of chick and quail embryos (Lutz-Ostertag and Kantelip, 1971).

The teratogenic activity of Toxaphene was studied on pregnant rats and mice treated from the 7th to 16th day *p.c.* (Chernoff and Carver, 1976). The tested doses (15, 25, and 35 mg/kg) were strongly toxic for females. In rats, a slightly decreased number of ossification centers was noted. In mice, the ossification centers were normal, but there was an increased incidence of encephaloceles.

## 5.2. Organophosphorus Insecticides

A large number of organophosphorus insecticides were reported to have teratogenic activity for avian embryos. This is the case for chicks treated by Azodrin (Schom *et al.*, 1979), Bidrin (Roger *et al.*, 1969), Diazinon (Khera, 1966; Ceausescu *et al.*, 1978; Eto *et al.*, 1980), Dichlorvos (Khera, 1966; Upshall *et al.*, 1968; Roger *et al.*, 1969), Dicrotophos (Eto *et al.*, 1980), Ethyl pirimiphos (Eto *et al.*, 1980), Ethyl parathion (Khera, 1966; Upshall *et al.*, 1968; Roger *et al.*, 1969; Reis *et al.*, 1971; Yamada, 1972; Meiniel, 1973), Etrimphos (Eto *et al.*, 1980), Fenitrothion (Paul and Vadlamudi, 1976), Methyl azinphos (Upshall *et al.*, 1968; Roger *et al.*, 1969). Methyl pirimiphos (Eto *et al.*, 1980), Malathion (Greenberg and La Ham, 1969; Walker, 1971), and Phosdrin (Roger *et al.*, 1969).

Positive results have also been obtained on duck embryos treated by Diazinon (Khera, 1966), Dichlorvos (Khera, 1966), and Ethyl parathion (Khera, 1966); on quail treated by Azodrin (Schom *et al.*, 1979), Bidrin (Meiniel, 1976), and Ethyl parathion (Meiniel, 1973); and on partridge treated by Azodrin (Schom *et al.*, 1979) and Ethyl azinphos (Lutz and Lutz-Ostertag, 1971). A few negative results were reported for Malathion in chicks (Upshall *et al.*, 1968; Roger *et al.*, 1969), and quail (Meiniel, 1977); for Mevinphos on chicks (Upshall *et al.*, 1968), and for Salithion on chicks (Eto *et al.*, 1980).

The teratogenic activity of organophosphorus insecticides was also tested in fishes. Positive results were obtained in *Seriola quinqueradiata* with Fenitrothion and Trichlorfon (Baba *et al.*, 1975); in medaka fish with Malathion and Ethyl parathion (Solomon and Weis, 1979), and in killifish with Ethyl parathion (Weis and Weis, 1974). No teratogenic effect was found after treatment of killifish by Malathion (Weis and Weis, 1974).

All the experiments attempting to demonstrate a teratogenic effect of Dichlorvos in mammals yielded negative results. Pregnant mice received 60 mg/kg/day from the 6th to 15th day *p.c.* and showed no fetal anomalies (Schwetz *et al.*, 1979). In rats fed for two years a diet containing 100 or 500 ppm, no effect on the number and size of litters was observed, and there was no anomaly of anatomical structure in any of more than 6000 offspring (Witherup *et al.*, 1971). Pregnant rats received a single i.p. dose (15 mg/kg) on day 11 *p.c.* The number of resorbed embryos was not increased and the weight of fetuses was normal (Kimbrough and Gaines, 1968). Similarly, a daily oral dose (25 mg/kg/day) from the 8th to 15th day *p.c.* produced no significant difference in gross, visceral, and skeletal anomalies (Baski, 1978), and 0.25 to 6.25 $\mu$g/air liter throughout pregnancy induced no teratogenic effect (Thrope *et al.*, 1972).

A treatment by inhalation also gave negative results for rabbits (Thorpe *et al.*, 1972). In the same species no teratogenic effect was obtained after treatment at the 5 mg/kg/day dose level from the 6th to 18th day *p.c.* (Schwetz *et al.*, 1979), which confirms the data of Vogin and Carson (1971).

Male and female pigs were fed for up to 36 months a diet containing 200 to 500 ppm Dichlorvos. No inhibitory effect on number, viability, and growth of offspring, and no gross anatomical abnormalities in any piglets were observed (Collins *et al.*, 1971a).

In a multigeneration study with rats fed 30, 100, or 300 ppm Chlorfenvinphos, Ambrose *et al.* (1970) observed a dose-related decrease of litter size, but there were no gross abnormalities in fetuses born dead or alive or in rats autopsied with fetuses *in situ*.

Methyl parathion was tested in mice and rats. In mice, a single i.p. dose on the 10th day *p.c.* gave negative results at 20 mg/kg, but 60 mg/kg induced an increased number of cleft palates (Tanimura *et al.*, 1967).

In Wistar rats, a single i.p. injection (5, 10, or 15 mg/kg) at the 12th day *p.c.* induced no embryotoxic or teratogenic effects (Tanimura *et al.*, 1967). Given orally during the whole gestation period (0.1 to 10 mg/kg/day), it decreased the number of neonates (Leibovich, 1973).

Ethyl parathion seems to be more embryotoxic than teratogenic. In mice, a single i.p. injection (12 mg/kg) on the 8th, 9th, or 10th day *p.c.* induced 27%

fetal deaths *in utero*. For injections on days 12, 13, or 14 *p.c.*, the percentage of mortality rose to 90% (Harbison, 1975).

In rats, subcutaneous treatment (1.4 mg/kg/day from the first to 7th day *p.c.*) decreased the number of implantations and increased the number of dead implants. Nevertheless, no teratogenic effect was observed (Noda *et al.*, 1972a). These data are in good agreement with the results obtained by Kimbrough and Gaines (1968) and Talens and Woolley (1973).

Oral treatment with Diazinon of pregnant rats (0.125 mg/kg on days 6, 7, and 8 *p.c.* or 0.25 mg/kg on days 7 or 8 *p.c.*) and rabbits (7 or 30 mg/kg from 5th to 15th day *p.c.*) did not produce either teratogenic or embryotoxic effects (Robens, 1969). In contrast, in beagle dogs (1, 2, or 5 mg/kg/day *per os*), Diazonin induced a high incidence of stillbirths (Earl *et al.*, 1973).

Mice were treated with Fenthion (60 ppm in drinking water) during five generations. The litter size was normal and no teratogenic potentiality was demonstrated (Budreau and Singh, 1973b). A single i.p. injection (40 or 80 mg/kg) on days 7 to 12 *p.c.* increased the number of malformations, especially at 40 mg/kg. The fetal weight was reduced but the mortality was not enhanced (Budreau and Singh, 1973a).

In Wistar rats, Fenthion (5 mg/kg/day from the first to 8th day *p.c.* and 10 mg/kg/day from 7th to 10th day *p.c.*) was embryotoxic but not teratogenic Fytizas-Danielidou, 1971).

At high doses, Chloropyrifos (1, 10, and 25 mg/kg/day by gavage from the 6th to 15th day *p.c.*) induced fetal toxicity (delayed ossification) in mice. No teratogenic effect was detected (Deacon *et al.*, 1980).

Studies performed in rats did not indicate a teratogenic activity of Ethyl bromophos (Vettorazzi, 1976) or Cyanophos (10 mg/kg/day from the 9th to 14th day *p.c.*) (Yamamoto *et al.*, 1972).

In mice, acute i.p. treatment with Ethyl demeton (7 to 10 mg/kg/day from the 7th to 12th day *p.c.*) decreased the fetal weight and had only a mild teratogenic effect. Pregnant mice treated for three consecutive days (7, 8, and 9 *p.c.*; 8, 9, and 10 *p.c.*, or 9, 10, and 11 *p.c.*) by Ethyl demeton (10 mg/kg) produced a small number of minor skeletal anomalies (Budreau and Singh, 1973a).

Oral treatment of rats with Malathion during two generations (4000 ppm in the diet), throughout the gestation period (0.1 to 100 mg/kg/day), from the 6th to 15th day *p.c.* (50 to 300 mg/kg) or i.p. injection on day 11 *p.c.* (600 or 900 mg/kg) gave negative results (Kalow and Marton, 1961; Kimbrough and Gaines, 1968; Leibovich, 1973; Khera *et al.*, 1978).

The effects of Dimethoate were studied in three different species. In mice, Dimethoate (60 ppm) in drinking water during five generations did not modify the litter size and fetus weight. No teratogenic effect was observed (Budreau and Singh, 1973b). In Wistar rats, Cygon 4E (47% Dimethoate) given orally from the 6th to 15th day *p.c.* was not embryotoxic or teratogenic at 3 and 6 mg/kg/day. Higher doses (12 and 24 mg/kg/day) were not embryotoxic, but the percentage of minor abnormalities such as waxy ribs was increased (Khera *et al.*, 1979).

In cats, daily oral treatment from the 14th to 22th day *p.c.* was not embryotoxic. A 12 mg/kg/day dose induced an increased number of polydactyls. The 3 and 6 mg/kg/day doses were ineffective (Khera, 1979).

Methyl azinphos (1.25, 2.5, and 5 mg/kg/day from the 6th to 15th day *p.c.*) was not teratogenic in rats and mice (Short *et al.*, 1980).

Aminophos (40 mg/kg/day from the first to 14th day *p.c.*) had no teratogenic effect in mice (Hashimoto *et al.*, 1972).

In rabbits, daily oral treatment with Formothion (6 to 30 mg/kg/day) or Thiometon (1 to 5 mg/kg/day) from the 6th to 18th day *p.c.* had no teratogenic or embryotoxic effect (Klotzsche, 1970).

Phosmet given in the diet had no teratogenic activity in rats even at very high doses (Staples *et al.*, 1976). A 30 mg/kg dose once on day 9 *p.c.* or 1.5 mg/kg daily throughout pregnancy increased the post-implantation mortality and caused developmental abnormalities. A 0.06 mg/kg dose had no reverse effect (Martson and Voronina, 1976).

Trichlorfon has been tested in different rodent species. In the golden hamster, daily doses of 400 mg/kg given by gavage 3 times a day from the 7th to 11th day *p.c.* induced teratogenic effects. Lower doses (100, 200, and 300 mg/kg/day) gave negative results (Staples and Goulding, 1979). In Wistar rats, a single oral dose (80 mg/kg) on day 9 *p.c.* or 13 *p.c.* caused embryotoxicity and teratogenicity, which were not observed when the females had been treated throughout gestation with a 8 mg/kg/day dose (Martson and Voronina, 1976). Pregnant rats received Trichlorfon by inhalation during the whole pregnancy. The 0.005 mg/m$^3$ and 0.02 mg/m$^3$ doses induced skeletal defects. At higher doses (0.2 and 9 mg/m$^3$), histopathological placental changes were also observed (Gofmekler and Tabakova, 1970).

The results obtained after oral treatments were very different depending upon whether the substance was given in the diet or by intubation. A treatment by gavage from the 6th to 15th day *p.c.* at doses ranging from 175 to 519 mg/kg/day had no teratogenic effect, even at dose levels producing maternal lethality (Staples *et al.*, 1976). The same doses were given in the diet; 375 mg/kg/day produced minor skeletal changes and 432 and 519 mg/kg/day induced major external and skeletal alterations (Staples *et al.*, 1976).

If, during the same gestation period, a 480 mg/kg/day dose given by intubation was split into three parts a day, the substance was also strongly teratogenic (Staples and Goulding, 1979). Treatment at lower doses (0.1 to 10 mg/kg/day) during the whole pregnancy was reported to decrease the number of neonates (Leibovich, 1973).

In mice, no serious embryonic malformations were observed after i.p. injection (360 mg/kg). The embryotoxicity was higher in the AB Iena/Halle strain than in the C57BL and DBA strains (Scheufler, 1975). Dental anomalies were induced by i.p. treatments (3 to 10 mg/kg) in AB Iena/Halle strain but not in C57BL strain (Freye and Scheufler, 1975).

The effects of oral treatments (by gavage 3 times a day) were dependent on the period of gestation. A 300, 400, 500, or 600 mg/kg/day dose from the 6th to 10th day *p.c.* was not teratogenic. When Trichlorfon was given from the 10th to 14th day *p.c.*, the two highest doses increased the percentage of malformations, which were largely cleft palates (Staples and Goulding, 1979).

A teratogenic study performed with Ruelene in pregnant cows (8.8 g into the jugular vein) revealed no fetal abnormalities (Rumsey *et al.*, 1974).

## 5.3. Carbamate Insecticides

As with other types of insecticides, the teratogenic activity of Carbaryl was first demonstrated in birds. According to Khera (1966) doses ranging from 10 to 1000 µg/egg are teratogenic for duck and chick embryos. These results were confirmed by Eto *et al.* (1980) for white Leghorn eggs. Nevertheless, after injection into the allantoic cavity of the chick egg at the 10th day of development of high doses of Carbaryl (1.95 to 6.75 mg/embryo), Tos-Luty *et al.* (1973) did not observe any histopathological changes in organs of surviving embryos.

In fishes, a high incidence of abnormalities was observed in Medaka fish (Solomon and Weis, 1979), *Fundulus heteroclitus* (Weis and Weis, 1974), and *Seriola quinqueradiata* (Baba *et al.*, 1975).

In pregnant mice, Carbaryl given by gavage (100 mg/kg/day) or in the diet (5660 ppm) from the 6th to 15th day *p.c.* revealed no teratogenic activity (Murray *et al.*, 1979).

Different long-term studies were carried out on rats during three generations. Weil *et al.* (1972, 1973) giving Carbaryl *per os* in the diet (2.5 to 200 mg/kg/day) or by intubation (3 to 100 mg/kg) observed no embryotoxic or teratogenic effects. In the Osborne–Mendel strain, rats receiving Carbaryl in the diet (5000 ppm) showed a slight decrease in litter size. At 10,000 ppm, the litter size was strongly decreased in the first generation and null in the second (Collins *et al.*, 1971b). Shtenberg and Ozhovan (1971), treating rats for six months at 2 and 5 mg/kg/day doses, observed an enhanced number of stillbirths. Carbaryl (200 and 350 mg/kg) given 3 times *per os* at different stages of development had only a slight teratogenic effect (Golbs *et al.*, 1975). Given from the first to 7th, the 5th to 15th, or the 19th to 20th day *p.c.* at doses of 20, 100, and 500 mg/kg/day, Carbaryl was neither embryotoxic nor teratogenic (Weil *et al.*, 1972).

The results obtained in Guinea pigs are contradictory. On the one hand, according to Robens (1969), Carbaryl at 300 mg/kg/day from the 11th to 20th day *p.c.* is slightly embryotoxic and gives rise to malformations of the vertebrae. On the other hand, Weil *et al.* (1973) observed no embryotoxic or teratogenic activity after oral treatment in the diet (100, 200, and 300 mg/kg/day), or by intubation (30, 100, and 200 mg/kg/day) from the 10th to 24th day *p.c.* A three-generation study was performed with Mongolian gerbils receiving 2000, 4000, 6000, and 10,000 ppm Carbaryl in the diet (Collins *et al.*, 1971b). At the highest dose the litter size was greatly decreased. No visible abnormalities were observed. The gerbils from the third generation receiving 10,000 ppm were studied histopathologically. No anomalies were seen.

Two experiments were performed with New Zealand rabbits. In the first, Carbaryl at 100 and 200 mg/kg/day from the 5th to 15th day *p.c.* had no embryotoxic or teratogenic effects (Robens, 1969). In the second, a 200 mg/kg/day dose from the 6th to 18th day *p.c.* increased the incidence of omphalocele (Murray *et al.*, 1979).

In golden hamsters, a single dose of 125 mg/kg on day 6, 7, or 8 *p.c.* was not embryotoxic or teratogenic (Robens, 1969), but a higher dose (250 mg/kg) on day 7 or 8 *p.c.* was both embryotoxic and teratogenic (Robens, 1969). This embryotoxicity was also found in miniature swine. Carbaryl at 4, 8 and 16 mg/kg/day in the diet produced a high incidence of resorptions (Earl *et al.*, 1973).

Beagle dogs received 3.125, 6.25, 12.5, 25, or 50 mg/kg/day in food throughout the gestation period. A teratogenic effect was observed for all but the lowest doses. Abdominal-thoracic fissures, brachygnathia, ecaudate pups, failure of skeletal formation, and superfluous phalanges were observed (Smalley *et al.*, 1968). The results obtained by Dougherty *et al.* (1971) with the *Maccacca mulatta* monkey are difficult to interpret due to the small number of individuals. In the control group, five monkeys conceived, 4 delivered normal infants and 1 aborted. In the group receiving 2 mg/kg/day *per os* throughout the gestation period, 2 monkeys conceived but aborted. In the group receiving 20 mg/kg/day, 6 conceived, 3 delivered normal infants, and 3 aborted. Examination of the live infants and of some aborted fetuses revealed no gross developmental abnormalities.

Very few data are available on the teratogenic activity of the other carbamate insecticides. In beagle dogs, albino rats, and albino rabbits fed a diet containing 50 ppm Carbofuran, Mc Carthy *et al.* (1971) observed no teratogenic effects. Vettorazzi (1976) reported that teratogenicity studies performed in rats with Propoxur gave negative results.

## 5.4. Miscellaneous Insecticides

To investigate potential teratogenic effects, nicotine and some derivatives were injected into the yolk sac of chick eggs after incubating 4 days at 1 or 2.5

mg/egg. Several abnormalities were observed which were correlated with the nicotinic activity of the compounds tested (Upshall, 1972).

The following pyrethroids were tested for their teratogenic potentialities in ICR mice, Sprague–Dawley rats, and rabbits: Allethrin, Fenothrin, Furamethrin, Permethrin (*per os*), Resmethrin, and Tetramethrin. The maximum dose was determined by growth supression and toxic symptoms in pregnant females. No significant adverse effects were observed (Miyamoto, 1976).

An investigation was specifically designed to detect teratogenic effects of Piperonyl butoxide in COBS Charles River rats (see also Section 4.4). No significant abnormalities could be observed even at the highest dose given *per os* (Kennedy *et al.*, 1977).


## 6. DISCUSSION AND CONCLUSIONS

There are various conditions by which insecticides can create human hazards. First, there are occupational risks for two groups of workers; those in manufacturing plants, and those occupied in agricultural areas. Secondly, there is the possibility of accidents, including suicide cases, leading to acute intoxications. Finally, there is a lower risk for the whole population through the trophic chain, and in this context the differences in biodegradation of various insecticides in the environment should be accounted for (see Section 1).

Whereas acute intoxication can result in toxic symptoms and possibly mutagenic and/or teratogenic effects, one can scarcely evaluate tumorigenic consequences, which arise only from long-term exposure at low doses. Such consequences should be mainly looked for in the two aforementioned groups of workers, i.e., manufacturing and agriculture. This difficulty explains why few epidemiological studies were performed, and those mostly after acute poisoning or chronic occupational exposures (Section 3.2.2d.).

If, on the one hand, these investigations revealed chromosome damage after acute doses, such damage decreased considerably with time. In all these reports, it is impossible to get an accurate or even approximate idea of the dose absorbed. The same can be said for epidemiological studies of chronic occupational exposures. Moreover, it is generally difficult to avoid the interaction of other drugs taken simultaneously or sporadically by the same investigated workers, and to determine the control level of damage in the nonoccupationally exposed population.

In the field of carcinogenesis, conclusions from epidemiological studies are even more difficult to draw. For insecticides, such investigations failed to establish a causal relation, as in clear-cut cases of bladder papilloma induced by aromatic amines, skin carcinomas of pitch and tar workers, mesotheliomas induced of asbestos workers, etc. (Section 4.1).

The conclusion to be drawn here is the need for more such epidemiological studies on large-size samples.

Serious methodological problems arise from the mutagenicity testing of insecticides. They involve answering the following questions: which organism should be used? How far should the battery of tests be taken? How should results be interpreted when contradictions between tests occur?

The methodology of the mutagenicity testing of insecticides is handicapped by the fact that no organism adequately allows us to detect all kinds of mutations, especially point mutations. *Drosophila*, for which elaborate tests have been developed, is not at all recommended to test such substances, since it is too sensitive. Tests performed on prokaryotes show great differences of response between species and between strains of the same species (Sections 3.1, 3.2.1, 3.3.1 and 3.4) so that no results can be generalized. One gets the impression that there are particular situations, e.g., with Dichlorvos or other organophosphates in *E. coli*, where DNA repair genes rec $A^+$ and exr $A^+$ are required for mutagenic activity (Section 3.2.1).

The real significance of some criteria from which genetic consequences could be predicted is not known, or only partly known. This is the case of the convertogenic effect observed in *Saccharomyces cerevisiae* and of the recombinogenic effects observed in *Aspergillus nidulans* after organo-phosphorus compounds (Section 3.2.2a.).

This is also the case of sister chromatid exchanges observed in animal tissue cultures [Section 3.2.2d.]. These data can scarcely be extrapolated to man. The tests of clastogenicity on plants usually yielded positive results for chlorinated insecticides [Sections 3.1.2 and 3.1.5], organophosphorus compounds [Section 3.2.2b.], Carbaryl (Section 3.3.1), and tobacco fumigations (Section 3.4).

The majority of the results of these experiments are in agreement. It should be pointed out that whenever positive effects were obtained, doses were very high and the commercial products containing solvents or impurities were generally used. These results are of importance, however, since they indicate clearly that excessive use of insecticides could genetically modify the structure of crop populations in an unpredictable manner. Indeed, the fact that they induce gross chromosome aberrations could reduce fertility, thus decreasing production.

Tests with mammalian cells *in vitro* sometimes revealed clastogenicity from insecticides, e.g., in the case of DDT (Section 3.1.1), cyclodienes (Section 3.1.2), organophosphates [Section 3.2.2d.], Carbaryl (Section 3.3.1) and, strangely, Allethrine (Section 3.4) for which it is the only positive effect recorded. In this latter case, however, clastogenicity is revealed only after activation by S9 microsomal fractions of rat liver, although such fractions generally rapidly detoxicate other insecticides. It should be stressed that in such *in vitro* tests, cells are directly in contact with the insecticide, which is generally dissolved in strongly cytotoxic solvents like DMSO. Therefore, this model does not accurately mimic *in vivo* situations.

In the *in vivo* experiments, clastogenic, or mutagenic effects were only observed at high and sometimes very high doses (e.g., 200–400 mg i.p. for DDT, Section 3.1.1., and also for organophosphates, Section 3.2.2d), and some results are conflicting. No genetic effect of carbamate insecticides in mammals has been reported, even at high doses (Sections 3.3.1 and 3.3.2), but few compounds other than Carbaryl have been thoroughly tested. The specific problem posed by carbamates is the possibility of reacting with nitrites, giving rise to nitrosocarbamates. Nevertheless, this reaction only occurs under quite specific conditions and seemingly never in the environment. It could only occur at the low stomach pH after simultaneous absorption of carbamates and nitrites, and it is known that under such conditions the amount of nitrosocarbamate actually formed is difficult to evaluate (Beraud *et al.*, 1979).

The picture which emerges from all these data on mutagenicity testing of insecticides is that these substances are weakly mutagenic, generally at high doses and with specific conditions.

However, since commercial insecticides are in general mixtures of different products, the possibility of synergistic effects should be systematically investigated in further experiments.

Apart from some recent short-term studies on bacteria, which attempt to correlate mutagenicity with carcinogenicity, all experiments have been performed with mammals *in vivo*. The difficulties encountered in the field of experimental cancer studies are finding an adequate strain of the tested animal, and selecting the type of tumors to be investigated. The long time which elapses between the beginning of the treatment and the appearance of detectable tumors is an additional difficulty.

Hepatocarcinomas have been frequently investigated, but sometimes in hybrid strains or in newborns, which are particularly susceptible. When the increase in tumor incidence is restricted to one specific strain of a single species, which shows a high spontaneous incidence of tumors, the meaning of the results should be considered doubtful, since, after treatments with such highly carcinogenic substances as polycyclic hydrocarbons or aflatoxin, all tested species, even nonmammalian, respond.

There is no evidence of a significant increase in tumor incidence after organophosphorus insecticides (Section 4.2), or pyrethroid-like substances (Section 4.4), at least in conditions comparable to those of manufacturing plants or agricultural areas. Chlorinated compounds have been by far the most thoroughly investigated in a variety of animals. There are discrepancies between the results, the most intricate case being DDT and its analogues.

Antitumorigenic effects were even suggested (Section 4.1.1). In Section 4.1, effects reported as tumorigenic should rather be described as premalignant, i.e., in some cases only nodules appeared in the liver parenchyma after long-term treatment. They do not infiltrate the liver and never produce metastases.

The case of Methoxychlor differs a bit from DDT. Although some discrepancies between results make it difficult to generalize, its carcinogenicity seems overt in some cases. However, Mazuchi et al. (1975) isolated three polycyclic aromatic molecules as impurities of Methoxychlor solutions, so that the possibility remains that these impurities were responsible for the tumor induction.

Due to the great variety of response of mammals to chlorinated insecticides, one can conclude that they show less tumorigenic activity than, e.g., polycyclic hydrocarbons, though quantitative conclusions are impossible to draw in this matter.

However, since tumors of glands, principally mammary or testis carcinomas, were induced in some experiments, the possibility of oestrogenic effects of DDT analogues, due to the structural similarity with diethylstilboestrol, should inspire new experiments along this line of research.

The problem of alterogenic properties of carbamates has been discussed before in this section. As with carcinogenicity, these properties limited to the formation of nitrosocarbamates, which have been shown to induce forestomach cancers under specific experimental conditions (Section 4.3). The circumstances under which such compounds could be formed in man as an occupational hazard should be evaluated.

It is sometimes difficult to interpret the results of teratogenicity tests. Some morphological modifications observed after treatments are so slight that they only indicate embryotoxicity or even some other features not related to the treatments. Experiments in which the animals had received only one treatment should be based on the exact knowledge of the sensitive embryological stages. It can be seen in Section 5 that a great many experiments for teratogenicity testing were performed on birds.

Though interesting for developmental studies, the data from birds could scarcely be extrapolated to mammals. Birds differ from mammals in that the effects are directly produced on embryos, ignoring the detoxication processes by the mother organism and also placental barriers.

True teratogenic effects of chlorinated insecticides have been observed in mammals only at high doses (up to 300 mg/kg body wt. for DDT), which kill a large percentage of the mothers (Section 5.1). This can happen in man only after exceptional acute poisoning, but not as a chronic occupational hazard. The most widely investigated organophosphorus insecticide, Dichlorvos, for all toxic effects yielded negative results in teratogenicity tests on mammals (Section 5.2). Some other compounds tested induced malformations at acute doses but there is a great variability of response, and the results could not be quantified. The same variability is observed after tests using carbamates, but some results cannot be interpreted due to the small number of animals tested (Section 5.3). No teratogenic adverse effects in mammals have been observed after exposure to naturally occurring insecticides.

The conclusion which emerges is that the teratogenic potentialities of all classes of insecticides tested in mammals are slight. Such capabilities can neither be generalized nor compared with the effects of well-known teratogenic substances, which should have been taken as positive controls, e.g., the dye amaranth and the sedative thalidomide, which are active in a large majority of the species tested. In almost all countries, there are rules which fix the maximum concentrations of each insecticide tolerated in several circumstances in occupational conditions as well as in food. There is a sharp contrast between these tolerated concentrations and the high doses used in animal experiments. However, if the use or abuse of insecticides makes us neglect other insect control methods, sometimes of lower toxicity, these latter should certainly be developed along with the older, more toxic, methods.

## REFERENCES

Agostini, S., 1957, L'azione citogenetica di un gruppo di derivati naftalenici, *Caryologia* **9(3)**:377–407.

Ahmed, F., Hart, R., and Lewis N., 1977, Pesticide induced DNA damage and its repair in cultured human cells, *Mutat. Res.* **42**:161–174.

Alam, M., and Kasatiya, S., 1974, Chromosomal aberrations induced by an organic phosphate pesticide, *Can. J. Genet. Cytol.* **16**:701.

Alam, M., and Kasatiya, S., 1975, Chromosome damage induced by an organic phosphate pesticide in human cells, *Can. J. Genet. Cytol.* **17**:455.

Alam, M., and Kasatiya, S., 1976, Cytological effects of an organic phosphate pesticide on human cells *in vitro*, *Can. J. Genet. Cytol.* **18**:665–671.

Alam, M., Corbeil, M., Chagnon, A., and Kasatiya, S., 1974, Chromosomal anomalies induced by the organic phosphate pesticide Guthion in Chinese hamster cells, *Chromosoma* **49**:77–86.

Ambrose, A., Larson, P., Borzelleca, J., and Hennigar, G., 1970, Toxicologic studies on diethyl-1-(2,4 dichlorophenyl)-2-chlorovinyl phosphate, *Toxicol. Appl. Pharmacol.* **17**:323–336.

Amer, S., and Farah, O., 1974, Cytological effects of pesticides VI. Effect of the insecticide "Rogor" on the mitosis of *Vicia faba* and *Gossypium barbadense*, *Cytologia* **39**:507–514.

Amer, S., and Farah, O., 1976, Cytological effects of pesticides, VIII. Effects of the carbamate pesticides "IPC", "Rogor" and "Duphar" on *Vicia faba*, *Cytologia* **41**:597–606.

Amer, S., Hammouda, M., and Farah, O., 1971, Cytological and morphological effects of the insecticide N-methyl-1-naphtyl carbamate "Sevin", *Flora* (Jena), *Abt . B*, **160**:433–439.

Anderson, D., and Styles, J., 1978, An evaluation of six short term tests for detecting organic chemical carcinogens, *Brit. J. Cancer* **37**:924–930.

Arnold, D., 1971, Mutagenic study with Guthion in albino male mice, *Industr. Bio Test Lab. Inc.*

Arnold, D., Kennedy, G., Keplinger, M., Calandra, J., and Calo, C., 1977, Dominant lethal studies of technical chlordane, HCS-3260 and heptachlor: heptachlor epoxide, *J. Toxicol. Environ. Health* **2**:547–555.

Ashwood-Smith, M., 1981, The genetic toxicology of aldrin and dieldrin, *Mutat. Res.* **86**:137–154.

Ashwood-Smith, M., Trevino, J., and Ring, R., 1972, Mutagenicity of dichlorvos, *Nature* (London) **240**:418–420.

Aulicino, F., Bignami, M., Carere, A., Conti, G., Morpurgo, G., and Velcich, A., 1976, Mutational studies with some pesticides in *Aspergillus nidulans, Mutat. Res.* **38**:138.

Baba, K., Nara, M., Iwahashi, Y., Matsushima, M., and Sasaki, T., 1975, Toxicity of agricultural chemicals on marine fishes. II. The vertebral deformation observed in young yellowtail during the determination of TLm, *Shizuokaken Suisan Shikenjo Kenkyu Hokoku* (Bull. Shizuoka Prefect. Fish. Exp. Str.) **9**:43–52.

Baksi, S., 1978, Effect of dichlorvos on embryonal and fetal development in thyroparathyroidectomized, thyroxine-treated and euthyroid rats, *Toxicol. Lett.* **2**:213–216.

Bartsch, H., Malaveille, C., Camus, A., Martel-Planche, G., Brun, G., Hautefeuille, A., Sabadie, N., Barbin, A., Kuroki, T., Drevon, C., Piccoli, C., and Montesano, R., 1980, Validation and comparative studies on 180 chemicals with *S. typhimurium* strains and V79 Chinese hamster cells in the presence of various metabolizing systems, *Mutat. Res.* **76**:1–50.

Beattie, K., 1975, N-nitrosocarbaryl-induced mutagenesis in *Haemophilus influenzae* strains deficient in repair and recombination, *Mutat. Res.* **27**:201–217.

Beattie, K., and Kimball, R., 1974, Involvement of DNA replication and repair in mutagenesis of *Haemophilus influenzae* induced by N-nitrosocarbaryl, *Mutat. Res.* **24**:105–115.

Becker, K., and Schöneich, J., 1980, Dominant lethal test with trichlorfon in male mice, *Mutat. Res.* **74**:224.

Benes, V., and Sram, R., 1969, Mutagenic activity of some pesticides in *Drosophila melanogaster, Ind. Med.* **38**:50–53.

Benes, V., Sram, R., and Tuscany, R., 1973, Testing of mutagenicity of fenitrothione, *Mutat. Res.* **21**:23–24.

Bennison, B., and Mostofi, F., 1950, Observations on inbred mice exposed to DDT, *J. Nat. Cancer Inst.* **10**:989–992.

Beraud, M., Pipy, B., Derache, R., and Gaillard, D., 1979, Formation d'un cancérigène, le N-nitrosocarbaryl par interactions entre un insecticide de la série des carbamates, le carbaryl et le nitrite, dans le suc gastrique de rat, *Food Cosmet. Toxicol.* **17**:579–583.

Bergenstal, D., Lipsett, M., Moy, R., and Hertz, R., 1960, in *Biological Activities of Steroids in Relation to Cancer*, (edited by G. Pincus and F. P. Vollmer), Academic Press, New York, pp. 463–473.

Bhan, A., and Kaul, B., 1975, Cytogenetic activity of dichlorvos in barley, *Ind. J. Exp. Biol.* **13**:403–405.

Bhunya, S., and Behera, J., 1975, Centromeric sensitivity of mouse chromosomes to the systemic insecticide dimethoate (Rogor), *Curr. Sci.* **44**:859–860.

Bhunya, S., and Dash, N., 1976, Effect of a systemic insecticide dimethoate on the spermatocytic chromosomes of a short-horned grasshopper *Poecilocerus pictus, Sci. Cult.* **42**:571–573.

Bidwell, K., Weber, E., Nienhold, I., Connor, T., and Legator, M., 1975, Comprehensive evaluation for mutagenic activity of dieldrin, *Mutat. Res.* **31**:314.

Bierbower, G., 1966, Histopathology in miniature swine fed methoxychlor in the diet, prepared as a memorandum to A. J. Lehman, Food and Drug Administration, May 27, Washington D.C.

Bierbower, G., 1967a, Histopathology in castrated male swine fed methoxychlor mixed in the diet, Prepared as a memorandum to A. J. Lehman, Food and Drug Administration, April 18, Washington D.C.

Bierbower, G., 1967b, Histopathology in young castrated miniature swine fed methoxychlor mixed in the diet, Prepared as a memorandum to A. J. Lehman, Food and Drug Administration, July 24, Washington D.C.

Bignami, M., Aulicino, F., Velcich, A., Carere, A., and Morpurgo, G., 1977, Mutagenic and recombinogenic action of pesticides in *Aspergillus nidulans*, *Mutat. Res.* **46**:395–402.

Bitman, J., and Cecil, H., 1970, Estrogenic activity of DDT analogs of polychlorinated biphenyls, *J. Agr. Food Chem.* **18**:1108–1112.

Blair, D., Hoadley, E., and Hutson, D., 1975, The distribution of dichlorvos in the tissues of mammals after its inhalation or intravenous administration, *Toxicol. Appl. Pharmacol.* **31**:243–253.

Blair, D., Dix, K., Hunt, P., Thorpe, E., Stevenson, D., and Walker, A., 1976, Dichlorvos: a two year inhalation carcinogenesis in rats, *Arch. Toxicol.* **35**:281–294.

Blevins, R., Lijinsky, W., and Regan, J., 1977a, Nitrosated methylcarbamate insecticides: effect on the DNA of human cells, *Mutat. Res.* **44**:1–7.

Blevins, R., Lee, M., and Regan, J., 1977b, Mutagenicity screening of five methyl carbamate insecticides and their nitroso derivatives using mutants of *Salmonella typhimurium* LT2, *Mutat. Res.* **56**:1–6.

Bond, H. W., and De Feo, J. J., 1969, Toxicity of pyrethrum in combination with certain common chemicals and drugs, Report of University of Rhode Island to Kenya Pyrethrum Company.

Boucard, M., Beaulaton, I., Mestres, R., and Allieu, M., 1970, Etude expérimentale de la tératogenèse: Influence de la période et de la durée du traitement, *Therapie* **25**:907–913.

Bridges, B., Mottershead, R., Green, M., and Gray, W., 1973, Mutagenicity of dichlorvos and methyl methanesulphonate for *Escherichia coli* WP2 and some derivatives deficient in DNA repair, *Mutat. Res.* **19**:295–303.

Brooks, G. T., 1974, *Chlorinated insecticides*, Volume II, Biological and environmental aspects, CRC Press, Inc.

Brown, A. W. A., 1969, Insect resistance, *Farm Chem.*

Brusick, D., Simmon, V., Rosenkranz, H., Ray, V., and Stafford, R., 1980, An evaluation of the *Escherichia coli* WP2 and WP2 uvr A reverse mutation assay, *Mutat. Res.* **76**:169–190.

Budreau, C., and Singh, R., 1973a, Teratogenicity and embryotoxicity of demeton and fenthion in CF-1 mouse embryos, *Toxicol. Appl. Pharmacol.* **24**:324–332.

Budreau, C., and Singh, R., 1973b, Effect of fenthion and dimethoate on reproduction in the mouse, *Toxicol. Appl. Pharmacol.* **26**:29–38.

Buselmaier, W., Röhrborn, G., and Propping, P., 1972, Mutagenitätsuntersuchungen mit Pestiziden im host-mediated assay und mit dem Dominanten Lethaltest an der Maus, *Biol. Zentralbl.* **9**:311–325.

Buselmaier, W., Röhrborn, G., and Propping, P., 1973, Comparative investigations on the mutagenicity of pesticides in mammalian test systems, *Mutat. Res.* **21**:25–26.

Cabral, J. P. R., and Shubik, P., 1977, Lack of carcinogenicity of DDT in hamster, *Fed. Proc.* **36**:1086.

Cabral, J. P. R., Hall, R. K., Bronczyk, S. A., and Shubik, P., 1979, A carcinogenicity study of the pesticide dieldrin in hamsters, *Cancer Lett.* **6**:241–246.

Carere, A., Ortali, V., Cardamone, G., and Morpurgo, G., 1978, Mutagenicity of dichlorvos and other structurally related pesticides in *Salmonella* and *Streptomyces*, *Chem. Biol. Interact.* **22**:297–308.

Carey, M. A., and McDonough, E. S., 1943, On the production of polyploidy in *Allium* with paradichlorobenzene, *J. Hered.* **34**:238–240.

Casarett, L. J., Fryer, G. C., Yauger, W. L. Jr., and Klemmer, H. W., 1968, Organochlorine pesticide residues in human tissue—Hawaii, *Arch. Environm. Health* **17**:306–311.

Ceausescu, S., Stancioiu, N., Stefan, A., and Ionita, E., 1978, Effects of diazinon on the formation and development of *Gallus domesticus* embryos, *Stud. Cercet. Biochim.* **21**:27–30.

Cerey, K., Izakovic, V., and Ruttkay–Nedecka, J., 1973, Effect of heptachlor on dominant lethality and bone marrow in rats, *Mutat. Res.* **21**:26.

Chen, H., Hsueh, J., Sirianni, S., and Huang, C., 1981, Induction of sister chromatid exchanges and cell cycle delay in cultured mammalian cells treated with eight organophosphorus pesticides, *Mutat. Res.* **88**:307–316.

Chen, H., Sirianni, S., and Huang, C., 1982, Sister chromatid exchanges in Chinese hamster cells treated with seventeen organophosphorus compounds in the presence of a metabolic act activation system. *Environmental Mutagenesis.* **4**:621–624.

Chernoff, N., and Carver, B., 1976, Fetal toxicity of toxaphene in rats and mice, *Bull. Environm. Contam. Toxicol.* **15**:660–664.

Chernoff, N., and Rogers, E., 1976, Fetal toxicity of kepone in rats and mice, *Toxicol. Appl. Pharmacol.* **38**:189–194.

Chernoff, N., Kavlock, R., Kathrein, J., Dunn, J., and Haseman, J., 1975, Prenatal effects of dieldrin and photodieldrin in mice and rats, *Toxicol. Appl. Pharmacol.* **31**:302–308.

Chernoff, N., Kavlock, R., Hanisch, R., Whitehouse, D., Gray, J., Gray, L., and Sovocool, G., 1979a, Perinatal toxicity of endrin in rodents. I. Fetotoxic effects of prenatal exposure in hamsters, *Toxicology* **13**:155–165.

Chernoff, N., Linder, R., Scotti, T., Rogers, E., Carver, B., and Kavlock, R., 1979b. Fetotoxicity and cataractogenicity of mirex in rats and mice with notes on kepone, *Environm. Res.* **18**:257–269.

Clark, J., 1974, Mutagenicity of DDT in mice, *Drosophila melanogaster and Neurospora crassa*, *Aust. J. Biol. Sci.* **27**:427–440.

Cohn, W. J., Boylan, J. J., Blanke, R. Y., Fariss, M. W., Howell, J. R., and Guzelian, P. S., 1978, Treatment of chlordecone (Kepone) toxicity with cholestyramine, *N. Engl. J. Med.* **298**:243–248.

Collins, J., Schooley, M., and Singh, V., 1971, The effect of dietary dichlorvos in swine reproduction and viability of their offspring, *Toxicol. Appl. Pharmacol.* **19**:377.

Collins, T., Hansen, W., and Keeler, H., 1971, The effect of carbaryl (Sevin) on reproduction of the rat and the gerbil, *Toxicol. Appl. Pharmacol.* **19**:202–216.

D'Amato, F., 1949, Early influence of m-inositol and sugars on gammexane induced C-mitosis, *Caryologia* **1**:223–228.

D'Amato, F., 1950, Notes on the chromosome breaks induced by pure gammexane, *Caryologia* **2**:361–364.

Darlington, C. D., and La Cour, F., 1969, *Handling of Chromosomes*, Unwin Brothers Limited, London.

David, D., and Lutz–Ostertag, Y., 1972, Etude comparative de l'action du DDT sur la mortalité, la morphologie externe et interne chez l'embryon de poulet et de caille, *C. R. Acad. Sci.* (*Paris*) **275**:2171–2173.

Davis, K. J., 1969, Histopathological diagnosis of lesions noted in mice fed DDT or Methoxychlor, Prepared as a memorandum to W. Hansen, Food and Drug Administration, January 30, Washington D.C.

Davis, K. J., and Fitzhugh, O. G., 1962, Tumorigenic potential of aldrin and dieldrin for mice, *Toxicol Appl. Pharmacol.* **4**:187–189.

Deacon, M., Murray, J., Pilny, M., Rao, K., Dittenber, D., Hanley, T., and John, J., 1980, Embryotoxicity and fetotoxicity of orally administered chlorpyrifos in mice, *Toxicol. Appl. Pharmacol.* **54**:31–40.

Dean, B., 1972a, The mutagenic effects of organophosphorus insecticides on micro-organisms, *Arch. Toxicol.* **30**:64–74.

Dean, B., 1972b, The effect of dichlorvos on cultured human lymphocytes, *Arch. Toxicol.* **30**:75–85.

Dean, B., and Blair, D., 1976, Dominant lethal assay in female mice after oral dosing with dichlorvos or exposure to atmospheres containing dichlorvos, *Mutat. Res.* **40**:67–72.

Dean, B., and Thorpe, E., 1972a, Cytogenetic studies with dichlorvos in mice and Chinese hamsters, *Arch. Toxicol.* **30**:39–49.

Dean, B., and Thorpe, E., 1972b, Studies with dichlorvos vapour in dominant lethal mutation tests on mice, *Arch. Toxicol.* **30**:51–59.

Dean, B., Doak, S., and Funnell, J., 1972, Genetic studies with dichlorvos in the host-mediated assay and in liquid medium using *Saccharomyces cerevisiae,. Arch. Toxicol.* **30**:61–66.

Dean, B., Doak, S., and Somerville, H., 1975, The potential mutagenicity of Dieldrin (HEOD) in mammals, *Food Cosmet. Toxicol.* **13**:317–323.

Dedek, W., Scheufler, H., and Fischer, G., 1975, Zur Mutagenität von Desmethyl-Trichlorfon im Dominanten-Lethal-Test an der Hausmaus, *Arch. Toxicol.* **33**:163–168.

Degraeve, N., Moutschen, J., Moutschen-Dahmen, M., Houbrechts, N., and Colizzi, A., 1976, A propos des risques d'un insecticide: le carbaryl utilisé seul et en combinaison avec les nitrites, *Bull. Soc. R. Sci. Liege* **45**:46–57.

Degraeve, N., Moutschen, J., Moutschen-Dahmen, M., Gilot-Delhalle, J., Houbrechts, N., and Colizzi, A., 1977, Cytogenetic and genetic effects of Phosan-plus, *Mutat. Res.* **46**:204.

Degraeve, N., Gilot-Delhalle, J., Moutschen, J., Moutschen-Dahmen, M., Colizzi, A., Chollet, M., and Houbrechts, N., 1980, Comparison of the mutagenic activity of organophosphorus insecticides in mouse and in the yeast *Schizosaccharomyces pombe*, *Mutat. Res.* **74**:201–202.

Degraeve, N., Gilot-Delhalle, J., Colizzi, A., Chollet, M., Moutschen, J., and Moutschen-Dahmen, M., 1981, Evaluation des risques génétiques d'un insecticide organophosphoré: le trichlorfon (O,O-dimethyl-(2,2,2-trichloro-1-hydroxy)-ethyl-phosphonate), *Bull. Soc. R. Sci. Liège* **50**:85–98.

Degraeve, N., and Moutschen, J., 1983, Genotoxicity of an organophosphorus insecticide, dimethoate, in the mouse. *Mutat. Res.* **119**:331–337.

Deichmann, W., and Keplinger, M., 1966, Effect of combinations of pesticides on reproduction of mice, *Toxicol. Appl. Pharmacol.* **8**:337.

Deichmann, W., Keplinger, M., Sala, F., and Glass, E., 1967, Synergism among oral carcinogens. IV. The simultaneous feeding of four tumorigens to rats, *Toxicol. Appl. Pharmacol.* **11**:88–103.

Deichmann, W., Mac Donald, W., Blum, E., Bevilacqua, M., Radomski J., Keplinger, M., and Balkus, M., 1970, Tumorigenicity of aldrin, dieldrin and endrin in the albino rat, *Ind. Med.* **39**:37–45.

Derman, H., and Scott, D. H., 1940, Chromosome count in apples and strawberry aided by paradichlorobenzene, *Proc. Am. Soc. Hortic. Sci.* **56**:145–148.

Dikshith, T., 1973, *In vivo* effects of parathion on Guinea pig chromosomes, *Environm. Physiol. Biochem.* **3**:161–168.

Dougherty, W., Golberg, L., and Coulston, F., 1971, The effect of carbaryl on reproduction in the monkey (*Maccacca mulatta*), *Toxicol. Appl. Pharmacol.* **19**:365.

Dulout, F., Larramendy, M., and Bianchi, N., 1978, Chromosome stickiness in mouse L-cells induced by the organophosphorous insecticide Malathion, *Abstr. 14th Int. Congr. Genet.* (Moscow) **II**:223.

Dyer, K., and Hanna, P., 1973, Comparative mutagenic activity and toxicity of triethylphosphate and dichlorvos in bacteria and *Drosophila*, *Mutat. Res.* **21**:175–177.

Earl, F., Miller, E., and Van Loon, E., 1973, Reproductive, teratogenic, and neonatal effects of some pesticides and related compounds in beagle dogs and miniature swine, *Pestic. Environm. Contin. Controversy*, Pap. Inter. Am. Conf. Toxicol. Occup. Med. **8th**:253–266.

Edwards, C. A., 1973, *Environmental Pollution by Pesticides*, Plenum Press, New York.

Eisenbrand, G., Ungerer, O., and Preussmann, R., 1975, The reaction of nitrite with pesticides. II. Formation, chemical properties and carcinogenic activity of the N-nitroso derivatives of N-methyl-1-naphtylcarbamate (carbaryl), *Food Cosmet. Toxicol.* **13**:365–367.

Eisenbrand, G., Schmäll, D., and Preussmann, R., 1976, Carcinogenicity in rats of high oral doses of N-nitrosocarbaryl, a nitrosated pesticide, *Cancer Lett.* **1**:281.

Elespuru, R., Lijinsky, W., and Setlow, J., 1974, Nitrosocarbaryl as a potent mutagen of environmental significance, *Nature* **247**:386–387.

Epstein, S. S., 1976, Carcinogenicity of heptachlor and chlordane, *Sci. Total Environm.* **6**:103–154.

Epstein, S., and Shafner, H., 1968, Chemical mutagens in the human environment, *Nature* **219**:385–387.

Epstein, S., Arnold, E., Andrea, J., Bass, W., and Bishop, Y., 1972, Detection of chemical mutagens by the dominant lethal assay in the mouse, *Toxicol. Appl. Pharmacol.* **23**:288–325.

Eto, M., 1974, Organophosphorus pesticides. Organic and biological chemistry, CRC Press.

Eto, M., Seifert, J., Engel, J., and Casida, J., 1980, Organophosphorus and methylcarbamate teratogens: structural requirements for inducing embryonic abnormalities in chickens and kynurenine formamidase inhibition in mouse liver, *Toxicol. Appl. Pharmacol.* **54**:20–30.

Fahrig, R., 1973, Nachweis einer genetischen Wirkung von Organophosphor-Insektiziden, *Naturwissenschaften* **60**:50–51.

Fahrig, R., 1974, Comparative mutagenicity studies with pesticides, *IARC Sci. Publ.* **10**:161–181.

Feaster, J., Van Middelem, C., and Davis, G., 1972, Zinc-DDT interrelationships in growth and reproduction in the rat, *J. Nutr.* **102**:523–527.

Federal Register, 1978, Reports on bioassays of aldrin and dieldrin for possible carcinogenicity, *Fed. Regist.* **43**:2450–2451.

Fischer, G., Schneider, P., and Scheufler, H., 1977, Zur Mutagenität von dichloracetaldehyd und 2,2-dichlor-1,1-dihydroxy-äthanphosphonsäuremethylester, möglichen Metaboliten des phosphororganischen Pestizides Trichlorforn, *Chem. Biol. Interact.* **19**:205–213.

Fitzhugh, O. G., and Nelson, A. A., 1947, Chronic oral toxicity of DDT (2,2-bis(p. chlorophenyl-1,1,1-trichloroethane)), *J. Pharmacol. Exp. Ther.* **89**:18–30.

Fitzhugh, O. G., Nelson, A. A., and Frawley, J. P., 1950, The chronic toxicities of technical hexachloride and its alpha, beta and gamma isomers, *J. Pharmacol. Exp. Ther.* **100**:59–66.

Fitzhugh, O. G., Nelson, A. A., and Quaife, M. L., 1964, Chronic oral toxicity of aldrin and dieldrin in rats and dogs, *Food Cosmet. Toxicol.* **2**:551–562.

Food and Agriculture Organization of the United States (F.A.O.), 1977, Evaluation of some pesticide residues in food, *Report* N° AGP:1975/M/13:379–392.

Food and Agriculture Organization of the United Nations (F.A.O.), 1979, Pesticide residues in food, *FAO Plant production and protection paper* **15 Rev.**:27.

Freye, H., and Scheufler, H., 1975, Experimentell ausgelöstes vorzeitiges Längenwachstum der Schneidezähne bei der Hausmaus, *Nova Acta Leopold.* **41**:183–190.

Fytizas-Danielidou, R., 1971, Effects des pesticides sur la reproduction des rats blancs. I. Lebaycide, *Meded. Fac. Landbouwwet. Rijskuniv. Gent* **36**:1146–1150.

Gentile, J., Gentile, G., Bultman, J., Sechriest, R., Wagner, E., and Plewa, M., 1982, An evaluation of the genotoxic properties of insecticides following plant and animal activation, *Mutat. Res.* **101**:19–29.

Georgian, L., 1975, The comparative cytogenetic effects of aldrin and phosphamidon, *Mutat. Res.* **31**:103–108.

Gerstengarbe, S., 1975, Die Mutagenität von Dimethoat-nachgewiesen mit dem Dominanten Letaltest an der Hausmaus (*Mus musculus* L.), *Wiss. Z. Martin-Luther-Univ. (Halle-Wittenber) Math. Naturwiss. Reihe* **24**:87–88.

Gibel, W., Lohs, Kh., Wildner, G. P., and Ziebarth, D., 1971, Tierexperimentelle Untersuchungen über hepatotoxische und kanzerogene Wirkung phosphororganischer Verbindungen, *Arch. Geschwulstforsch.* **37**:303–312.

Gibel, W., Lohs, Kh., Wildner, G. P. Ziebarth, D., and Stieglitz, R., 1973, Über die Kanzerogene hämatologische und hepatotoxische Wirkung pestizider organischer Phosphoverbindungen, *Arch. Geschwulstforsch.* **41**:311–328.

Gilot-Delhalle, J., Colizzi, A., Moutschen, J., and Moutschen-Dahmen, M., 1983, Mutagenicity of some organophosphorus compounds at the ade 6 locus of *Schizosaccharomyces pombe*. *Mutat. Res.* **117**:139–148.

Gofmekler, V., and Tabakova, S., 1970, Action of chlorophos on the embryogenesis of rats, *Farmakol. Toksikol.* **33:**735–737.

Golbs, S., Kuehnert, M., and Leue, F., 1975, Prenatal toxicological study of Sevin (carbaryl) for Wistar Rats, *Arch. Exp. Veterinaermed.* **29:**607–614.

Grant, E., Mitchell, R., West, P., Mazuch, L., and Ashwood-Smith, M., 1976, Mutagenicity and putative carcinogenicity tests of several polycyclic aromatic compounds associated with impurities of the insecticide methoxychlor, *Mutat. Res.* **40:**225–228.

Greenberg, J., and La Han, Q., 1969, Malathion-induced teratisms in the developing chick, *Can. J. Zool.* **47:**539–542.

Griffin, D., and Hill, W., 1978, *In vitro* breakage of plasmid DNA by mutagens and pesticides, *Mutat. Res.* **52:**161–169.

Grosch, D., and Valcovic, L., 1967, Chlorinated hydrocarbon insecticides are not mutagenic in *Bracon hebetor* tests, *J. Econ. Entomol.* **60:**1177–1179.

Grover, I., and Tyagi, P., 1980, Cytological effects of some common pesticides in barley, *Environm. Exp. Bot.* **20:**243–245.

Guerzoni, M., Del Cupolo, L., and Ponti, I., 1976, Attivita mutagenica degli antiparassitari, *Riv. Sci. Tecn. Alim. Nutr. Um.* **6:**161–165.

Gupta, A., and Singh, J., 1974, Dichlorvos (DDVP) induced breaks in the salivary gland chromosomes of *Drosophila melanogaster*, *Curr. Sci.* **43:**661–662.

Haag, H. B., Finnegan, J. K., Larson, P. S., Riese, W., and Dreyfuss, M. L., 1950, Comparative chronic toxicity for warmblooded animals of 2,2-bis(p chlorophenyl)-1,1,1-trichloroethane (DDT) and 2,2-bis(p methoxyphenyl)-1,1,1-trichloroethane (DMDT, methoxychlor), *Arch. Int. Pharmacodyn. Ther.* **83:**491–504.

Hanna, P., and Dyer, K., 1975, Mutagenicity of organophosphorus compounds in bacteria and *Drosophila*, *Mutat. Res.* **28:**405–420.

Harbison, R., 1975, Parathion-induced toxicity and phenobarbital-induced protection against parathion during prenatal development, *Toxicol. Appl. Pharmacol.* **32:**482–493.

Hart, N., Whang-Peng, J., Sieber, S., Fabro, S., and Adamson, R., 1972, Distribution and effects of DDT in the pregnant rabbit, *Xenobiotica* **2:**567–574.

Hashimoto, Y., Makita, T., and Noguchi, T., 1972, Teratogenic studies of O,O dimethyl S-(2 acetylaminoethyl)dithiophosphate (DAEP) in ICR-strain mice, *Oyo Yakuri* **6:**621–626.

Hodge, H. C., Maynard, E. A., and Blanchet, H. J., Jr., 1952, Chronic oral toxicity tests of methoxychlor (2,2 di-p-methoxyphenyl)-1,1,1-trichloroethane) in rats and dogs, *J. Pharmacol. Exp. Therap.* **104:**60–66.

Hodge, H. C., Maynard, E. A., Downs, W. C., Ashton, J. K., and Salerno, L. L., 1966, Tests on mice for evaluating carcinogenicity, *Toxicol. Appl. Pharmacol.* **9:**583–596.

Hoffman, W. S., Adler, H., Fishbein, W., and Bauer, F. C., 1967, Relation of pesticide concentrations in fat to pathological changes in tissues, *Arch. Environm. Health* **15:**758–765.

Holan, G., 1969, New halocyclopropane insecticides and the mode of action of DDT, *Nature* **221:**1025–1029.

Huang, C., 1972, Effect on growth but not on chromosome of the mammalian cells after treatment with three organophosphorus insecticides, *Proc. Soc. Exp. Biol. Med.* **142:**36–40.

Huff, J. E., and Gerstner, H. B., 1977, A litterature summary, Black, S. A. Kepone II. An abstract litterature collection 1952–1977, Bethesda, Maryland, National Library of Medicine, Toxicology Information Program, Toxicology Information Center ORNL/TIRC-7613.

I.A.R.C., 1974, Monographs on the evaluation of the carcinogenic risk of chemicals to man. Some organochlorine pesticides. Lyon, Vol. 5.

I.A.R.C., 1976, Monographs on the evaluation of the carcinogenic risk of chemicals to man. Some carbamates, thiocarbamates and carbazides, Lyon, vol. 12.

Innes, J., Ulland, B., Valerio, M., Petrucelli, L., Fishbein, L., Hart, E., Pallotta, R., Bates, R., Falk, H., Gart, J., Klein, M., Mitchell, J., and Peters, J., 1969, Bioassay of pesticides and industrial chemicals for tumorigenicity in mice: A preliminary note, *J. Natl. Cancer Inst.* **42**:1101–1114.

Ishidate, M., and Odashima, S., 1977, Chromosome tests with 134 compounds in Chinese hamster cells *in vitro*. A screening for chemical carcinogens, *Mutat. Res.* **48**:337–354.

Jager, K. W., 1970, *Aldrin, Dieldrin, Endrin and Telodrin: An Epidemiological and Toxicological Study of Long-Term Occupational Exposure*, Elsevier, Amsterdam, 234 p.

Jain, A., and Goswami, H. K., 1977, A comparative response to chemicals by *Allium cepa* and *Allium sativum*, *Genet. Iber.* **29**:151–161.

Jenssen, D., and Ramel, C., 1980, The micronucleus test as part of a short-term mutagenicity test program for the prediction of carcinogenicity evaluated by 143 agents tested, *Mutat. Res.* **75**:191–202.

Johnson, G., and Jalal, S., 1973, DDT-induced chromosomal damage in mice, *J. Hered.* **64**:7–8.

Jorgenson, T., Rushbrook, C., and Newell, G., 1976, *In vivo* mutagenesis investigations of ten commercial pesticides, *Toxicol. Appl. Pharmacol.* **37**:109.

Kalow, W., and Marton, A., 1961, Second-generation toxicity of malathion in rats, *Nature* **192**:464–465.

Kelly-Garvert, F., and Legator, M., 1973, Cytogenetic and mutagenic effects of DDT and DDE in a Chinese hamster cell line, *Mutat. Res.* **17**:223–229.

Kemèny, T., and Tarján, R., 1966, Investigations on the effects of chronically administered small amounts of DDT in mice, *Experientia* **22**:748–749.

Kennedy, G. L., Jr., Smith, S. H., Kinoshita, F. K., Keplinger, M. L., and Calandra, J. C., 1977, Teratogenic evaluation of piperonyl butoxide in the rat, *Food Cosmet. Toxicol.* **15**:337–339.

Khera, K., 1966, Toxic and teratogenic effects of insecticides in duck and chick embryos, *Toxicol. Appl. Pharmacol.* **8**:345.

Khera, K., 1979, Evaluation of dimethoate (Cygon 4E) for teratogenic activity in the cat, *J. Environ. Pathol. Toxicol.* **2**:1283–1288.

Khera, K., Villeneuve, D., Terry, G., Panopio, L., Nash, L., and Trivett, G., 1976, Mirex: A teratogenicity, dominant lethal and tissue distribution study in rats, *Food Cosmet. Toxicol.* **14**:25–29.

Khera, K., Whallen, C., and Trivett, G., 1978, Teratogenicity studies on linuron, malathion and methoxychlor in rats, *Toxicol. Appl. Pharmacol.* **45**:435–444.

Khera, K., Whalen, C., Trivett, G., and Angers, G., 1979, Teratogenicity studies on pesticidal formulations of dimethoate, diuron and lindane in rats, *Bull. Environ. Contam. Toxicol.* **22**:522–529.

Kimbrough, R., and Gaines, T., 1968, Effect of organic phosphorus compounds and alkylating agents on the rat fetus, *Arch. Environ. Health.* **16**:805–808.

Kimbrough, R., Gaines, T. B., and Scherman, J. D., 1964, Nutritional factors, long-term DDT intake, and chloroleukemia in rats, *J. Nat. Cancer Inst.* **33**:215–225.

Kimbrough, R. D., Gaines, T. B., and Hayes, W. S., Jr., 1968, Combined effects of DDT, pyrethrum and piperonyl butoxide on rat liver, *Arch. Environ. Health* **16**:333–341.

Kimbrough, R. D., Gaines, T. B., and Liwder, R. E., 1971, The ultrastructure of livers of rats fed DDT and dieldrin, *Arch. Environ. Health* **22**:460–467.

Kiraly, J., Szentesi, I., Ruzicska, M., and Czeizel, A., 1979, Chromosome studies in workers producing organophosphate insecticides, *Arch. Environ. Contamin. Toxicol.* **8**:309–319.

Klotzsche, C., 1970, Teratologic and embryotoxic investigations with formothion and thiometon, *Pharm. Acta Helv.* **45**:434–440.

Kostoff, D., 1931, Heteroploidy in *Nicotiana tabacum* and *Solanum melongena* caused by fumigation with nicotine sulphate, *Bull. Soc. Bot. Bulg.* **4**:87–92.

Kostoff, D., 1948, Cytogenetic changes and atypical growth induced by hexachlorocyclohexane ($C_6H_6Cl_6$), *Curr. Sci.* **17**:294–295.

Kramers, P., and Knaap, A., 1975, Absence of a mutagenic effect after feeding dichlorvos to larvae of *Drosophila melanogaster*, *Mutat. Res.* **57**:103–105.

Kuhr, J., and Dorough, H. W., 1976, *Carbamate Insecticides: Chemistry, Biochemistry, and Toxicology*, CRC Press.

Kurinniy, A., and Pilinskaya, M., 1977, Cytogenetic activity of pesticides Imidan, Dipterex and Gardona in cultured human lymphocytes, *Genetika* **13**:337–339.

Lamb, M., 1977, Mutagenicity tests with metrifonate in *Drosophila melanogaster*, *Mutat. Res.* **56**:157–162.

Larsen, C. D., 1947, Evaluation of carcinogenicity of a series of esters of carbamic acid, *J. Nat. Cancer Inst.* **8**:99–101.

Larsen, K., and Jalal, S., 1974, DDT induced chromosome mutations in mice. Further testing, *Can. J. Genet. Cytol.* **16**:491–497.

Lawley, P., Shah, S., and Orr, D., 1974, Methylation of nucleic acid by 2,2-dichlorovinyl dimethyl phosphate, *Chem. Biol. Interact.* **8**:171–182.

Laws, E. R., 1971, Evidence of antitumorigenic effects of DDT, *Arch. Environ. Health* **23**:181–184.

Laws, E. R., and Biros, F. J., 1967, Men with intensive occupational exposure to DDT, *Arch. Environ. Health* **15**:766–775.

Laws, E. R., Jr., Maddrey, W. C., Curley, A., and Burse, V. W., 1973, Long-term occupational exposure to DDT. Effect on the human liver, *Arch. Environ. Health* **27**:318–321.

Lehman, A. J., 1948, The toxicology of the newer agricultural chemicals, *Q. Bull. Ass. Food Drug Off. U.S.* **13**:82.

Lehman, A. J., 1952, Chemicals in foods: A report to the association of Food and Drug Officials on current developments, Part II, Pesticides, Section III, *Q. Bull. Ass. Food Drug Off. U.S.* **26**:47–53.

Leibovich, D., 1973, Embryotropic action of small doses of the organophosphorous pesticides Chlorophos, metaphos, and carbophos, *Gig. Sanit.* **8**:21–24.

Lessa, J., Beçak, W., Rabello, M., Pereira, C., and Ungaro, M., 1976, Cytogenetic study of DDT on human lymphocytes *in vitro*, *Mutat. Res.* **40**:131–138.

Lijinsky, W., and Schmähl, D., 1978, Carcinogenicity of N-nitroso derivatives of N-methylcarbamate insecticides in rats, *Ecotoxicol. Environ. Safety* **2**:413–419.

Lijinsky, W., and Taylor, H. W., 1976, Carcinogenesis in Sprague–Dawley rats of N-nitroso-N-alkylcarbamate esters. *Cancer Lett.* **1**:275.

Lijinsky, W., and Taylor, H. W., 1977, Transplacental chronic toxicity test of carbaryl with nitrite in rats, *Food Cosmet. Toxicol.* **15**:229–232.

Löfroth, G., 1970, Alkylation of DNA by dichlorvos, *Naturwissenschaften* **57**:393–394.

Löfroth, G., Kim, C., and Hussain, S., 1969, Alkylating property of 2,2-dichlorovinyl dimethyl phosphate: A disregarded hazard, *EMS Newslett.* **2**:21–26.

Logvinenko, V., and Morgun, V., 1978, Study of the mutagenic effect of some pesticides on spring durum wheat, *Tsitol. Genet.* **12**:207–212.

Lorke, D., and Löser, E., 1965, BAY 15922, Chronische toxikologische Untersuchungen an Ratten, *Unveröff. Bericht* **29**:7.

Lutz, H., and Lutz-Ostertag, Y., 1971, Action de l'azinphos (insecticide organo-phosphoré) sur l'embryon de faisan, de perdrix grise et de perdrix rouge, *Bull. Soc. Zool. Fr.* **96**:265–271.

Lutz–Ostertag, Y., and David, D., 1973, Action du DDT sur le tractus urogénital de l'embryon de poulet et de caille, *C. R. Acad. Sci.* (*Paris*) **276**:1213–1216.

Lutz-Ostertag, Y., and Kantelip, J., 1971, Action stérilisante de l'endosulfan (Thiodan) (insecticide organo-chloré) sur les gonades de l'embryon de poulet et de caille "*in vivo*" et "*in vitro*," *C. R. Soc. Biol.* **165**:844–848.

Lutz-Ostertag, Y., and Lutz, H., 1969, Note préliminaire sur les effets "oestrogenes" de l'aldrine sur le tractus uro-genital de l'embryon d'oiseau, *C. R. Acad. Sci.* (*Paris*) **269**:484–486.

Mahr, U., and Miltenburger, H., 1976, The effect of insecticides on Chinese hamster cell cultures, *Mutat. Res.* **40**:107–118.

Maier-Bode, H., 1960, DDT im Körperfett des Menschen, *Med. Exp.* **1**:146–152.

Majumdar, S., Kopelman, H., and Schnitman, M., 1976, Dieldrin-induced chromosome damage in mouse bone-marrow and W1-38 human lung cells, *J. Hered.* **67**:303–307.

Marshall, T., Dorough, H., and Swim, H., 1976, Screening of pesticides for mutagenic potential using *Salmonella typhimurium*, *J. Agric. Food Chem.* **24**:560–563.

Martson, L., and Voronina, V., 1976, Experimental study of the effect of a series of phosphoroorganic pesticides (Dipterex and Imidan) on embryogenesis, *Environ. Health Perspect.* **13**:121–125.

Matsuoka, A., Hayashi, M., and Ishidate, M. Jr., 1979, Chromosomal aberration tests on 29 chemicals combined with S9 mix *in vitro*, *Mutat. Res.* **66**:277–290.

Mazuch, L., Mitchell, R. H., and West, P. R., 1975, Isolation of tetrakis (p-methoxyphenyl) ethylene from commercial methoxychlor (2,2-bis(4 methoxyphenyl)-1,1,1-trichlorethane), DMDT, *Chem. Ind.* **1**:399–400.

McCann, J., Choi, E., Yamasaki, E., and Ames, B., 1975, Detection of carcinogens as mutagens in the *Salmonella*/microsome test: Assay of 300 chemicals, *Proc. Nat. Acad. Sci. (USA)* **72**:5135–5139.

McCarthy, J., Fancher, O., Kennedy, G., Keplinger, M., and Calandra, J., 1971, Reproduction and teratology studies with the insecticide carbofuran, *Toxicol. Appl. Pharmacol.* **19**:370.

Meiniel, R., 1973, L'action tératogene d'un insecticide organophosphoré(le parathion) chez l'embryon d'oiseau, *Arch. Anat. Histol. Embryol. Norm. Exp.* **56**:97–110.

Meiniel, R., 1976, Pluralité dans le déterminisme des effets tératogènes des composés organophosphorés, *Experientia* **32**:920–921.

Meiniel, R., 1977, Activites cholinestérasiques et expression de la tératogenèse axiale chez l'embryon de caille exposé aux organophosphores, *C. R. Acad. Sci. (Paris)* **285**:401–404.

Meyer, J. R., 1945, Prefixing with para-dichlorobenzene to facilitate chromosome study, *Stain Technol.* **20**:121–125.

Michalek, S., and Brockman, H., 1969, A test for mutagenicity of Shell No-Pest Strip insecticide in *Neurospora crassa*, *Neurospora Newslett.* **14**:8.

Miyamoto, J., 1976, Degradation, metabolism and toxicity of synthetic pyrethroids, *Environ. Health Perspect.* **14**:15–28.

Mizusaki, S., Okamoto, H., Akiyama, A., and Fukuhara, Y., 1977, Relation between chemical constitutents of tobacco and mutagenic activity of cigarette smoke condensate, *Mutat. Res.* **48**:319–326.

Mohn, G., 1973a, 5-methyltryptophan resistance mutations in *Escherichia coli* K-12. Mutagenic activity of monofunctional alkylating agents including organophosphorus insecticides, *Mutat. Res.* **20**:7–15.

Mohn, G., 1973b, Comparison of the mutagenic activity of eight organophosphorus insecticides in *Escherichia coli*, *Mutat. Res.* **21**:196.

Molina, L., Rinkus, S., and Legator, M., 1978, Evaluation of the micronucleus procedure over a 2-year period, *Mutat. Res.* **53**:125.

Morpurgo, G., Aulicino, F., Bignami, M., Conti, L., and Velcich, A., 1977, Relationship between structure and mutagenicity of dichlorvos and other pesticides, *Atti Accad. Naz. Lincei Mem. Cl. Sci. Fis. Mat. Nat.* **62**:692–701.

Moutschen-Dahmen, J., Degraeve, N., Houbrechts, N., and Colizzi, A., 1976, Cytotoxicity of carbaryl alone and combined with nitrites, *Mutat. Res.* **38**:122–123.

Moutschen, J., Moutschen-Dahmen, M., Gilot-Delhalle, J., Colizzi, A., and Degraeve, N., 1979, Comparison of the efficiency of different tests to evaluate mutagenicity of organophosphates, *Mutat. Res.* **64**:114.

Moutschen, J., Moutschen-Dahmen, M., and Degraeve, N., 1981, Metrifonate and dichlorvos: cytogenetic investigations, *Acta Pharmacol. Toxicol.* **49**(Suppt. 5):29–39.

Murray, F., Staples, R., and Schwetz, B., 1979, Teratogenic potential of carbaryl given to rabbits
and mice by gavage or by dietary inclusion, *Toxicol. Appl. Pharmacol.* **51**:81–89.

Nagasaki, H., Tomii, S., Mega, T., Marugami, M., and Ito, N., 1972a, Carcinogenicity of benzene
hexachloride (BHC), in *Topics in Chemical Carcinogenesis*, (edited by W. Nakahara, S.
Takayama, T, Sugimura, and S. Odashima), University of Tokyo Press, Tokyo.

Nagasaki, H., Tomii, S., Mega, T., Marugami, M., and Ito, N., 1972b, Hepatocarcinogenic effet
of alpha-, beta-, gamma-, and sigma-isomers of benzene hexachloride in mice, *Gann*
**63**:393.

Naithani, S., and Sarbhoy, R., 1973, Cytological studies in *Lens esculenta* Moench, *Cytologia*
**38**:195–203.

National Cancer Institute, 1976, Report on carcinogenesis bioassay of technical grade Chlordecone (Kepone) availability, *Clin. Toxicol.* **9**:603–607.

National Cancer Institute, 1977, Carcinogenesis bioassay of dichlorvos, (*NCI-CG-TR10*) *DHEW
Public. No.* (*NIH*):77–810.

National Cancer Institute, 1978, Carcinogenesis bioassay of tetrachlorvinphos, (*NCI-CG-TR33*)
*DHEW Public. No.* (NIH):78–833.

National Cancer Institute, 1978b, Carcinogenesis Technical Reports. Bioassay of methoxychlor
for possible carcinogenicity, Series No. 35.

National Cancer Institute, 1979, Carcinogenesis bioassay of parathion, (*NCI-CG-TR70*) *DHEW
Public. No.* (*NIH*):78–1340.

Nelson, A. A., 1942, Pathological changes in rabbits produced by inunction of methoxy DDT,
30% in NTM, Prepared as memorandum to A. J. Lehman, Food and Drug Administration,
Washington D.C., December 9.

Nelson, A. A., 1951, Pathological changes produced in rats by feeding of methoxychlor at levels
up to 0.2% of diet for two years, Prepared as a memorandum to A. J. Lehman, Food and
Drug Administration, Washington D.C., October 23.

Nelson, A. A., 1953, Pathological changes produced in dogs by feeding of methoxychlor 300
mg/kg/day for 3-½ years, Prepared as a memorandum to A. J. Lehman, Food and Drug
Administration, Washington D.C., June 9.

Nelson, D., 1974, Pharmacology and toxicology of Guthion, *Residue Rev.* **51**:136–139.

Nicholas, A., Vienne, M., and Van Den Berghe, H., 1978, Sister chromatid exchange frequencies
in cultured human cells exposed to an organophosphorus insecticide—dichlorvos, *Toxicol.
Lett.* **2**:271–276.

Nicholas, A., Vienne, M., and Van Den Berghe, H., 1979, Induction of sister chromatid
exchanges in cultured human cells by an organophosphorus insecticide: malathion, *Mutat.
Res.* **67**:167–172.

Nishio, A., and Uyeki, E., 1981. Induction of sister chromatid exchanges in Chinese hamster
ovary cells by organophosphate insecticides and their oxygen analogs. *J. Toxicol. Environ.
Health* **8**:939–946.

Noda, K., Numata, H., Hirabayashi, M., and Endo, I., 1972a, Effect of pesticides on embryos. 1.
Effect of organophosphorus pesticides, *Oyo Yakuri* **6**:667–672.

Noda, K., Hirabayashi, M., Yonemura, I., Maruyama, M., and Endo, I., 1972b, Effect of
pesticides on embryos. 2. Effect of organochlorine pesticides, *Oyo Yakuri* **6**:673–679.

Nybom, N., and Knutsson, B., 1947, Investigations on C-mitosis in *Allium cepa*, *Hereditas*
**33**:220–234.

Oehlkers, F., 1952, Chromosome breaks induced by chemicals, *J. Heredity* (*Suppl.*) **6**:95–105.

Ortega, P., Hayes, W. J., and Durham, W. F., 1957, Pathologic changes in liver of rats after
feeding low levels of various insecticides, *Arch. Pathol.* **64**:614–622.

Ortelee, M. F., 1958, Study of men with prolonged intensive occupational exposure to DDT,
*Arch. Ind. Health* **18**:433–440.

Ottoboni, A., 1969, Effect of DDT on reproduction in the rat, *Toxicol. Appl. Pharmacol.*
**14**:74–81.

Ottolenghi, A., Haseman, J., and Suggs, F., 1974, Teratogenic effects of aldrin, dieldrin, and endrin in hamsters and mice, *Teratology* 9:11–16.

Palmer, A., Bottomley, A., Worden, A., Frohberg, H., and Bauer, A., 1978a, Effect of lindane on pregnancy in the rabbit and rat, *Toxicology* 9:239–247.

Palmer, A., Cozens, D., Spicer, E., and Worden, A., 1978b, Effects of lindane upon reproductive function in a 3-generation study in rats, *Toxicology* 10:45–54.

Palmer, K., Green, S., and Legator, M., 1972, Cytogenetic effects of DDT and derivatives of DDT in cultured mammalian cell line, *Toxicol. Appl. Pharmacol.* 22:355–364.

Palmer, K., Green, S., and Legator, M., 1973, Dominant lethal study of *p-p′*-DDT in rats, *Food Cosmet. Toxicol.* 11:53–62.

Panda, B., and Sharma, C., 1979, Organophosphate induced chlorophyll mutations in *Hordeum vulgare*, *Theor. Appl. Genet.* 55:253–255.

Panda, B., and Sharma, C., 1980, Cytogenetic hazards from agricultural chemicals. 3. Monitoring the cytogenetic activity of trichlorfon and dichlorvos in *Hordeum vulgare*, *Mutat. Res.* 78:341–345.

Park, S., and Lee, S., 1977, Genetic effects of pesticides in the mammalian cells. I. Induction of micronucleus, *Korean J. Zool.* 20:19–28.

Paul, B., and Vadlamudi, V., 1976, Teratogenic studies of fenitrothion on White Leghorn chick embryos, *Bull. Environ. Contam. Toxicol.* 15:223–229.

Poland, A., 1970, Effect of intensive occupational exposure to DDT on phenylbutazone and cortisol metabolism in human subjects, *Clin. Pharmacol. Ther.* 11:724–732.

Poole, D., Simmon, V., and Newell, G., 1977, *In vitro* mutagenic activity of fourteen pesticides, *Toxicol. Appl. Pharmacol.* 41:196.

Poussel, H., 1948, Mecanisme de quelques actions toxiques exercées par les dérivés chlorés des carbures aliphatiques et les hexachlorocyclohexanes, *Gallica Biol. Acta* 1:11–23.

Probst, G., Mc Mahon, R., Hill, L., Thompson, C., Epp, J., and Neal, S., 1981, Chemically induced unscheduled DNA synthesis in primary rat hepatocyte cultures: A comparison with bacterial mutagenicity using 218 compounds. *Environ. Mutagenesis.* 3:11–32.

Quinto, I., Martire, G., Vricella, G., Riccardi, F., Perfumo, A., Giulivo, R., and De Lorenzo, F., 1981, Screening of 24 pesticides by *Salmonella*/microsome assay: mutagenicity of benazolin, mctoxuron and paraoxon, *Mutat. Res.* 85:265.

Rubello, M., Becak, W., De Almeida, W., Pigati, P., Ungaro, M., Murata, T., and Pereira, C., 1975, Cytogenetic study on individuals occupationally exposed to DDT, *Mutat. Res.* 28:449–454.

Radomski, J. L., Deichmann, W. B., Mac Donald, W. E., and Glass, E. M., 1965, Synergism among oral carcinogens. I. Results of the simultaneous feeding of four tumorigens to rats, *Toxicol. Appl. Pharmacol.* 7:652–656.

Radomski, J. L., Deichmann, W. B., Clizer, E. E., and Rey, A., 1968, Pesticide concentrations in the liver, brain and adipose tissue of terminal hospital patients, *Food Cosmet. Toxicol.* 6:209–220.

Ravindran, P., 1971, Cytological effects of folidol, *Cytologia* 36:504–508.

Reddy, M., and Rao, B., 1969, The cytological effects of insecticides (Dimecron-100 and Rogor-40) on *Vicia faba*, *Cytologia* 34:408–417.

Reddy, P., Reddy, G., and Subramanyan, S., 1974, Cytological effects of the insecticide "Sevin" on the meiotic cells of *Poecilocerus pictus*, *Curr. Sci.* 43:187–189.

Regan, J., Setlow, R., Francis, A., and Lijinsky, W., 1976, Nitrosocarbaryl: its effect on human DNA, *Mutat. Res.* 38:293–302.

Reis, C., Pellegatti, I., Oga, S., and Zanini, A., 1971, Toxic and teratogenic activities of anticholinesterase substances. I. Teratogenic activity of parathion in chick embryos, *Rev. Farm. Bioquim. Univ. Sao Paulo* 9:343–355.

Reuber, M. D., 1979, Interstitial cell carcinomas of the testis in BALB/c male mice ingesting methoxychlor, *J. Cancer Res. Clin. Oncol.* 93:173.

Reuber, M. D., 1980, Carcinogenicity and toxicity of methoxychlor, *Environ. Health Perspect.* **36**:205–219.

Reuber, M., 1981, Carcinogenicity of Dichlorvos. *Clin. Toxicol.* **18**:47–84.

Rivett, K. F., Chesterman, H., Kellett, D. N., Newman, A. J., and Worden, A. N., 1978, Effects of feeding lindane to dogs for periods of up to 2 years, *Toxicology* **7**:273–289.

Robens, J., 1969, Teratologic studies of carbaryl, diazinon, norea, disulfiram, and thiram in small laboratory animals, *Toxicol. Appl. Pharmacol.* **15**:152–163.

Robinson, J., Richardson, A., Hunter, C. G., and Crabtree, A. N., 1965, Organochlorine insecticide content of human adipose tissue in southeastern England, *Br. J. Ind. Med.* **22**:220–229.

Roger, J., Upshall, D., and Casida, J., 1969, Structure, activity and metabolism studies on organophosphate teratogens and their alleviating agents in developing hen eggs, with special emphasis on bidrin, *Biochem. Pharmacol.* **18**:373–392.

Rossi, L., Ravera, M., Repi, G. III, and Santi, L., 1977, Long term administration of DDT or phenobarbital-Na in Wistar rats, *Int. J. Cancer* **19**(2):179–185.

Rumsey, T. S., Samuelson, G., Bowd, J., and Daniels, F. L., 1974, Teratogenicity to 35-day excretion patterns and placental transfer in beef heifers administered 4-tert-butyl-2 chlorophenyl methyl methylphosphoramidate (Ruelene®), *J. Anim. Sci.* **39**:386–391.

Sarbhoy, R., 1971, Cytogenetical studies of some pulses and beans, *D. Phil. Thesis* Allahabad Univ.

Sarbhoy, R., 1980, Effect of paradichlorobenzene on the somatic chromosomes and mitosis of *Lens esculenta* (L) Moench, *Cytologia* **45**:381–388.

Sax, K., and Sax, H., 1968, Possible mutagenic hazards of some food additives, beverages and insecticides, *Jpn. J. Genet.* **43**:89–94.

Scheufler, H., 1975, Effect of relatively high doses of dimethoate and trichlorfon on the embryogenesis of laboratory mice, *Biol. Rundsch.* **13**:238–240.

Schiemann, S., 1975, Untersuchungen zur mutagenen Wirkung von Trichlorfon auf die Hausmaus unter besonderer Berücksichtigung des dominanten Letaltestes, *Wiss. Z. Martin-Luther Univ. (Halle-Wittenberg) Math. Naturwiss. Reihe* **24**:85–86.

Schmidt, R., 1975, Zur Wirkung von 1,1,1-Trichlor-2,2-bis(p-chlorphenyl)-äthan (DDT) auf die Praenatalentwicklung der Hausmaus, *Nova Acta Leopold.* **41**:271–344.

Schoeny, R., Smith, C., and Loper, J., 1979, Non-mutagenicity for *Salmonella* of the chlorinated hydrocarbons Arachlor 1254, 1,2,4-trichlorobenzene, mirex and kepone, *Mutat. Res.* **68**:125–132.

Schom, C., Abbott, U., and Walker, N., 1979, Adult and embryo responses to organophosphate pesticide: Azodrin, *Poult. Sci.* **58**:60–66.

Schwetz, B., Ioset, H., Leong, B., and Staples, R., 1979, Teratogenic potential of dichlorvos given by inhalation and gavage to mice and rabbits, *Teratology* **20**:383–387.

Segerbäck, D., 1981, Estimation of genetic risks of alkylating agents. V. Methylation of DNA in the mouse by DDVP (2,2-dichlorovinyl dimethyl phosphate), *Hereditas* **94**:73–76.

Seiler, J., 1977a, Inhibition of testicular DNA synthesis by chemical mutagens and carcinogens. Preliminary results in the validation of a novel short-term test, *Mutat. Res.* **46**:305–310.

Seiler, J., 1977b, Nitrosation *in vitro* and *in vivo* by sodium nitrite, and mutagenicity of nitrogenous pesticides, *Mutat. Res.* **48**:225–236.

Sharma, A. K., and Bhattacharya, N. K., 1956, Chromosome breakage through para-dichlorobenzene treatment, *Cytologia* **21**:253–260.

Sharma, A. K., and Mookerjea, A., 1955, Paradichlorobenzene and other chemicals in chromosome work, *Stain Technol.* **30**:1–7.

Shiau, S., Huff, R., Wells, B., and Felkner, I., 1980, Mutagenicity and DNA-damaging activity for several pesticides tested with *Bacillus subtilis* mutants, *Mutat. Res.* **71**:169–179.

Shimkin, M. B., Wieder, R., McDonough, M., Fischbein, L., and Swern, D., 1969, Lung tumor response in strain A mice as a quantitative bioassay of carcinogenic activity of some carbamates and aziridines, *Cancer Res.* **29**:2184–2190.

Shirasu, Y., Moriya, M., Kato, K., and Kada, T., 1975, Mutagenicity screening of pesticides in microbial systems, II, *Mutat. Res.* **31**:268–269.

Shirasu, y., Moriya, M., Kato, K., Furumashi, A., and Kada, T., 1976, Mutagenicity screening of pesticides in microbial system, *Mutat. Res.* **40**:19–30.

Shirasu, Y., Moriya, M., Tezuka, H., Teramoto, S., Ohta, T., and Inoue, T., 1982, Mutagenicity screening studies on pesticides, in *Environmental Mutagens and Carcinogens* (Sugimura, T., Kondo, S., and Takabe, H., eds.) pp. 331–335, Alan Liss, New York.

Short, R., Minor, J., Lee, C., Chernoff, N., and Baron, R., 1980, Developmental toxicity of guthion in rats and mice, *Arch. Toxicol.* **43**:177–186.

Shtenberg, A., and Ozhovan, M., 1971, Effect of low sevin doses in the reproductive function of animals in a number of generations, *Vop. Pitan.* **30**:42–49.

Siebert, D., and Eisenbrand, G., 1974, Induction of mitotic gene conversion in *Saccharomyces cerevisiae* by N-nitrosated pesticides, *Mutat. Res.* **22**:121–126.

Siebert, D., and Lemperle, E., 1974, Genetic effects of herbicides: Induction of mitotic gene conversion in *Saccharomyces cerevisiae*, *Mutat. Res.* **22**:111–120.

Simmon, V., and Kauhanen, K., 1978a, *In vitro* microbiological mutagenicity assays of aldrin, *Stanford Res. Inst. Rept.*, 15 pp.

Simmon, V., and Kauhanen, K., 1978b, *In vitro* microbiological mutagenicity assays of dieldrin, *Stanford Res. Inst. Rept.*, 14 pp.

Simmon, V., Poole, D., and Newell, G., 1976, *In vitro* mutagenic studies of twenty pesticides, *Toxicol. Appl. Pharmacol.* **37**:109.

Simmon, V., Kauhanen, K., and Tardiff, R., 1977, Mutagenic activity of chemicals identified in drinking water, *Develop. Toxicol. Environ. Sci.* **2**:249–258.

Singh, B. Singh, R., Singh, R. Singh, Y., and Singh, J., 1979, Effect of insecticides on germination, early growth and cytogenetic behaviour of barley (*Hordeum vulgare*), *Environ. Exp. Bot.* **19**:127–132.

Smalley, H., Curtis, J., and Earl, F., 1968, Teratogenic action of carbaryl in beagle dogs, *Toxicol. Appl. Pharmacol.* **13**:392–403.

Sobels, F., and Todd, N., 1979, Absence of a mutagenic effect of dichlorvos in *Drosophila melanogaster*, *Mutat. Res.* **67**:89–92.

Solomon, H., and Weis, J., 1979, Abnormal circulatory development in medaka caused by the insecticides carbaryl, malathion and parathion, *Teratology* **19**:51–62.

Srivastava, L. M., 1966, Induction of mitotic abnormalities in certain genera of Tribe *Vicieae* by para-dichlorobenzene, *Cytologia* **31**:166–171.

Staples, R., and Goulding, E., 1979, Dipterex teratogenicity in the rat, hamster, and mouse when given by gavage, *Environ. Health Perspect.* **30**:105–113.

Staples, R., Kellam, R., and Haseman, J., 1976, Developmental toxicity in the rat after ingestion or gavage of organophosphate pesticides (Dipterex, Imidan) during pregnancy, *Environ. Health Perspect.* **13**:133–140.

Stieglitz, R., Gibel, W., and Werner, W., 1974, Experimental study on haematotoxic and leukaemogenic effects on trichlorfon and dimethoate, *Acta Haemat* (*Basel*) **52(2)**:70–76.

Sternberg, S. S., 1979, The carcinogenesis, mutagenesis and teratogenesis of insecticides, Reviews of studies in animals and man, *Pharmacol. Ther.* **6(1)**:147–166.

Stevenson, D. E., Thorpe, E., Hunt, P. F., and Walker, A. I. T., 1976, The toxic effects of dieldrin in rats: A reevaluation of data obtained in a two-year feeding study, *Toxicol. Appl. Pharmacol.* **36**:247–254.

Talens, G., and Wooley, D., 1973, Effects of parathion administration during gestation in the rat on development of the young, *Proc. West. Pharmacol. Soc.* **16**:141–145.

Tanimura, T., Katsuya, T., and Nishimura, H., 1967, Embryotoxicity of acute exposure to methyl parathion in rats and mice, *Arch. Environ. Health* **15:**609–613.

Tarján, R., and Kemèny, T., 1969, Multigeneration studies on DDT in mice, *Food Cosmet, Toxicol.* **7:**215–222.

Taylor, J. R., Selhorst, J. B., Houff, S. A., and Martinez, A. J., 1978, Chlordecone intoxication in man. I. Clinical observations, *Neurology* **28:**626–630.

Tezuka, H., Ando, N., Suzuki, R., Terahata, M., Moriya, M., and Shirasu, Y., 1980, Sister-chromatid exchanges and chromosomal aberrations in cultured Chinese hamster cells treated with pesticides positive in microbial reversion assays, *Mutat. Res.* **78:**177–191.

Thorpe, E., and Walker, A. I. T., 1973, The toxicology of dieldrin (HEOD). II. Comparative oral toxicity of long term oral toxicity studies in mice with dieldrin, DDT, phenobarbitone, $\beta$BHC and $\gamma$BHC, *Food Cosmet. Toxicol.* **11:**433.

Thorpe, E., Wilson, A., Dix, K., and Blair, D., 1972, Teratological studies with dichlorvos vapor in rabbits and rats, *Arch. Toxicol.* **30:**29–38.

Tomatis, L., Turosov, V., Day, N., and Charles, R. T., 1972, The effect of long term exposure to DDT on DF1 mice, *Int. J. Cancer* **10:**489–506.

Tos-Luty, S., Puchala-Matysek, W., and Latuszynska, J., 1973, Carbaryl toxicity in chick embryo, *Bromatol. Chem. Toksykol.* **6:**409–411.

Trepanier, G., Marchessault, F., Bansal, J., and Chagnon, A., 1977, Cytological effects of insecticides on a human lymphoblastoid cell line, *In Vitro* **13:**201.

Trinh Van Bao, Szabo, I., Ruzicska, P., and Czeizel, A., 1974, Chromosome aberrations in patients suffering acute organic phosphate insecticide intoxication, *Humangenetik* **24:**33–57.

Truhaut, R., 1954, Communication au Symposium International de la Prévention du Cancer, Sao Paulo, Cited by FAO/WHO Expert Committee on Pesticide Residues, 1968, Evaluation of Some Pesticide Residues, *WHO/FOOD Add.* **67.32:**130.

Turosov, V. S., Day, N., Tomatis, L., Gati, E., and Charles, R. T., 1973, Tumors in CF1 mice exposed for six consecutive generations to DDT, *J. Nat. Cancer Inst.* **51:**983–997.

Tyrkiel, E., 1977, Mutagenic action of O-isopropoxyphenyl-N-methyl-carbamate (Propoxur) on mouse gametes, *Rocz. Pzh.* **28:**601–613.

Ulland, B. M., Page, N. P., Squire, R. A., Weisburger, E. K., and Cypher, R. L., 1977, A carcinogenicity assay of mirex in Charles River CD rats, *J. Nat. Cancer Inst.* **58:**133–140.

Upshall, D. G., 1972, Correlation of chick embryo teratogenicity with the nicotinic activity of a series of tetrahydropyrimidines, *Teratology* **5:**287–294.

Upshall, D., Roger, J., and Casida, J. 1968, Biochemical studies on the teratogenic action of bidrin and other neuroactive agents in the developing hen egg, *Biochem. Pharmacol.* **17:**1529–1542.

Usha Rani, M., Reddy, O., and Reddy, P., 1980, Mutagenicity studies involving aldrin, endosulfan, dimethoate, phosphamidon, carbaryl and ceresan, *Bull. Environ. Contam. Toxicol.* **25:**277–282.

Vaarama, A., 1947, Experimental studies on the influence of DDT insecticide upon plant mitosis, *Hereditas* **33:**191–219.

Van Raalte, H. G. S., 1977, Human experience with dieldrin in perspective, *Ecotoxicol. Environ. Safety* **1:**203–210.

Vettorazzi, G., 1976, State of the art of the toxicological evaluation carried out by the Joint FAO/WHO Meeting on pesticide residues. II. Carbamate and organophosphorus pesticides used in agriculture and public health, *Residue Rev.* **63:**1–44.

Vogel, E., 1972, Mutagenitätsuntersuchugen mit DDT und den DDT-Metaboliten DDE, DDD, DDOM und DDA an *Drosophila melanogaster*, *Mutat. Res.* **16:**157–164.

Vogel, E., 1974, Mutagenic activity of the insecticide oxydemeton methyl in a resistant strain of *Drosophila melanogaster*, *Experientia* **30:**396–397.

Vogin, E., and Carson, S., 1971, Teratology studies with dichlorvos in rabbits, *Toxicol. Appl. Pharmacol.* **19:**377–378.

Voogd, C., Jacobs, J., and Van Der Stel, J., 1972, On the mutagenic action of dichlorvos, *Mutat. Res.* **16:**413–416.

Wade, M., Moyer, J., and Hine, C., 1979, Mutagenic action of a series of epoxides, *Mutat. Res.* **66:**367–371.

Walker, A. I. T., Stevenson, D. E., Robinson, J., Thorpe, E., and Roberts, M., 1969, The toxicology and pharmacodynamics of dieldrin (HEOD): Two year oral exposures of rats and dogs, *Toxicol. Appl. Pharmacol.* **15:**345–373.

Walker, N., 1971, The effect of malathion and malaoxon on esterases and gross development of the chick embryo, *Toxicol. Appl. Pharmacol.* **19:**590–601.

Wallace, M., Knights, P., and Dye, A., 1976, Pilot study of the mutagenicity of DDT in mice, *Environ. Pollut.* **11:**217–222.

Ware, G., and Good, E., 1967, Effects of insecticides on reproduction in the laboratory mouse. II. Mirex, telodrin and DDT, *Toxicol. Appl. Pharmacol.* **10:**54–61.

Weil, C., Woodside, M., Carpenter, C., and Smyth, H., 1972, Current status of tests of carbaryl for reproductive and teratogenic effect, *Toxicol. Appl. Pharmacol.* **21:**390–404.

Weil, C., Woodside, M., Bernard, J., Condra, N., King, J., and Carpenter, C., 1973, Comparative effect of carbaryl on rat reproduction and guinea pig teratology when fed either in the diet or by stomach intubation, *Toxicol. Appl. Pharmacol.* **26:**621–638.

Weis, P., and Weis, J., 1974, Cardiac malformations and other effects due to insecticides in embryos of the killifish, *Fundulus heteroclitus, Teratology* **10:**263–268.

Weisse, I., and Herbst, M., 1977, Carcinogenicity study of lindane in the mouse, *Toxicology* **7:**233–238.

Wild, D., 1973, Chemical induction of streptomycin-resistant mutations in *Escherichia coli.* Dose and mutagenic effects of dichlorvos and methyl methanesulfonate, *Mutat. Res.* **19:**33–41.

Wild, D., 1975, Mutagenicity studies on organophosphorus insecticides, *Mutat. Res.* **32:**133–150.

Witherup, S., Jolley, W., Stemmer, R., and Pfitzer, E., 1971, Chronic toxicity studies with 2,2-dichlorovinyl dimethyl phosphate (DDVP) in dogs and rats including observations on rat reproduction, *Toxicol. Appl. Pharmacol.* **19:**377.

Wuu, K., and Grant, W., 1966, Morphological and somatic chromosomal aberrations induced by pesticides in barley (*Hordeum vulgare*), *Can. J. Genet. Cytol.* **8:**481–501.

Wuu, K., and Grant, W. 1967, Chromosomal aberrations induced by pesticides in meiotic cells of barley, *Cytologia* **32:**31–41.

Wyrobek, A., and Bruce, W., 1975, Chemical induction of sperm abnormalities in mice, *Proc. Nat. Acad. Sci. (USA)* **72:**4425–4429.

Yadav, A., Vashishat, R., and Kakar, S., 1982, Testing of Endosulfan and Fenitrothion for genotoxicity in *Saccharomyces cerevisiae. Mutat. Res.* **105:**403–407.

Yamada, A., 1972, Teratogenic effects of organophosphorous insecticides in the chick embryo, *Osaka Shiritsu Diagaku Igaku Zasshi* **21:**345–355.

Yamamoto, H., Yano, I., Nishino, H., Furata, H., and Masuda, M., 1972, Effects of the organophosphorus insecticide Cyanox on rat fetuses and offspring, *Oyo Yakuri* **6:**523–528.

Yamamoto, I., 1970, Mode of action of pyrethroids, nicotinoids, and rotenoids, *Annu. Rev. Entomol.* **15:**257–272.

Yoder, J., Watson, M., and Benson, W., 1973, Lymphocyte chromosome analysis of agricultural workers during extensive occupational exposure to pesticides, *Mutat. Res.* **21:**335–340.

Zavon, M. R., 1970, The effect of long continued ingestion of Dieldrin in *Rhesus* monkeys: A six year study. Preliminary draft, Kettering laboratory.

Zeller, F., and Häuser, H., 1974, Polyploidisierung von Getreidearten durch Lindan-haltige Beizmittel, *Experientia* **30:**345–348.

*Chapter 4*

# Mutagenicity, Carcinogenicity, and Teratogenicity of Industrially Important Monomers

F. Poncelet, M. Duverger-van Bogaert,
M. Lambotte-Vandepaer, and C. de Meester

## 1. INTRODUCTION

Owing to their widespread use and occurrence in the environment, and their toxicological hazards, the group vinyl chloride (VCM), vinylidene chloride (VDC), acrylonitrile (ACN), styrene (STY), butadiene (BUT), and chlorobutadiene (CBD) form an important category of industrial chemicals. These so-called monomers are extensively used in the production of homo- and copolymeric materials utilized in the manufacture of many and various products, such as food packaging (VCM, VDC, STY), synthetic textile fibers (ACN, VDC), synthetic rubber goods (CBD, BUT), resins, and elastomers (VCM, VDC, BUT, etc.) and, according to published reports, world annual production varies from 7000 million kg for STY to 300 million kg for chlorobutadiene. All of them are gaseous or volatile and are generally poorly soluble in water.

The exposure of workers in working areas, the atmosphere of which is contaminated by these chemicals, may consequently be a major threat to health. People living in the neighborhood of such establishments are also highly exposed to environmental contamination by the volatile monomers; exposure to lower doses, either by inhalation of air polluted by cigarette smoke or by consumption of contaminated beverages and foodstuffs, is not

E. Poncelet, M. Duverger-van Bogaert, M. Lambotte-Vandepaer, and C. de Meester • Laboratory of Toxicology, Tour Ehrlich, 72.37 Av Emm. Mouner, B-1200 Brussels, Belgium.

negligible. Exposure to very low but chronic levels is also a risk to human health since toxic, carcinogenic, teratogenic, embryotoxic, and mutagenic effects have been reported.

Their properties, production, use, and occurrence, as well as the work environment standards for exposure to them, are summarized in Tables I–IV.


## 2. VINYL CHLORIDE

### 2.1. Toxicity

Experimental exposure to vinyl chloride (VCM) by inhalation causes degenerative and neoplastic changes in the liver and other organs in several species. The early VCM effects in rats that inhaled 5000 ppm, 7 hours/day, 5 days/week for 52 weeks were: growth retardation, shortened blood-clotting time, increased potassium content of the blood serum, and mitochondria in the hepatocytes, which appeared swollen and malformed. At a later stage, the blood urea nitrogen content increased, and enlargement of the kidneys, liver, and spleen was observed. At this latter stage foci of cellular alteration appeared in the liver (Feron *et al.*, 1979a).

VCM is not acutely hepatotoxic in normal rats. Small doses of VCM (671 ppm) given simultaneously with 1,1-dichloroethylene (200 ppm) significantly protect against hepatic injury induced by 1,1-dichloroethylene (Jaeger *et al.*, 1975a).

When mice inhaled 50 and 500 ppm VCM, lactate dehydrogenase activity was elevated in both dose groups; alkaline phosphatase was increased in animals exposed to 500 ppm, but the transaminases were unchanged. These changes occurred after the appearance of tumors (Winell *et al.*, 1976). A decrease in the growth rate of male rats exposed to VCM (13,500 and 17,300 ppm) and treated with phenobarbital appeared on the third day of exposure. Morphological changes ranging from slight swelling of hepatocytes to vacuolization and necrosis (Drew *et al.*, 1975) were observed in the livers of the animals treated with phenobarbital and exposed to 13,500 ppm VCM. The acute liver injury due to VCM exposure in rats pretreated with phenobarbital or Arochlor 1254 was related to morphologic changes in the endoplasmic reticulum (Reynold *et al.*, 1975c).

Liver injury in male rats exposed to 50,000 ppm VCM for 6 hours was found only in animals pretreated with phenobarbital and Arochlor 1254, while cytochrome $P_{450}$ content and oxidative $N$-demethylation of amino-antipyrine and ethylmorphine were markedly decreased (Reynolds *et al.*, 1975a).

The initial exposure of rats to VCM seems to protect against acute injury from subsequent exposures for at least 5 days. An initial exposure alters the activation pathway of VCM in a manner similar to that proposed for CCl₄ (Jaeger *et al.*, 1974). The hepatotoxicity of VCM in male rats is enhanced by treatment with sodium phenobarbital or Arochlor 1254. Disulfiram given prior to VCM exposure potentiated VCM toxicity, as did fasting, but not diethylmaleate pretreatment.

SKF 525-A, given prior to exposure, prevented the liver injury produced by VCM (Jaeger *et al.*, 1977).

Nonprotein sulfhydryl levels (glutathione and/or cysteine) showed a slight but progessive increase. A 50–60% rise in glutathione reductase activity was noted after exposure of rats to 15,000 ppm VCM. This observation has been proposed as one of the earliest biochemical manifestations of injury (Du *et al.*, 1979). Serum alanine-α-ketoglutarate transaminase (SAKT) activity of the serum was significantly increased in male rats pretreated with Aroclor 1254 and exposed by inhalation to VCM (24,000 ppm, 4 hours); severe degeneration and necrosis of the liver were simultaneously observed (Conolly *et al.*, 1978). The biotransformation of VCM by rats is a dose-dependent process characterized by Michaelis–Menten type kinetics (Gehring *et al.*, 1978). The interaction of VCM with uninduced, phenobarbital, or 3-methylcholanthrene pretreated rat microsomes indicates that the binding of VCM is catalyzed by more than one type of cytochrome $P_{450}$. The metabolites of VCM decreased the levels of cytochrome $P_{450}$ (Ivanetich *et al.*, 1977). Trichloropropene oxide, which depleted hepatic glutathione and inhibited epoxide hydratase, significantly increased VCM toxicity in fasting but not in replete rats. Diethylmaleate pretreatment, which lowers hepatic glutathione, did not increase the hepatotoxicity of VCM (Conolly and Jaeger, 1979). The 2-hour $LC_{50}$ of VCM for mice and rabbits was 113,000 ppm, for rats 150,000 ppm, and for guinea pigs, 230,000 ppm (Prodan *et al.*, 1975).

In humans, the following groups are likely to be exposed to VCM:

(1) Workers engaged in the production of VCM, PVC, or using VCM for other industrial purposes.
(2) Workers manufacturing PVC.
(3) Residents in areas where VCM or PVC are produced.
(4) People using products containing VCM (propellant sprays).
(5) People having contact with resins made with VCM.
(6) Populations consuming food contained in plastics made with VCM (Maltoni, 1976a).

VCM has anesthetic properties and causes respiratory tract irritation in humans. Repeated exposure leads to neurological asthenia. Other toxic effects include hepatomegaly, spenomegaly, hepatitis without jaundice, ulcers, Raynaud's syndrome, allergic dermatitis, and scleroderma (Suciu *et al.*, 1963). Sensitization dermatitis has also been reported in VCM workers (Morris, 1953).

**Table I**
**Properties**

| | Physical properties | Boiling point | Solubility | Volatility |
|---|---|---|---|---|
| Vinyl chloride <br> (Cl/H C=C H/H) | Colorless gas | −13.37° C | Slightly soluble in water <br> Soluble in ethanol <br> Very soluble in ether, carbon tetrachloride, and benzene | Vapor pressure: 2,530 mm at 20° C |
| Acrylonitrile <br> (CN/H C=C H/H) | Clear—colorless liquid (Fasset, 1963) | 77.5–79° C | Soluble in water, acetone and benzene <br> Miscible with ethanol and ether | Vapor pressure: 100 at 23° C |
| Styrene <br> (⬡/H C=C H/H) | Colorless viscous liquid | 145.2° C | Insoluble in water; soluble in ethanol, ether and acetone. Very soluble in benzene and petroleum ether | Vapor pressure: 10 mm at 35° C |
| Vinylidene chloride <br> (Cl/Cl C=C H/H) | Clear liquid with a sweet odor | 32° C | Insoluble in water, miscible with most organic solvents | Vapor pressure is 400 mm at 14.8° C |
| Butadiene 1-3 <br> (H/H C=C H/H C=C H/H) | Colorless gas | — | Soluble in organic solvents (alcohol) | |
| 2-chlorobutadiene 1-3 <br> (H/H C=C H/H C=C Cl/H) | Colorless, inflammable liquid | 59.4° C | Partially soluble in water; soluble ether, acetone, benzene | Vapor pressure in 300 mm at 32.8° C |

| Stability | Conversion factor | Impurities |
|---|---|---|
| Flash point: $-78°C$ Polymerizes in light or in the presence of a catalyst. Degrades by combustion to hydrogen chloride, carbon monoxide, carbon dioxide, and traces of phosgene (O'Mara et al., 1971) | 1 ppm in air = 2.6 mg/m$^3$ (IARC, 1979) | Purity: 99.90%. No inhibitor is usually added Water, acetaldehyde, acetylene, iron, hydrogen chloride, hydrogen peroxide, nonvolatile residues Chlorinated hydrocarbons may be present (IARC, 1979) |
| Flash point: $0°C$ May release cyanide. Polymerizes spontaneously, particularly in the absence of oxygen, on exposure to visible light and in contact with concentrated alkali (Windholz, 1976) | 1 ppm in air = 1,2 mg/m$^3$ (IARC, 1979) | Purity: 99.9% Water, acetic acid, acetaldehyde, acrolein divinylacetylene, hydrogen cyanide, iron, methyl vinyl ketone, peroxides, nonvolatile matter; hydroquinone monomethyl ether is present as an inhibitor at concentrations of 35–45 mg/kg |
| Flash point: $32°C$ Polymerizes slowly and oxidizes on exposure to light and air (Windholz, 1976) | 1 ppm in air $-$ 4.2 mg/m$^3$ (IARC, 1979) | Purity: 99.6% min Polymer, sulfur, chlorine, hydrogen peroxide, benzaldehyde, ethyl benzene Tertiary butylcatechol is added as an inhibitor (12–15 mg/kg) (IARC, 1979) |
| Flash point—$17°C$ Polymerizes at temperatures above $0°C$ in the presence of oxygen or other catalysts (Windholz, 1976) | 1 ppm in air = 4 mg/m$^3$ | Purity: 99.6% Acetylene—other chlorinated hydrocarbons hydrogen chloride hydrogen peroxide water Hydroquinone monomethyl ether is added as inhibitor (180–220 mg/kg) |
| Polymerizes easily | | Stabilized with O-dihydroxybenzene or with aliphatic mercaptans |
| Flash point = $-20°C$ (Hawley, 1971) Polymerizes on standing (Pollock and Stevens, 1965) | 1 ppm in air = 3.6 mg/m$^3$ | Min. purity: 95%. Inhibitors as hydroquinone or phenothiazine are added |

## Table II
## Production and Use[a]

|  | Use | Production (million kg) | | |
|---|---|---|---|---|
|  |  | U.S. | Western Europe | Japan |
| Vinyl chloride | Homo- and copolymer resins (floor coverings, electrical and transport applications, food containers) | 2580 (1976) | 3925 (1976) | 1281 (1976) |
|  | Production of methylchloroform |  |  |  |
| Acrylonitrile | Acrylic and modacrylic fibers (clothing) | 690 (1976) | 915 (1976) | 633 (1976) |
|  | ABS and styrene–acrylonitrile resins (pipe fitting, automotive vehicle, drinking tumblers, packaging, toys) |  |  |  |
|  | Production of adiponitrile |  |  |  |
|  | Elastomers, acrylamide |  |  |  |
|  | Tobacco fumigant, pesticide |  |  |  |
| Styrene | Polystyrene, ABS and styrene–acrylonitrile resins (packaging, houseware toys, construction) | 2864 (1976) | 2340 (1976) | 1090 (1976) |
|  | Styrene butadiene rubber (tires, latex applications) |  |  |  |
|  | Unsaturated polyesters (construction materials) |  |  |  |
| Vinylidene chloride | Copolymers with vinyl chloride (films for food packaging, fibers, tubes, and pipes, coating of other polymer films) | 70 | — | 28.1 |
|  | Manufacture of modacrylic fibers (clothing, home furnishing) |  |  |  |
| Butadiene | Copolymeric resins (ABS), (food packaging). |  |  |  |
|  | Synthetic rubber. | 1707 (1976) | 1300 | — |
| Chlorobutadiene | Polychloroprene elastomers (industrial and automotive rubber goods, consumer products) | 164 (1976) | 100 (1977) | 80 (1976) |

[a](IARC 1979).

A rare clinical syndrome named acro-osteolysis has been reported in workers engaged in handcleaning the polymerization vessels of VCM. Hepatic fibrosis of a noncirrhotic type, frequently associated with splenomegaly and portal hypertension, has been reported in workers exposed to VCM (Binns, 1979). Reduced pulmonary function has also been observed (Miller *et al.*, 1975).

The presence of aberrant immune complexes has been reported in workers exposed to VCM. It is suggested that the so-called VCM disease may be an immune complex disorder, and that the immune response may be initiated by the adsorption of VCM or its metabolite on tissue or plasma protein (Ward *et al.*, 1976). Most industries have reduced the exposure level to 50 ppm, a concentration which has not produced liver pathology in experimental animals (Haley, 1975a).

## 2.2. Metabolism

The *in vivo* and *in vitro* vinyl chloride metabolism has been reviewed (Figure 1) (Antweiler, 1976; Bartsch and Montesano, 1975; Plugge and Safe, 1977; IARC, 1979).

The primary step in the metabolic activation of vinyl chloride is oxidation catalyzed by mixed-function oxidases (Reynolds *et al.*, 1975a; Salmon, 1976); however, some metabolism seems to occur in a nitrogen atmosphere (Kappus *et al.*, 1976). Chloroethylene oxide, which transforms spontaneously into chloroacetaldehyde, is proposed as the primary reactive intermediate (Gross and Freiberg, 1969) and indirect evidence for its formation exists *in vitro* (Barbin *et al.*, 1975; Gothe *et al.*, 1974) and *in vivo* (Muller *et al.*, 1978). Pretreatment of the animals with mixed-function-oxidase inhibitors such as 6-bromobenzothiazine (Radwan and Henschler, 1977), $CoCl_2$ (Pessayre *et al.*, 1979), or 3-bromophenyl-4-(5)imidazole (Bolt *et al.*, 1976), inhibited VCM metabolism.

Pretreatment of rats with pyrazole caused an important decrease in the rate of VCM metabolism. Ethanol was also an inhibitor, but was less effective when rats were exposed to high concentrations of VCM. SKF 525-A was without effect when the exposure dose to VCM was low (Hefner *et al.*, 1975).

Chloroethylene oxide and/or chloroacetaldehyde behaved as bifunctional alkylating agents to the deoxyadenosine and the deoxycitidin residues of DNA (Green and Hathway, 1978). They were also able to alkylate adenosine and cytosine, producing 1-$N^6$-ethenoadenosine (Barbin *et al.*, 1975; Barrio *et al.*, 1972) and 3-$N^4$-ethenocytidine (Laib and Bolt, 1978).

Exposure to VCM caused progressive depression of the hepatic non-protein sulfhydryl content (Watanabe *et al.*, 1976). Chloroethylene oxide and/or chloroacetaldehyde reacted with glutathione, directly or enzymatically, to form S-formylmethylglutathione, which was recovered in the urine as N-acetyl-S(2-hydroxy-ethyl)-cysteine, a major urinary VCM metabolite. N-acetyl-S-(2-chloro-ethyl)cysteine is also reported to be a VCM urinary metabolite. These two metabolites are probably connected by a reversible reaction via the formation of the episulfonium ion (Green and Hathway, 1977).

Chloroacetic acid has been found in the urine of rats exposed to VCM

Table III
Occurrence

| | Occupational exposure | Air | Water | Food | Other |
|---|---|---|---|---|---|
| Vinyl chloride | In working place of PVC industries, air concentrations range from 0.15 ppm (Murdoch and Hammond, 1977) and 312 ppm (Filatova and Gronsberg, 1957). Residual vinyl chloride in the polymer = 1–2 ppm (U.S.–F.D.A., 1975) | Prior to 1975, 110 million kg/year emitted from U.S. PVC industries (U.S. Environmental Protection Agency, 1975c) | 10 $\mu$g/liter of vinyl chloride detected in finished drinking water in U.S. (U.S. Environmental Protection Agency, 1975c) | Present in alcoholic beverages, vinegars, butter and margarines packed in PVC (Williams and Miles, 1975; Fuchs *et al.*, 1975) | Detected in new automobile interiors, cigarettes and little cigars (Hedley *et al.*, 1976, Hoffman *et al.*, (1976) |
| Acrylonitrile | Total emission in 1974 in U.S. Residual acrylonitrile in polymers: from 1 to 50 mg/kg | 14.1 million kg | 0.1 g/liter detected in effluent discharged from a U.S. acrylic fiber industry (Eurocop-Cost, 1976) | | In the smoke of US cigarettes (Guerin *et al.*, 1974) |
| Styrene | Detected in the workplace air during the production of polymeric materials in USSR (Martynenko, 1973) | Detected at a maximum concentration of 0.7 ppb in Delft, the Netherlands (Bos *et al.*, 1977) | Less than 1 $\mu$g/liter detected in finished drinking water in the US (US | Present in yogurt, butter fat cream, cottage cheese and honey packaged in polystyrene containers (Withey, 1976; | In the smoke of American cigarettes (Baggett *et al.*, 1974) |

| | | | | | | |
|---|---|---|---|---|---|---|
| | Detected in the subcutaneous fat tissues of styrene-exposed workers (0.1 at 1.2 μg/l (Wolff. 1976). | | | Environmental Protection Agency, 1975b) | Withey and Collins, 1978) | |
| Vinylidene chloride | Workers exposed in trace amounts (Kramer and Mutchler, 1972) Emission of 308 thousands kg from polymer synthesis (Hushon and Kornreich, 1976) | See occupational exposure | — | 0.1 μg/l detected in U.S. finished drinking water (U.S. Environmental Protection Agency, 1975a) | — | Impurity in vinyl chloride, chloroprene, and trichloroethylene (IARC, 1979) |
| Butadiene | — | | — | — | — | — |
| Chlorobutadiene | Concentration in the workplace varies between 6 and 6.760 ppm (Infante et al., 1977) Polychloroprene may contain 0.01–0.5% free chloroprene (NIOSH, 1977). | — | | — | | Impurity in vinyl chloride (Sassu et al., 1968) |

Table IV
Work Environment Hygiene Standards for Exposure to Monomers

|                      | TLV                                       | MAC          |
|----------------------|-------------------------------------------|--------------|
| Vinyl chloride       | 1 ppm (max. 5 ppm for 15 min.)            | 12 ppm       |
| Acrylonitrile        | 2 ppm (max. 10 ppm for 15 min.)           | —            |
| Styrene              | 100 ppm (max. 200 ppm for 5 min.)         | $5 \, mg/m^3$ |
| Vinylidene chloride  | 10 ppm                                    | —            |
| Butadiene            | $2,200 \, mg/m^3$ (1000 ppm)              | $100 \, mg/m^3$ |
| Chloroprene          | 25 ppm ($90 \, mg/m^3$)                   | $2 \, mg/m^3$ |

(IARC, 1979); (Fishbein, 1979)

and in the urine of exposed workers (Grigorescu and Toba, 1966; Hefner *et al.*, 1975).

The detection of $S$-(carboxymethyl)cysteine and thiodiglycolic acid in the urine of rats (Muller *et al.*, 1976) could result from the conjugation of chloroacetic acid with GSH. This has also been suggested by Yllner who recovered glycolic acid, $S$-(carboxy-methyl)-cysteine and thiodiglycolic acid

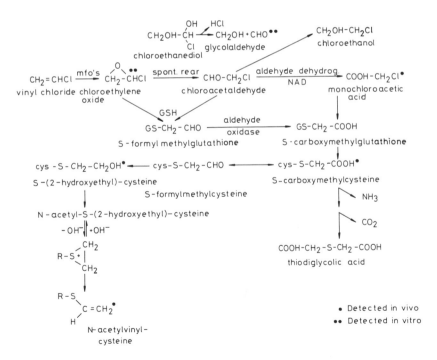

Figure 1. Metabolic pathway of vinyl chloride.

in the urine of rats treated with chloroacetic acid (Yllner, 1971). These metabolites could also result from the oxidation of the conjugation product of the epoxide or aldehyde: $S$-formylmethylglutathione (Green and Hathway, 1977).

The 2-chloroethylene oxide can be hydrolyzed by the epoxide hydratase after dechlorination of chloroethanediol and glycolaldehyde has been identified in aqueous buffer. This pathway seems to be negligible in vinyl chloride metabolism.

In a microsomal enzymatic system, 50% of the covalent binding is inhibited by epoxide hydratase, and 98% by alcohol or aldehyde dehydrogenase (Guengerich et al., 1979), suggesting the important role of those enzymes in VCM detoxification. Chloroacetaldehyde can be reduced to chloroethanol (Muller et al., 1976).

Hefner postulates that in rats exposed to VCM below 100 ppm, alcohol dehydrogenase is the main factor in metabolism; this is a saturable process.

This oxidative pathway gave rise to chloroethanol, chloroacetaldehyde, and monochloracetic acid (Hefner et al., 1975). The lungs appear to be the main elimination route for vinyl chloride after oral, intravenous, or intraperitoneal administration. Unchanged vinyl chloride and $CO_2$ were expired; the other metabolites were excreted via the kidneys (Green and Hathway, 1975).

After oral administration of $^{14}C$ vinyl chloride, $^{14}C$ $CO_2$, $^{14}C$-labeled urea, and glutamic acid were also identified as minor metabolites (Green and Hathway, 1975).

Following exposure to $^{14}C$ vinyl chloride, covalent protein binding was concentrated in the liver; smaller amounts were found in the kidneys, small intestine, lungs, and spleen (Bolt and Filser, 1977).

## 2.3. Mutagenicity

The mutagenic properties of vinyl chloride (VCM) have been studied using various short-term tests and have been reviewed (IARC, 1979; Fishbein, 1979) (Table V). The *Salmonella typhimurium* histidine-dependent strains developed by Ames have been very extensively used to predict the carcinogenic potency of suspected compounds. Exposure to vapors of vinyl chloride monomer increased the mutation rate of *Salmonella typhimurium* strains sensitive to base pair substitutions (G 46, TA 1530, TA 1535, TA 100). Such activity has been observed even in the absence of a metabolic-activating system and is dependent on dose and exposure time (Malaveille et al., 1975; McCann et al., 1975a; de Meester et al., 1980a; Garro et al., 1976; Bartsch et al., 1975a; Bartsch and Montesano, 1975; Bartsch et al., 1976; Elmore et al., 1976).

The addition of liver homogenates from rats or mice, fortified with an

## Table V
## Mutagenicity of Vinyl Chloride

| Test | Conditions[a] | Response | References |
|------|------------|----------|------------|
| *S. typhimurium* | B,C | + | Malaveille *et al.*, 1975; McCann *et al.*, 1975a; de Meester *et al.* 1980a; Garro *et al.*, 1976; Bartsch *et al.*, 1975a, Bartsch *et al.*, 1976; Bartsch and Montesano, 1975; Elmore *et al.*, 1976; Andrews *et al.*, 1976 |
| | A,C | + | Malaveille *et al.*, 1975 Bartsch *et al.*, 1975a, 1976; Bartsch and Montesano, 1976; de Meester *et al.*, 1980a; Rannug *et al.*, 1976; Andrews *et al.*, 1976 |
| | B,C | − | Rannug *et al.*, 1976 |
| | A,B,D | − | Rannug *et al.*, 1974; Bartsch *et al.*, 1975a, 1976; |
| | A,B,D | + | Bartsch and Montesano, 1975; Duverger–van Bogaert *et al.*, 1981 |
| | E,B,D | − | Mattern *et al.*, 1977 |
| *E. coli* K12 | A,D | + | Greim *et al.*, 1975 |
| *S. cerevisiae* | B,D | − | Shahin, 1976 |
| | A,D | + | Loprieno *et al.*, 1976a |
| *S. pombe* | A,D | + | Loprieno *et al.*, 1976a |
| *S. pombe* | Host mediated assay | + | Loprieno *et al.*, 1976a |
| *Neurospora crassa* | A,B,C,D | + | Drozdowicz and Huang, 1977 |
| V79 Chinese hamster cells | A,C | + | Huberman *et al.*, 1975 |
| *Drosophila melanogaster* | C | + | Verburgt and Bogel, 1977 Magnusson and Ramel, 1978 |
| Chromosomal aberrations | | | |
|   in rats | C | + | Muratov and Gus'Kova, 1978 |
|   in Chinese hamsters | C | + | Basler and Röhrborn, 1980 |
| Sister chromatid exchanges in Chinese | | | |
|   hamsters | C | + | Basler and Röhrborn, 1980 |

[a] A: + fortified liver fraction; B: − fortified liver fraction; C: Gas phase; D: Liquid medium; E: Urine.

NADPH-generating system, increased the mutagenicity of VCM in *Salmonella typhimurium* strains G 46, TA 1530, and TA 1535 (Malaveille *et al.*, 1975; Bartsch *et al.*, 1975a and 1976; Bartsch and Montesano, 1975). The presence of S9 obtained with phenobarbital-pretreated animals exacerbated the mutagenic response of VCM (Bartsch *et al.*, 1975a, 1976; Bartsch and Montesano, 1975).

Similarly, induction of the mixed-function-oxidase system by Aroclor 1254 increased the mutagenicity of VCM in *Salmonella typhimurium* strain TA 1530 (de Meester *et al.*, 1980a). On the other hand, pretreatment with either aminoacetonitrile or pregnenolone 16 $\alpha$ carbonitrile reduced the mutagenicity of VCM (Bartsch *et al.*, 1976).

The addition of kidney and lung fractions from rats and mice gave a negligible response in the Ames test (Malaveille *et al.*, 1975; Bartsch *et al.*, 1975a and 1976; Bartsch and Montesano, 1975). Liver homogenates from human biopsy samples were able to activate VCM vapors in mutagenic metabolite(s); large variations were observed in intensity of effect (Malaveille *et al.*, 1975; Bartsch *et al.*, 1975a, 1976; Bartsch and Montesano, 1975). Subcellular fractions have been assayed for their ability to transform VCM into mutagenic metabolite(s): purified liver microsomes played an important role, but the best results were obtained in the presence of both microsomal and soluble proteins (Bartsch *et al.*, 1975a, 1976; Bartsch and Montesano, 1975).

The activation process could involve a two-step mechanism located in two different cell compartments; the protective activity of soluble proteins against microsomal lipid peroxidation, and the consequent increased viability of microsomal enzymes could also be implicated.

Using *Salmonella typhimurium* strain TA 1535, Rannug *et al.* (1976) reported a liver-mediated mutagenicity of gaseous VCM; the absence of an S9 or NADPH generating system did not increase the mutation rate over spontaneous reversion rate.

On the other hand, Garro *et al.* (1976) showed that VCM (75% in the air) acted as a direct mutagen in *Salmonella typhimurium* strain TA 1530, and that mutagenicity was increased by the addition of S9 obtained from variously pretreated mice, although, neither the type of pretreatment or the presence of NADPH seemed to influence the intensity of the effect. Moreover, the use of heated liver fraction was able to produce a mutagenic response.

The addition of riboflavin associated with UV irradiation increased the mutagenicity of VCM, suggesting the intervention of a free radical mechanism. The increasing effect of liver homogenate was due neither to a nonspecific effect of lipid or protein nor to an exacerbating effect on VCM concentration in the reaction mixture.

Andrews *et al.* (1976) have similarly described a significant mutagenic effect of VCM in *S. typhimurium* strain TA 1535, both in the absence and presence of liver fractions. A positive mutagenic response in plates containing only bacteria, co-incubated with plates containing only liver homogenates—suggesting the formation of a volatile mutagenic intermediate—has been demonstrated by de Meester *et al.* (1980a). This observation may partly explain the direct mutagenic effect of VCM when tested in these conditions. All these studies were performed using VCM in a gas phase (from 0.2 to 20%).

When tested in the liquid medium, negative results were observed both in the presence and absence of a metabolism activating system (Rannug *et al.*, 1974; Bartsch *et al.*, 1975a; Bartsch *et al.*, 1976; Bartsch and Montesano, 1975; Elmore *et al.*, 1976). Recently, Duverger-van Bogaert *et al.* (1981) observed both direct and indirect mutagenic responses using a modified preincubation method and an ethanolic VCM dilution. From their results, it may be concluded that VCM acts as a direct and an indirect mutagen.

Its direct mutagenicity may be due to a bacterial activation or to the formation of breakdown products (Bartsch *et al.*, 1975, 1976), and partly also to the formation of volatile metabolites (de Meester *et al.*, 1980a). The intervention of a radical formation has been proposed by Garro *et al.* (1976) and by Duverger-van Bogaert *et al.* (1981a). On the other hand, the liver-mediated mutagenicity of VCM suggests its activation by the mixed-function-oxidase system.

The primary reactive metabolite is most probably chloroethylene oxide, which spontaneously transforms into chloroacetaldehyde. Chloroethanol and chloroactic acid are also formed and these four molecules have been studied for their mutagenic properties in the Ames test.

Chloroethylene oxide acted as a direct and strong mutagen in *Salmonella typhimurium* strains TA 1530 (Malaveille *et al.*, 1975; Bartsch *et al.*, 1975a, 1976; Bartsch and Montesano, 1975), TA 1535 (Bartsch *et al.*, 1976; Rannug *et al.*, 1976), and TA 100 (Elmore *et al.*, 1976).

This molecule is characterized by low bacterial cytotoxicity, a very short lifetime and high electrophilic reactivity (Malaveille *et al.*, 1975; Bartsch and Montesano, 1975; Bartsch *et al.*, 976).

Chloroacetaldehyde was highly cytotoxic and caused direct and indirect mutagenic effects in *Salmonella typhimurium* strains TA 1530 (Malaveille *et al.*, 1975; Bartsch *et al.*, 1975a, and 1976; Bartsch and Montesano, 1975) TA 1535 (Rannug *et al.*, 1976; Bartsch *et al.*, 1976), and TA 100 (McCann *et al.*, 1975a; Bartsch *et al.*, 1976; Elmore *et al.*, 1976). Several hydrates, derivatives of chloroacetaldehyde, were tested by Elmore *et al.* (1976); they acted as direct mutagens. The monomer hydrate may be formed in an aqueous solution containing chloroacetaldehyde and may be considered as the ultimate carcinogenic metabolite of VCM.

The results obtained with chloroethanol have drawn high bacterial cytotoxicity as well as weak mutagenic activity in *Salmonella typhimurium* strains TA 1530 (Malaveille *et al.*, 1975; Bartsch *et al.*, 1975a, and 1976; Bartsch and Montesano, 1975), TA 1535 (Rannug *et al.*, 1976; Bartsch and Montesano, 1975; Bartsch *et al.*, 1976), and TA 100 (Bartsch *et al.*, 1976; McCann *et al.*, 1975). Elmore *et al.* (1976) obtained a negative response with *Salmonella typhimurium* strain TA 100. Monochloroacetic acid, excreted in urine as a VCM metabolite, showed toxic effects but was devoid of mutagenic properties in any tester strains (Malaveille *et al.*, 1975; Bartsch *et al.*, 1975a, 1976; Bartsch and Montesano, 1975; Rannug *et al.*, 1976; Elmore *et al.*, 1976).

Chloroethylene oxide, chloroacctaldehyde, and its monomer hydrate inhibited the growth of *Bacillus subtilis* MC-1, a mutant lacking recombination repair, but had no effect on mutant strains having the capacity for recombination repair (Elmore *et al.*, 1976). Chloroethanol and chloroacetic acid did not inhibit the growth of any tester strains.

Negative results were reported by Mattern *et al.* (1977) when urine from VCM-treated rats was tested using the *Salmonella typhimurium* strains TA 100, TA 1535, and TA 98. The addition to the test of rat liver homogenates or $\beta$-glucuronidase did not influence the results.

From all these data, chloroethylene oxide and chloroacetaldehyde must be considered the mutagenic metabolites of VCM. VCM has been assayed using *Escherichia coli* K12 which can be used in four mutation systems: three back mutation systems ($gal^+$, $arg^+$, and $nad^+$), and a forward mutation system leading to resistance to 5-methyl-DL-tryptophane (MTR system). VCM was tested by bubbling into the incubation medium at $15°C$ in order to obtain a final concentration of 10.6 mM. The authors suggest that the mutagenicity of VCM is related to the instability of its epoxide (Greim *et al.*, 1975). The presence of a microsomal suspension obtained from phenobarbital-pretreated mice is indispensable to note mutations in the four systems. At a concentration of 0.55% in the incubation mixture, VCM was neither mutagenic nor recombingenic in *Saccharomyces cerevisiae* strains D5 (recombination) and XV185-14C (mutation) in the absence of a metabolic activation system (Shahih, 1976). VCM in solution at concentrations of 16 and 48 mM was able to produce a significant increase of the forward mutation frequency in *Schizosaccharomyces pombe*, only in the presence of mouse liver microsomes (Loprieno *et al.*, 1976a). In the same experimental conditions, the gene conversion frequency of *Saccharomyces cerevisiae* (ade 2 and trp 5 loci) was increased. In none of the experiments did VCM treatment produce any detectable decrease in cell survival (Loprieno *et al.*, 1976a).

In a host-mediated assay in mice treated with an oral dose of 700 mg/kg VCM and in intraperitoneal injection of *Schizosaccharomyces pombe*, genetic effects were detected; they confirm the need for metabolic activation (Loprieno *et al.*, 1976a). These results have been further confirmed by studying the mutagenic properties of several VCM metabolites in yeast.

Chloroethylene oxide, at a dose of 0.1 mM, proposed as the first reactive metabolite of VCM, induced either forward mutations in *Schizosaccharomyces pombe* or gene conversion in *Saccharomyces cerevisiae*. In either the absence or presence of mouse liver microsomes, chloroacetaldehyde showed borderline genetic activity and chloroethanol was completely inactive. Chloroacetaldehyde, when assayed in a host-mediated assay, was unable to induce forward mutations in *Schizosaccharomyces pombe*; these negative results suggest that this molecule does not contribute to the mutagenicity of VCM in yeast (Loprieno *et al.*, 1977). VCM, whether in ethanol solution or in the gas phase, did not induce mutations in strains of *Neurospora crassa* that were not repair-deficient. The addition of liver microsome from control and phenobarbital-pretreated mice had no effect on the mutation frequency (Drozdowicz and Huang, 1977).

Mutations in V 79 Chinese hamster cells in terms of 8-azaguanine and ouabain resistance were induced by VCM vapors (20%), in the presence of liver fractions from phenobarbital-pretreated mice (Huberman *et al.*, 1975). Under the same conditions, cytotoxicity was noted but, in the absence of liver fraction, neither mutagenicity nor cytotoxicity appeared. Using the same test, chloroethylene oxide and its transformation product, chloroacetaldehyde, were able to increase the number of 8-azaguanine and ouabain resistants. For chloroacetaldehyde, cytotoxicity was noted. On the other hand, 2-chloroethanol and monochloroacetic acid were ineffective in inducing mutations in V 79 Chinese hamster cells (Huberman *et al.*, 1975).

In *Drosophila* males exposed to VCM by inhalation at concentrations ranging from 200 up to 50,000 ppm for either 2 or 17 days, VCM was mutagenic in the recessive lethal test. The mutagenic frequency increased with concentration; however, negative results were obtained when tests on dominant lethals, translocations, entire and partial sex chromosome loss were carried out with VCM at 30,000 ppm for 2 days; this reinforces the nonreliability of the link between chromosome breakage and mutagenic activity (Verburgt and Vogel, 1977).

The same increase of recessive lethals after inhalation exposure to 1 to 20% VCM for 3 days has been reported by Magnusson and Ramel (1978); a more pronounced effect was observed by these authors when *Drosophila* were pretreated with phenobarbitone.

When rats inhaled VCM for $3\frac{1}{2}$ months, they showed an increase in the chromosome aberration rate (chromosome bridges and chromosome fragments) (Muratov & Gus'kova, 1978). On the other hand, bone marrow chromsome aberrations have been reported for Chinese hamsters inhaling VCM, as a function of both time and dose of exposure (Fleig and Thiess, 1978; Basler and Röhrborn, 1980). Most of the aberrations were breaks and fragments followed by exchanges, multiple aberrations, gaps, and deletions.

An increase of the sister chromatid exchange (SCE) frequency was noted in the same experiment as dependent on dose and duration of exposure (Basler and Röhrborn, 1980).

Male mice exposed by inhalation to VCM (3,000, 10,000, or 30,000 ppm) for 5 days did not develop mutagenic alterations at any maturation stage or spermatogenesis. Furthermore, no reduction of fertility was observed, nor were post-implantational early fetal deaths or preimplantational egg losses noted after such treatment (Anderson *et al.*, 1976).

In female mice (C57BL/6 J Han) exposed to VCM (5,600 ppm for 5 h) after mating to rotated bred males, no difference could be observed in the average litter size at birth or 3–5 weeks after birth, nor were there any offspring with abnormal morphology among the exposed animals (Peter and Ungvary, 1980). Vinyl chloride and its two presumed metabolites depress the first wave of DNA synthesis by approximatively 50% after intravenous injection to partially hepatectomized rats. The second peak of DNA synthesis was similar to that in the controls after vinyl chloride injection, but desynchronization of this second peak was noted for chloroacetaldehyde. The three molecules were thus able to retard DNA replication, probably due to an alkylation of DNA (Border and Webster, 1977).

Several studies have been performed on lymphocyte cultures from VCM-exposed workers in order to estimate the genetic risk associated with this molecule (Table VI). The equivocal results reported have recently been discussed by Hopkins (1980). In 1975, the first evidence of chormosomal

**Table VI**
**Mutagenicity of Vinyl Chloride in Man**

| Test | Response | References |
|------|----------|-----------|
| Chromosomal aberrations of lymphocytes | + | Ducatman *et al.*, 1975; Funes-Cravioto *et al.*, 1975; Purchase, 1975; Szentesi *et al.*, 1976; Léonard *et al.*, 1977; Heath *et al.*, 1977; Fleig and Thiess, 1978; Kucerova, 1979; Hansteen *et al.*, 1978; Purchase *et al.*, 1978 |
| | − | Picciano *et al.*, 1977 |
| Sister chromatid exchanges | + | Kucerova, 1979 |
| | − | Hansteen *et al.*, 1978 |
| Chromosomal aberrations in the bone marrow cells | + | Hansteen *et al.*, 1978 |
| Urines from VC-exposed workers/*S. typhimurium* | + | Mattern *et al.*, 1977 |

aberrations caused by VCM was reported by Ducatman et al. in the U.S.A., by Funes-Cravioto in Sweden, and by Purchase in the U.K. The anomalies were described as fragments, rearrangements, and break events. Afterwards, other studies confirmed these results. Szentesi et al. (1976) reported an increased frequency of chromatid type aberrations in lymphocytes from VCM-exposed men; Leónard et al. (1977) described chromsomal anomalies such as dicentrics, fragments, rings, and translocations, but underlined the frequent x-ray exposures of the workers, and concluded that the cytogenetic effects were probably attributable to x-rays rather than to VCM. However, a previous report of Purchase et al. (1975), in which an x-ray exposed control group had been included, revealed a significant increase in chromosomal aberrations due to VCM exposure.

An increase of chromatid gaps was described in blood lymphocytes from VCM-exposed workers; this effect did not seem to be dose-related, but it must be noted that the workers were exposed to other chemicals, such as solvents (Heath, 1977).

In a group of workers, Fleig and Thiess (1978) reported a correlation between the symptoms of VCM illness (a case of living angiosarcoma) and a significant increase in the rate of chromosomal aberrations; Kucerova et al. (1979) revealed an increased incidence of chromatid and chromosome breaks in blood samples from workers exposed to high levels of VCM, and Hansteen et al. (1978) described the increased frequency of chromosomal aberrations in exposed workers, and the return to normal values after two years of reduced contact with VCM.

Purchase et al. (1978) suggested a relationship between the increased incidence of chromsomal anomalies and both dose and duration of exposure, but smoking habits seem also to be implicated in these effects.

Hopkins (1980) underlined that some of these studies were open to criticism, since they involved small groups of workers. In a study at the Dow Chemical Company, no statistical difference was noted for chromatid and chromsomal aberrations and the proportion of abnormal cells, when VCM-exposed workers and unexposed people were compared. It must be noted that the VCM-exposure level did not exceed 15 ppm, and thus probably explains the lack of effect. It was suggested that such chromosomal aberrations could be avoided by minimal exposure environments (Picciano et al., 1977).

A significant increase in the SCE rate was noted in lymphocyte cultures from VCM-exposed workers (Kucerova, 1979); on the other hand, no increase of this anomaly was noted by Hansteen et al. (1978).

In the bone marrow cells of VCM-exposed men, the frequency of chromosome breakage was higher than that reported for normal samples (Hansteen et al., 1978), but the urine of workers exposed to VCM did not induce mutations in the Salmonella typhimurium strain TA 100, even in the presence of rat liver homogenate or $\beta$-glucuronidase (Mattern et al., 1977).

## 2.4. Carcinogenicity

Various studies on experimental animals have proved the carcinogenic properties of VCM (Table VII).

The first of these studies reported by Viola *et al.* (1971) revealed a high frequency of tumors, principally in the liver, among rats exposed to VCM vapors (from 500 up to 20,000 ppm for 8 to 13 months). Other authors (see Table VIII) have confirmed and completed these data. From these results, it appears that VCM induces various types of tumors in different animal species after inhalation or oral administration, and that the intensity of tumor incidence depends on dose and duration of treatment (Maltoni, 1977b). The association of ethanol treatment with VCM inhalation increased the incidence of liver angiosarcoma in rats (Radike *et al.*, 1977), and newborn rats seemed to be more sensitive to the carcinogenic effects of VCM than adults (Maltoni, 1977b). The liver alterations in rats due to VCM exposure claim most attention, since they have also been described for VCM-exposed workers.

Feron *et al.* (1979b) described their evolution and underlined that parenchymal cell alterations preceded those of nonparenchymal tissue.

**Table VII**
**Carcinogenicity of VCM in Animals**

| References | Conditions | Observations |
|---|---|---|
| Viola *et al.* (1971) | Rats—inhalation | High frequency of tumors, mainly in the liver |
| Caputo *et al.*, (1974) | Rats—inhalation | Increased incidence of cutaneous tumors, lung carcinomas, and, less frequently, osteochondromas |
| Maltoni *et al.*, (1974) | Rats—inhalation | Zymbal gland carcinomas, nephroblastomas, angiosarcomas and angiomas of the liver and other sites, skin carcinomas, hepatomas, brain neuroblastomas, and possibly mammary carcinomas |
| Lee *et al.* (1977) | Rats—inhalation | Angiosarcomas of the liver |
| Maltoni *et al.* (1974) | Mice—inhalation | Lung adenomas, mammary carcinomas, angiosarcomas, and angiomas of the liver and other sites, and skin epithelial tumors |
| Keplinger *et al.* (1975) Holmberg *et al.* (1976) Lee *et al.* (1977, 1978) | Mice—inhalation | Liver angiosarcomas, pulmonary adenomas, and mammary gland carcinomas |
| Suzuki (1978) | Mice—inhalation | Pulmonary tumors (alveologenic cancers) |
| Maltoni *et al.*, (1974) | Hamsters—inhalation | Liver angiosarcomas, skin trichoepitheliomas, lymphomas, forestomach papillomas, and acanthomas |
| Maltoni *et al.*, (1974) | Rabbits—inhalation | Skin acanthomas and lung adenocarcinomas |
| Maltoni (1977a) | Rats—oral administration | Liver angiosarcomas, nephroblastomas, and zymbal gland carcinomas |

The first parenchymal damages observed are foci of cellular alterations, neoplastic nodules and hepatocellular carcinomas. At the cellular level, the alterations were described as swelling of the mitochondria, decrease in rough endoplasmic reticulum, and loss of ribosomes in rough endoplasmic reticulum. The nonparenchymal damges comprised focal dilatation of sinusoids, focal proliferation of atypical sinusoidal cells and multicentric angiosarcomas. A marked fibrosis accompanied only the fully developed angiosarcomas (Feron *et al.*, 1979b). A considerable increase in proliferative activity of the endothelial cells was described for partly hepatectomized rats exposed to VCM vapors (50, 125 or 500 ppm for 28 hr). However, increased activity of alkaline phosphatase occurred in the bile duct canaliculi, but not in the liver sinosoids (Norpoth *et al.*, 1980).

The nonreactivity of VCM, as well as the results of mutagenicity and metabolism studies, strongly suggest the intervention of a metabolic intermediate as carcinogen, mutagen, and toxic. Hydroperoxides, peroxides, and free radical intermediates may be involved, but the epoxide form is the most probable candidate as the activated carcinogenic intermediate, particularly in the liver (Van Duuren, 1975). Chloroethylene oxide acted as a highly reactive alkylating agent (Bartsch *et al.*, 1979). Chloroacetaldehyde, spontaneously formed from chloroethylene oxide, reacted with adenine to give triheterocyclic products (Bartsch *et al.*, 1979). Furthermore, chloroethylene oxide, repeatedly administered subcutaneously to mice, induced local tumors (Fibrosarcomas, squamous cells carcinomas), but no tumors distant from the injection site. On the other hand, skin applications of chloroethylene oxide followed by applications three times weekly of 12-O-n-tetradecanoylforbol (initiation–promotion experiment) induced skin tumors in mice (papillomas, carcinomas). Chloroacetaldehyde tested in the same conditions did not produce either benign or malignant tumors (Zajdela *et al.*, 1980).

Observations of the oncogenic effect of VCM in experimental animals have promoted the clinical observations which, in 1973, for the first time identified a liver angiosarcoma in a VCM-exposed worker as occupational in origin (Creech and Johnson, 1974). Afterwards, systematic medical screening revealed the association of angiosarcomas of the liver and VCM exposure in various countries: Canada (Delorme and Thierault, 1978; Noria *et al.*, 1976); the Federal Republic of Germany (Lange *et al.*, 1975); France (Couderc *et al.*, 1976; Ravier *et al.*, 1975; Roche *et al.*, 1978); Italy, (Maltoni, 1974); Norway (Lloyd, 1975); Sweden (Byren and Holmberg, 1975); the U.K. (Lee and Harry, 1974; Smith *et al.*, 1976; Baxter *et al.*, 1977; the U.S. (Block, 1974; Falk *et al.*, 1974; Makk *et al.*, 1974).

In 1978, 64 known VCM-associated angiosarcomas were recorded among exposed workers (Spirtas and Kaminski, 1978). In exposed workers, fibrosis would seem to be an early step in the development of neoplasia. The first changes were foci of subcapsular and portal fibrosis. Neoplasia began as an activation of sinusoid lining cells accompanied by megalocytosis of hepatocytes. The neoplasm was ordinarily multicentric; angiosarcomas could be observed in the spleen, lungs, kidneys, heart, and intestine, and were interpreted as multicentric origins rather than metastases (Lingeman, 1976; Popper and Thomas, 1975; Popper, 1979; Thomas and Popper, 1975).

Delorme (1978) described an association between liver angiosarcoma and hepatoma in a worker exposed for 23 years to VCM vapors and suggested, in agreement with Popper and Thomas (1975), that VCM could act on the hepatic cell itself and that the liver angiosarcoma could be a consequence of this attack. An excess of other types of cancers has been described among workers exposed to VCM (Table VIII).

From these mortality studies, an increased risk of death associated with all forms of cancer must be noted (Monson *et al.*, 1974; Nicholson *et al.*, 1975; Ott *et al.*, 1975; Buffler *et al.*, 1979).

Furthermore, an increased incidence of cancers has been described for people living in the neighborhood of PVC manufacturing plants (Infante *et al.*, 1976; Brady *et al.*, 1977; Locker *et al.*, 1979).

Several screening procedures have been proposed to detect and prevent VCM-associated disease: measurement of the carcino-embryonic antigen titer (increased by VCM exposure, Pagé *et al.*, 1976); examination by *in vivo* microscopy of the hands of exposed workers (Maricq *et al.*, 1976), and scintigraphy of the liver and spleen of VCM-exposed workers (Biersack *et al.*, 1977). However, longer observation periods are required to provide information on the full spectrum of VCM malignancies and their incidence on exposed humans.

## 2.5. Teratogenicity and Embryotoxicity

The offspring of breeders exposed to VCM vapors during pregnancy for seven days developed two subcutaneous angiosarcomas and one zymbal gland carcinoma, indicating a possible transplacental effect of VCM (Maltoni *et al.*, 1974).

Mice, rats, and rabbits were exposed to VCM vapors at a dose of 500 ppm, 7 hours daily during the period of major organogenesis. While maternal toxicity was noted (in mice more than in rats and rabbits), vinyl chloride did not cause significant embryonic or fetal toxicity and was not teratogenic in any of the species at the concentration tested (John *et al.*, 1977). Vinyl chloride was present in fetal and maternal blood and in the amniotic fluid after exposure of pregnant CFY rats to vapors (2,000, 7,000, and 12,000 ppm, for 2.5 h on the 18th day of pregnancy). The placenta is thus permeable to this substance, but pregnant rats inhaling VCM vapors (1500 ppm) showed

## Table VIII
## Cancers Developed as a Consequence of VCM Exposure

| References | Observations |
| --- | --- |
| Tabershaw and Gaffey (1974) U.S. | Increased incidence of digestive and respiratory systems, brain, lymphatomas and cancers of unknown sites among workers exposed to the highest doses of VC |
| | Excess of cancers of the buccal cavity and of unspecified sites at lower exposure levels |
| Monson *et al.* (1974) U.S. | Excess of deaths due to cancer of the liver and biliary tract, brain, digestive tract, and lung |
| Nicholson *et al.* (1975) U.S. | Excess of deaths due to liver angiosarcoma, brain tumors, and lymphomas |
| Duck and Carter (1976) U.K. | Increased risk of cancer of the digestive system |
| Ott *et al.* (1975) U.S. | Increased risk of death due to all malignancies |
| Maltoni, 1976b | Higher incidence of abnormal sputum cytology in workers exposed to VC |
| Saric *et al.* (1976) Yugoslavia | Increased risk of liver angiosarcoma |
| Chiazze *et al.* (1977) U.S. | Excess of cancers of the digestive system (intestine) among white male employees |
| | Increased risk of breast and urinary cancers among white female employees |
| Locker *et al.* (1979) U.K. | Excess of liver angiosarcomas |
| Buffler *et al.* (1979) U.S. | Increased incidence of cancer of the respiratory system |
| Wagoner (1978) | Excess of cancers of the respiratory system |
| Waxweiller *et al.* (1976) U.S. | Excess of cancer of brain and central nervous system, respiratory system, hepatic system, lymphatic, and haematopoietic systems |
| Byren *et al.* (1976) Sweden | Excess of cancers of the liver and pancreas |
| | Increase of brain and lung cancers (not significant) |
| Fox and Collier (1976) U.K. | Excess of lung cancers for workers having terminated their employment less than 15 years since initial exposure |
| Fox and Collier (1977) U.K. | High incidence of liver cancers; increase of lungs and brain cancers (not significant) |
| von Reinl *et al.* (1977) G.F.R. | Excess of cancers of the liver, brain, lung, and lymphatic organs |
| Infante *et al.* (1976) U.S. | Increased incidence of cancers of the liver, lung, and brain |
| | Increased risk of C.N.S. cancers for population residing near PVC industries |

neither teratogenic nor embryotoxic effects when exposed during the second or the last third of pregnancy.

However, increased fetal mortality and embryotoxic manifestations (microphthalmia and anophthalmia) were described after exposure during the first period (Ungvary *et al.*, 1978). An increased incidence of birth defects was described for children born to parents residing near VCM polymerization plants. This study revealed that the most severe and largest number of defects were malformations of the DNS, cleft lip and palate, club foot, and malformations of the genital organs. On the other hand, an increased frequency of fetal deaths was described among the wives of VCM-exposed workers (mainly the men under 30 years of age), indicating that VCM could induce germinal mutations (Infante *et al.*, 1976). Afterwards, an increased incidence of CNS malformations was described in children born to parents living near PVC industries, but there was no relationship between a decreased atmospheric VCM level and the CNS malformation rate, so that other organic compounds discharged into the air of this region were perhaps partly responsible (Edmonds *et al.*, 1978).

## 3. ACRYLONITRILE

### 3.1. Toxicity

Acrylonitrile (ACN) caused congestion in all organs of mice, rats, and guinea pigs, as well as CNS, liver, and kidney damage (Paulet and Desnos, 1961).

Intravenous administration of 200 mg/kg to rats induced massive bilateral apoplexy of the adrenal glands (Szabo *et al.*, 1976), the rats showing signs of acute acrylonitrile poisoning characterized by cyanosis, excitement, tremor, convulsion, paralysis, and respiratory failure (Paulet and Desnos, 1961). A lethal dose of ACN (144 mg/kg) given subcutaneously to rats resulted in the formation of cyanomethemoglobin (Magos, 1962).

When male guinea pigs received an intraperitoneal administration of 100 mg/kg ($2 \times LD_{50}$) or when treated with an intrevenous administration of 30 mg/kg ($LD_{50} = 50$ mg/kg), protein and nonprotein sulfhydryls (especially the latter in the liver and brain) greatly decreased. The sulfhydryls in blood decreased at an early stage of intoxication (Hushimoto and Kanai, 1977; Szabo *et al.*, 1977a). Depression of the hepatic nonprotein sulfhydryls content in rat, mice, hamsters, and guinea pigs was also noted after an i.p. administration of ACN (20–80 mg/kg). Mice were the most vulnerable species and rats the most resistant to ACN effects (Vainio and Mäkinen, 1977).

When ACN was chronically administered to rats in drinking water at 20, 100, or 500 ppm, a dose-dependent increase of the liver GSH concentration was observed (Szabo *et al.*, 1977a). ACN affected the pyruvate oxidation in tissues, above all in the brain, and this excess level of pyruvate in the brain might explain cerebral dysfunction (Hashimoto and Kanai, 1972). High malonaldehyde levels were found in the liver after subcutaneous administration of 160 mg/kg ($2 \times LD_{50}$) to rats, indicating an increase in lipid peroxide concentration (Dinu, 1975). Acrylonitrile stimulated lipid peroxidation in isolated microsomes (Ivanov *et al.*, 1978).

Glutathione peroxidase was significantly increased following on the high peroxide levels, but remained ineffective because of a decrease in the glutathione levels.

After ACN intoxication, catalase failed to compensate glutathione ineffectiveness, probably due to lactic acid accumulation (Dinu, 1975; Dinu and Klein, 1976). An accumulation of lactate seemed to result from disturbance of the pyruvate oxidation (Hashimoto and Kanai, 1972).

A single intraperitoneal dose of ACN (3, 10 or 30 mg/kg) caused a decrease in liver cytochrome $P_{450}$ content to 50% of the control value and a decrease in microsomal aldrin oxide-synthetase activity. These effects were prevented by pretreatment of the animals with phenobarbital, 3-methylcholanthrene, Aroclor 1254, or L cystein. Pretreatment with diethylmaleate did not reinforce the effects of cytochrome $P_{450}$ or of aldrin oxide synthetase (Duverger *et al.*, 1978a).

The protective role exerted by the mixed-function-oxidase inducers on hepatic effects have to be correlated with the observations that adrenal lesions and mortality induced by ACN can be prevented by pretreatment with phenobarbital (Szabo and Selye, 1972).

Intraperitoneal injection of ACN (33 mg/kg) into male rats daily for three consecutive days resulted in a 20% decrease in the liver microsomal content of cytochrom $P_{450}$. Formation of 9-hydroxy and 9,10 dihydrodiol metabolites of benzo($\alpha$)pyrene *in vitro* in liver microsomes was inhibited. Serum corticosterone and prolactine decreased. Luteinizing hormone was unchanged. The follicle-stimulating hormone level was doubled. These results suggest impaired spermatogenesis in the exposed animals (Nilsen *et al.*, 1980). Sodium thiosulfate significantly reduced the hydrogen cyanide liberated in the blood.

*L*-cysteine greatly reduced both the ACN and cyanide concentration in the blood and greatly attenuated the signs of poisoning (Hashimoto and Kanai, 1965).

The distribution pattern of ($1$-$^{14}$C) ACN in rats after intravenous administration was characterized by an accumulation of radioactivity in the liver, kidneys, lungs, adrenal cortex, and blood. No significant difference could be observed in the distribution pattern after intravenous or oral administration. The localization of labeling corresponded well with ACN-induced injuries in those organs (Sandberg and Slanina, 1980).

### 3.2. Metabolism

The metabolic fate of acrylonitrile (Figure 2) appears to be strongly bound to the route of administration. When a single dose of ACN (0.75 nmol/kg) was administered orally to rats, 23% of the dose was found in the

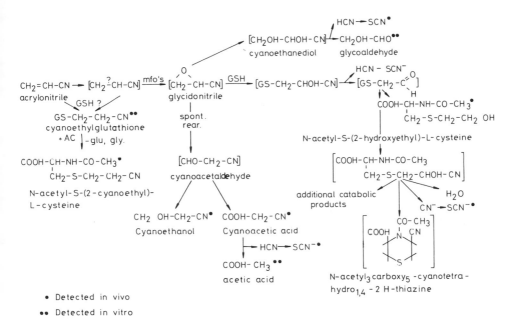

**Figure 2.** Metabolic pathway of acrylonitrile

urine as thiocyanate. After intravenous, subcutaneous, or intraperitoneal administration, only 1 to 4% of the dose was recovered as thiocyanate (Gut *et al.*, 1975); Nerudova *et al.*, 1978; Gut *et al.*, 1981). The excretion of radioactive metabolites of acrylonitrile-$^{14}$C seems to be little influenced by the rout of administration and was maximal four hours after administration; that of thiocyanate reached a maximum 8 to 14 hours after oral or intraperitoneal administration.

Less than 1% of radioactivity was eliminated in feces (Gut *et al.*, 1981).

The nonthiocyanate metabolites of acrylonitrile might result from the reaction of acrylonitrile with cysteine and/or glutathione; they represented approximatively $\frac{2}{3}$ of all the metabolites (Kopecky *et al.*, 1980a, b).

The metabolism into cyanide was higher after oral administration, indicating that the liver was probably the primary site of biotransformation (Nerudova *et al.*, 1978). This metabolic process was localized in the microsomal fraction and was NADPH and $O_2$-dependent and proportional to the microsomal protein and Cyt-$P_{450}$ concentrations (Abreu and Ahmed, 1980; Kopecky *et al.*, 1980a).

The cyanide formation was significantly enhanced when microsomes were obtained from phenobarbital, Aroclor 1254, or 3-methylcholanthrene treated rats. Phenobarbital pretreatment of rats did not significantly influence the excretion of thiocyanate in urine (Gut *et al.*, 1975; Nerudova *et al.*, 1978), and did not stimulate acrylonitrile metabolism in perfused rat liver (Nerudova *et al.*, 1978). The same pretreatment did not intensify the S9 mediated mutagenic response of acrylonitrile and suppressed the mutagenic activity detected in urine (de Meester *et al.*, 1979a, Lambotte-Vandepaer *et al.*, 1980). Pretreatment with $COCl_2$ or addition of SKF 525-A or CO to the incubation mixture inhibited acrylonitrile metabolism to cyanide. Addition of trichloropropene oxide decreased cyanide formation. (Abreu and Ahmed, 1980; Kopecky *et al.*, 1980a, b). When rats were pretreated with SKF 525-A, the elimination of thiocyanate was not modified (Gut *et al.*, 1975), but the mutagenic activity of urine was decreased (Lambotte-Vandepaer *et al.*, 1981).

The addition of SKF 525-A or metyrapone (another inhibitor of the mixed-function oxidases) to the incubation mixture, reduced the S9-mediated mutagenic activity of ACN (Duverger-van Bogaert *et al.*, 1981). In view of the conflicting results obtained with cyt-$P_{450}$ inducers and inhibitors, the exact role of cyt-$P_{450}$-dependent mixed-function oxidase in the activation of ACN remains unclear. However, six metabolites which have been identified can very easily be explained as originating from an epoxide type intermediate. The identification of glycolaldehyde can be explained as resulting from the hydration of the epoxide by epoxide hydratase. Cyanoethanediol decomposes spontaneously to glycolaldehyde and cyanide (Kopecky *et al.*, 1980a; Duverger-van Bogaert *et al.*, 1981b). Cyanoacetaldehyde, which would result from the spontaneous rearrangement of the epoxide, could subsequently be reduced either to cyanoethanol by the action of alcohol dehydrogenae or oxidized to cyanoacetic acid by aldehyde dehydrogenase (Duverger-van Bogaert *et al.*, 1981b).

ACN is postulated to react directly with GSH giving a Michael adduct, *N*-acetyl-*S*-2-cyanoethyl-L-cysteine which has been isolated in urine of rats treated with ACN (Kopecky *et al.*, 1980b; Langvardt and Putzig, 1980; Van Bladeren *et al.*, in press). The action of GSH on glycidonitrile results in the formation of a cyanohydrin, which has tentatively been identified (Langvardt and Putzig, 1980). This compound could then cyclize with loss of water to form *N*-acetyl-3-carboxy-5-cyanotetrahydro 1,4-2H-thiazine, which is in equilibrium with the corresponding aldehyde under extrusion of the cyanide ion. The aldehyde is then reduced enzymatically to the alcohol leading to the formation of *N*-acetyl-*S*-2-hydroxyethyl-L-cysteine. Pretreatment of rats with 1-phenylimidazole before administering ACN results in disappearance of the hydroxymercapturic acid, thus increasing the cyanoethyl mercapturic acid excretion. These observations indicate that the hydroxy mercapturic acid results from an oxidative process and probably from an epoxide (Van Bladeren *et al.*, in press).

## 3.3. Mutagenicity

ACN induced reverse mutations in *S. typhimurium* strains TA 1535, 1538, and 1978 in the presence of Aroclor 1254 pretreated mouse liver homogenate (See Table IX). In the aqueous phase, the ACN concentrations tested were 5, 10, and 20 $\mu$l in the incubation mixture. A mutagenic response was observed in the gas phase when the bacteria were exposed to an atmosphere containing 57 ppm of ACN (Milvy and Wolff, 1977).

The results described above were discussed; it seems that some mutagenic effects are still apparent but they are limited to only a few doses. The mutagenic effects in TA 1538 and TA 1978 are not substantiated (Venitt, 1978).

ACN in solution (5 and 10 $\mu$l/plate) caused a dose-related enhancement of the number of the revertant colonies in *E. coli* strains WP2, WP2 uvra, and WP2 uvra Pol. A. This mutagenic activity was observed without S9. Addition of S9 mix from Aroclor 1254 pretreated rat liver had no detectable effect on the mutagenic activity of ACN (Venitt *et al.*, 1977). These results suggest that ACN causes nonexcisable misrepair DNA damage. Incubation of *S.*

**Table IX.**
**Acrylonitrile Mutagenicity**

| Test | Conditions[a] | Response | References |
|------|-----------|----------|------------|
| *S. typhimurium* | A,C,D | ± | Milvy and Wolff (1977) |
| | A,C | + | de Meester *et al.* (1978a) |
| | A,C | + | de Meester *et al.* (1979a) |
| | A,D | + | Duverger-van Bogaert *et al.* (1981) |
| | E | + | Lambotte-Vandepaer *et al.* (1980) |
| | E | + | Lambotte-Vandepaer *et al.* (1981) |
| *E. coli* | B,D | + | Venitt *et al.* (1977) |
| Mammalian cells (*in vivo*) | Cytogenetic aberration in mice bone marrow cells | ⊖ | Rabello, Gay, and Ahmed (1980) |
| | Aberration metaphases in rat bone marrow cells | ⊖ | |
| | Chromosome aberration in mice bone marrow cells | ⊖ | Lèonard *et al.* (1981) |
| | Micronuclei | ⊖ | |
| | Chromosome aberration in human lymphocyte | ⊖ | Thiess and Fleig (1978) |

[a] A: + fortified liver fraction; B: = fortified liver fraction; C: gas phase; D: liquid medium; E: urines.

*typhimurium* strains in an atmosphere containing 0.2% ACN increased the number of revertants only in the presence of a fortified S9 liver fraction.

The mutagenic activity was more pronounced with strains Ta 1530, 1535, and TA 1950, and weaker with strains TA 100, TA 98, and TA 1978 (de Meester *et al.*, 1978a).

The reversion rate varied according to the animal species from which the S9 fraction was obtained, as well as according to the pretreatment of the animals. Pretreatment of mice with phenobarbital had an exacerbating effect on the S9-mediated mutagenicity of ACN. No similar increase was observed when rats were used.

Pretreatment of the animals with monomers had an exacerbating effect on the mutagenic activity of ACN; this effect raises the problem of possible comutagenic effects associated with simultaneous or consecutive exposures of such chemicals (de Meester *et al.*, 1979a).

The mutagenic activity of ACN has been tested in a modified method of incubation in liquid medium with *S. typhimurium* strain TA 1530. Pretreatment of the animals with diethylmaleat, phenobarbital, 3-methylcholanthrene, and Aroclor 1254 did not significantly affect the mutagenic activity of ACN. When inhibitors of the mixed-function-oxidase system (metyrapone, SKF 525-A) were added to the incubation mixture, a decreased mutagenic response was observed. The presence of light was an absolute prerequisite for obtaining liver-mediated mutagenic activity of ACN. When the preincubation was performed in the dark or in the presence of trichloroacetonitrile a radical trapping agent), the number of revertants/plate never exceeded the spontaneous reversion rate; on the other hand, when the preincubation was carried out under UV light (210 nm) or in the presence of $FeSo_4 \cdot 7H_2O$, a significant increase in the mutagenic response was observed. These results suggest a radicalar preactivation followed by the formation of an epoxide type intermediate (Duverger-van Bogaert *et al.*, 1981a).

Urine collected from rats and mice treated with ACN (30 mg/kg i.p.) had a direct mutagenic activity in *S. typhimurium* strain TA 1530. Pretreatment of the animals with phenobarbital abolished the direct mutagenicity of the urine from ACN-treated rats and reduced the activity observed in urine from mice. The addition of $\beta$-glucuronidase to the incubation mixture exacerbated the mutagenicity of the urine from both phenobarbital-treated and untreated rats, and from mice injected with ACN (Lambotte-Vandepaer *et al.*, 1980). Pretreatment of the animals with pyrazole, an inhibitor of alcohol dehydro-genase, reduced the mutagenic activity of the urine which was then completely suppressed after pretreatment of the animals with $COCl_2$ or SKF 525-A, inhibitors of the mixed-function-oxydase system, or in the presence of trichloroacetonitrile, a radical trapping agent (Lambotte-Vandepaer *et al.*, 1981). No chromosome aberrations have been detected in the bone marrow cells of rats and mice treated with ACN (Rabello-Gay and Ahmed, 1980;

Léonard *et al.*, 1981), or in the lymphocytes of chronically exposed workers (Thiess and Fleig, 1978a). ACN induced cell transformation in Syrian golden hamster embryo cell culture; an enhancement of virus transformation was obtained in similar cells pretreated with simian adenovirus (Parent and Casto, 1979). Breakage of the cellular DNA was observed after treatment of Syrian golden hamster embryo cells by ACN (Parent and Casto, 1979). These results suggest that ACN may be carcinogenic.

### 3.4. Carcinogenicity

The carcinogenic risk associated with ACN has been tested on rats exposed to inhalation or oral administration (Table X). A significantly increased incidence of various types of tumor was observed: microgliome of CNS, zymbal gland carcinoma, squamous cell papillomas of the forestomach, carcinoma and fibro-adenoma of the mammary gland, small intestinal carcinoma, and ear canal gland tumor (Maltoni *et al.*, 1977b; U.S. Department of Labor, 1978; Food and Drug Packaging, 1980). On the other hand, an increased incidence of cancer of the lung and large intestine seems to occur among workers occupationally exposed to ACN (IARC,.1979).

### 3.5. Teratogenicity and Embryotoxicity

The teratogenic potential of ingested or inhaled ACN has been evaluated in Sprague–Dawley rats, to whom 0, 10, 25, or 65 mg ACN/kg/day was administered by gavage to pregnant rats from days 6 to 15 of gestation. Oral administration of 65 mg/kg/day, the maternally toxic level of ACN, resulted in significant embryotoxic effects including an increased incidence of fetal malformations (short tail and trunk, missing vertebrae, right-sided aortic arch). Such effects were less apparent at 25 mg/kg/day or after inhlalation of an atmosphere containing 80 ppm ACN. No evidence of embryotoxicity or teratogenicity was detected in rats given 10 mg/kg/day orally, or in those inhaling 40 ppm (Murray *et al.*, 1978a).

Embryotoxicity has been studied in chicken eggs treated on day 3 and examined on day 14 of incubation. The $LD_{50}$ value is estimated to be in the range of 1–10 $\mu$mol (approx. 2.5 $\mu$mol/egg). No evidence of induced teratogenicity has been observed (Kankaanpää *et al.*, 1979a).

## 4. STYRENE

### 4.1. Toxicity

The oral $LD_{50}$ of styrene in rats is approximately 15 g/kg (Wolf *et al.*, 1956) and the $LD_{50}$ by intraperitoneal injection is 2–3 g/kg (Ohtsuji and Ikeda, 1971). The $LC_{50}$ concentration in rats was 2800 ppm for a 4-hour exposure and in mice 5000 ppm for a 2-hour exposure (Shugaev, 1969).

## Table X
### Carcinogenicity Studies of ACN in Animals

| Tumor Incidence | Response | Conditions | References |
|---|---|---|---|
| Squamous cell papillomas of forestomach | + in (a) ⊕ (e) ⊕ (i) <br> (b) (f) <br> ⊕ in (c) ⊕ (h) <br> (b) | (a) 35, 100, 300 mg/liter in drinking water (1) <br> (b) Examined after 12 months <br> (c) 100 and 300 mg/kg for 12 months (1) | (1) U.S. Department of Labor (1978) <br><br> (2) Maltoni et al. (1977) |
| Microgliome of CNS | ⊕ in (a) ⊖ (e) ⊕ (g) ⊕ (h) ⊕ (i) <br> (b) (f) (b) <br> ⊕ in (c) | (e) 5 mg/kg by gavage 3 times/week, for 52 weeks (2) | (3) U.S. Consumer Product Safety Commission (1978) U.S. Department of Labor (1978) |
| Zymbal gland carcinoma | ⊕ in (a) ⊕ (e) ⊕ (h) <br> (b) (f) (b) <br> ⊕ in (c) ⊕ (g) <br> (b) | (f) Examined after 131 weeks, (2) <br> (g) 20, 30 ppm for 6 hours a day, 5 days/week (3) <br> (h) 5, 10, 20, 40 ppm, 4 hours a day, 5 days/week (4) | (4) Maltoni et al., (1977) <br><br> (5) Anonymous Food and Drug Packaging (1980) |
| Fibroadenome of mammary gland (benign) | ⊕ (e) ⊕ (i) <br> (f) | (i) Drinking water 35, 85 210 ppm for 21 days and then 35, 100, 300 ppm (5) | |
| Carcinoma of mammary gland (malignant) | ⊕ (e) ⊕ (i) <br> (f) | | |
| Ear canal gland | ⊕⊕ (i) | | |
| Small intestine carcinoma | ⊕⊕ (i) | | |

The organ toxicity of styrene has been studied on several animal species: rats, guinea pigs, rabbits, and monkeys, exposed to 1300 ppm styrene vapors for 7–8 hours/day, 5 days a week for 6 months. Death occured in guinea pigs, 10% of which developed acute lung inflammation, edema, and hemorrhage; a slight increase in the weight of liver and kidneys was observed for rats. No abnormal microscopic tissue changes or alterations of the blood picture occured (Spencer et al., 1942). The deaths of rats and guinea pigs were due to lung irritation followed by pneumonia; lungs, kidneys and liver showed congestion (Spencer et al., 1942; Wilson et al., 1948).

A slight increase in the weight of liver and kidneys was noted when rats were treated with peroral doses of 400 mg/kg for 185 days; a dose of 133 mg/kg caused no change (Wolf et al., 1956). One year of styrene inhalation at a level of 1300 ppm produced no changes in rabbits or in rhesus monkeys (Wolf et al., 1956). When rats were exposed to 300 ppm styrene vapors for 2–11 weeks, 6 days a week, 6 hours daily, a marked accumulation of styrene in the brain and perinephric fat occurred. Furthermore, increased activity of lysosomal acid proteinase was detected after 9 weeks (Savolainen and Pfäffli, 1977). The same treatment increased ethoxycoumarine-deethylase, cytochrom-$P_{450}$, epoxide-hydratase, and UDP-glucuronosyl-transferase activity in the liver and kidney. A dose-dependent decrease of glutathione level occurred after four days of exposure, followed by a glutathione rebound.

Degenerative morphological lesions were observed in the liver parenchymal cells after a 2 week exposure (Vainio et al., 1979). Inhalation exposure of mice to 300 ppm styrene (5 hours/day, 5 days/week for 6 weeks) induced bronchiolar epithelial changes in 10% of the animals and thickened the bronchiolar walls (by stratification of the bronchiolar epithelium) in 90% of the animals. This last observation could be interpreted as a defense mechanism aiming at a higher production of glutathione-S-epoxide transferase and epoxide hydratase (Morisset et al., 1979). Styrene inhalation appeared to have an effect on body weight, which was probably related to tissue protein destruction: Styrene has been described as combining with thiol groups in rats, mice, guinea pigs, and hamsters after i.p. administration. Mice were the most sensitive species and rats the more resistant (Leibman, 1975; Vainio and Mäkinen, 1977). For this reason, styrene should accelerate the catabolism of proteins in the organism. These data are supported by the fact that the brain tissue of styrene-exposed rats showed a decrease in free amino acids (Gadzhiev and Aliev, 1974), while the serum albumin levels of workers handling styrene were low (Lukoshkina and Alekperov, 1973). An increase in the activity of epoxide hydratase and UDP glucuronosyl transferase was described for rats injected i.p. with 3 or 6 doses of 500 m/gkg styrene (Parkki et al., 1976) and for rats exposed to 450 ppm styrene vapor for 7 days (Sandell et al., 1979). No change in these enzymes was described for mice exposed to styrene oxide vapor (Vainio and Elovaara, 1979). Cutaneous administration of styrene to rats (0.5 and 3 g/kg for 7 days) depressed epoxide hydratase activity but did not affect UDP glucuronosyl transferase activity (Sandell *et al.*, 1979). Intraperitoneal injection of 10, 100, or 500 mg/kg styrene in rats caused a decrease of the Km of styrene oxide hydratase (increasing the affinity of the enzyme for its substrate) (Lambotte-Vandepaer *et al.*, 1978).

In these conditions, neither acute toxic effects nor cytochrome $P_{450}$ changes were noted, but other perturbations of the mixed function oxidases were described. There was a decrease in the Km of aldrin epoxidase and benzpyrene hydroxylase, but styrene epoxidase was not affected.

Increase of paranitroanisole $O$-demethylase activity was observed in styrene intraperitoneally treated rats (Parkii *et al.*, 1976). Styrene inhalation (450 ppm—8 hours daily for 7 days) increased the activity of ethoxycoumarine deethylase in the kidney, but did not alter hepatic cytochrome $P_{450}$, hepatic and renal NADPH cyc.c reductase, benzpyrene hydroxylase, and glutathione-S-transferase. No changes in enzymatic activity in the lungs were described (Sandell *et al.*, 1978).

The exposure of female CB-20 mice to styrene oxide inhalation produced acute intoxication, as shown both by clinical manifestations and depression of nonprotein sulfhydryl content in the liver and kidneys. Ethoxycoumarine deethylase activity and the cytochrom $P_{450}$ level were simultaneously induced in the liver and kidneys. Furthermore, a type-I difference spectrum was produced when styrene oxide was incubated in the presence of phenobarbital-induced microsomes, suggesting that the binding of styrene oxide is predominantly catalyzed by phenobarbital-induced cytochrome $P_{450}$ (Vainio and Elovaara, 1979).

Increased serum alanine aminotransferase activity and histological examinations, which are signs of hepatic necrosis, are observed in hamsters injected with i.p. doses of 2–3 g/kg styrene. Pretreatment with phenobarbital increased the acute lethality (Parkki *et al.*, 1979).

A study of 494 workers exposed to styrene revealed neurotoxic symptoms in 13% of them. The prenarcotic symptoms noted were distal hypoesthesia in the lower extremities and decreased radical and peroneal nerve-conduction velocity (Lillis *et al.*, 1978; Seppäläinen, 1978). Other data confirm the neurotoxic effects of styrene: EEG abnormalities (Klimkova-Deutschova *et al.*, 1973; Götell *et al.*, 1972; Kolmierski *et al.*, 1976; Seppäläinen and Härkönen, 1976) and prolonged reaction time in styrene-exposed workers (Götell *et al.*, 1972).

On the other hand, in a Finnish study, measurement of nerve conduction velocity carried out on 40 subjects revealed no relationship between styrene exposure and neuropathy (Savolainen and Vainio, 1977).

A morbidity study carried out at the BASF did not report a significantly higher incidence of abnormal values for hemoglobin, erithrocytes, leucocytes, SGOT, SGPT, and $\gamma$-GT in the styrene-exposed workers, but it should be noted that the styrene vapor concentrations were lower than the maximum allowable in the Federal Republic of Germany (Thiess and Friedheim, 1978). When examined with a psychological test battery, styrene-exposed workers showed only slight differences and only in visuomotor accuracy (Lindström *et al.*, 1976; Härkönen *et al.*, 1978).

The opthalmological examination of 300 styrene exposed workers revealed no sign of optic neuritis of fundal abnormality (Lorimer *et al.*, 1976).

In a Polish study, symptoms of the respiratory tract (obstructive changes) were described (Chmielewski and Renke, 1976). Screening by liver function tests did not suggest liver lesions (Chielewsky and Hac, 1976). Higher $\alpha$ and $\beta$ lipoprotein levels and higher cholesterol concentrations in serum were noted in the group exposed for more than 10 years (Chmielewski, 1976). The most common toxic effects in styrene-exposed workers were irritations of the skin, eyes, and respiratory tract and CNS depression.

At or below the TLV, there were no symptoms or objective signs in man on short exposure; with continued exposure, mild eye and throat irritation occured and there was a slight impairment of coordination and balance. At higher air concentration, nasal, air, throat, and skin irritation became more pronounced and there was decreased coordination, balance, and manual dexterity.

Nausea, headache, fatigue, and a feeling of drunkenness have been reported. As with other hydrocarbons, chemical pneumonitis is a great hazard if aspiration occurs after ingestion of styrene (Leibman, 1975; Härkönnen, 1978).

## 4.2. Metabolism

Styrene is metabolically transformed into styrene 7,8 oxide (Figure 3). This has been directly demonstrated *in vitro* using rat and rabbit liver microsomes (Leibman and Ortiz, 1969; Leibman, 1975; Watabe *et al.*, 1978a; Belvedere, 1977; Duverger-van Bogaert *et al.*, 1978b), extrahepatic tissue microsomes from rats, mice, guinea pigs, and rabbits (Cantoni *et al.*, 1978), rat liver nuclei (Gazzotti *et al.*, 1980), and human lymphocyte cultures (Norppa *et al.*, 1980b).

This metabolic step was catalyzed by the cytochrom-$P_{450}$ mixed-function-oxidase system, and indirect confirmation of this metabolic pathway has been obtained by *in vivo* studies. Phenobarbital pretreatment increased styrene metabolism while SKF 525-A showed an inhibiting effect, as measured by the excretion of urinary metabolites (Ohtsuji and Ikeda, 1971; Ikeda *et al.*, 1972). On the other hand, tests using radioactive styrene have

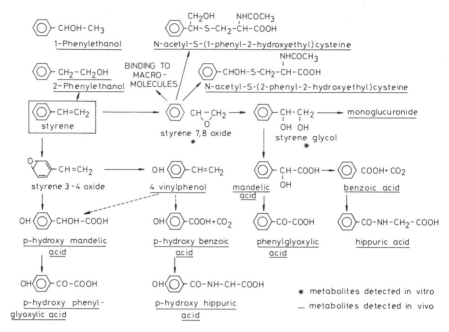

**Figure 3.** Metabolic pathway of styrene.

demonstrated its ability to bind to microsomal proteins in the presence of NADPH. Phenobarbital pretreatment intensifies this NADPH-dependent binding, while carbon tetrachloride pretreatment significantly decreased the amount of radioactivity bound to microsomal proteins from male rats (Watabe *et al.*, 1978b). Furthermore, styrene oxide has been described as binding covalently to macromolecules *in vivo* and *in vitro* (Marniemi *et al.*, 1976).

Styrene oxide may be detoxified by different routes: conjugation with glutathione is the first, leading to the formation of mercapturic acids excreted, as such, in the urine of styrene-treated rats and rabbits (James and White, 1967; Seutter-Berlage *et al.*, 1978; Yagen *et al.*, 1981).

It has been demonstrated that glutathione-*S*-epoxide-transferase, using styrene oxide as a substrate, has various specific activities in hepatic and extrahepatic tissues (lung, kidney, intestinal mucosa) from rat, guinea pig, and rabbit (James *et al.*, 1975; Boyland and Williams, 1965).

The other possibility for the metabolic detoxication of styrene oxide is via the epoxide hydratase (Oesch *et al.*, 1971; Belvedere *et al.*, 1977; Duverger-van Bogaert *et al.*, 1978; James *et al.*, 1975; Ryan *et al.*, 1975). The resulting styrene glycol was described as an *in vitro* styrene metabolite (El Masri *et al.*, 1958; Leibman and Ortiz, 1969). It was partly transformed into glucuronide detected in the urine of treated animals (El Masri, 1958), but the major metabolic pathway led to the formation of benzoic and hippuric acids or mandelic and phenylglyoxilic acids, which were excreted in the urine of treated animals (El Masri et al., 1958; James and White, 1967; Ohtsuji and Ikeda, 1971).

Mandelic and phenylglyoxilic acids have also been excreted in the urine of styrene-exposed workers and have been proposed as an exposure index in industry (Philippe et al., 1971; Bardodej and Bardodejova, 1970; Sollenberg et al., 1977; Engström et al., 1978; Wolff et al., 1978; Ogata and Sugishara, 1978; Ramsey et al., 1979; Caperos et al., 1979; Guillemin and Bauer, 1979). Only a small proportion is metabolized into hippuric acid in man (Guillemin and Bauer, 1979).

Minor metabolic pathways of styrene in the rat are represented by the formation of phenylethanol and the hydroxylation of the phenyl moiety (4-vinyl phenol) (El Masri et al., 158; Bakke and Sheline, 1970, Pantarotto et al., 1978).

The formation of 4-vinyl phenol could involve the intervention of an oxide in the 3,4-position and could explain the urinary excretion of p-hydroxy mandelic, p-hydroxy benzoic, and p-hydroxy hippuric acids (Pantarotto et al., 1978).

Styrene is principally absorbed via the lungs with an influence of alveolar ventilation and, to a lesser extent, through the skin (Härkönen, 1978).

Quantitative analysis revealed that, after administration, styrene was rapidly cleared from the blood, according to a 2-compartment model, in man (Ramsey et al., 1980) and in animals (Withey and Collins, 1977 and 1979; Danishefsky and Willhite, 1954). Accumulation occured only when the styrene exposure level was above 200 ppm (Ramsey and Young, 1978). Ninety percent of the administered dose is eliminated in the urine after metabolization in man (Ramsey et al., 1980; Caperos et al., 1979, Engström et al., 1978) and animals (Leibman, 975; Plotnick and Weigel, 1979), while small proportions were excreted in the feces and in expired air.

It has been noted that styrene largely accumulates in fat in proportion to the exposure level and to a small extent in the liver, kidney and brain (Withey and Collins, 1979; Danishefsky and Willhite, 1954; Savolainen and Pfäffli, 1978; Engström et al., 1978; Savolainen and Vainio, 1977; Wolff, 1976). In conclusion, styrene 7,8 epoxide is considered as the major reactive metabolite, capable of producing mutagenic, carcinogenic, and toxic effects. The intervention of styrene 3,4 oxide, recently proposed as another styrene pathway, must also be considered as potentialy mutagenic, carcinogenic, and toxic. It may further be pointed out that, in rats, the affinity of mono-oxygenase for styrene is 20 times lower than that of oxide hydratase for styrene oxide; this consequently reduces the lifetime of the epoxide (Duverger-van Bogaert et al., 1978; Cantoni et al., 1978) and is probably responsible for the weak mutagenic, carcinogenic, and toxic potentialities of styrene. Mice and rabbits seem to be the species least able to inactivate styrene oxide (Cantoni *et al.*, 1978).

## 4.3. Mutagenicity

When assayed in the Ames test, styrene is reported as able to induce reverse mutations from 0.1 μmole up to 10 μmole/plate in *Salmonella typhimurium* TA 1535 and TA 100 (base pair substitution), in the presence of a metabolic activating system in the plate incorporation assay (Vainio *et al.*, 1976; de Meester *et al.*, 1977; Watabe, 1978a,b) or in the gas phase (de Meester *et al.*, 1981) (Table XI).

These effects were intensified by the addition of trichloropropene oxide (inhibition of epoxide hydratase) or diethylmaleate (decrease of the glutathione level) (Vainio *et al.*, 1976; Watabe, 1978a,b).

Styrene caused a highly toxic effect on *Salmonella typhimurium*, making the detection of a mutagenic effect difficult (Vainio *et al.*, 1976; de Meester *et al.*, 1977; Watabe, 1978a,b; Loprieno *et al.*, 1978).

On the other hand, negative results have been observed with styrene using *Salmonella typhimurium* as target cells in the absence or presence of liver homogenates (Stoltz and Withey, 1977; Milvy and Garro, 1976; Busk, 1979; Loprieno *et al.*, 1978), even when epoxide hydratase or glutathione conjugation was inhibited (Busk, 1979).

Styrene oxide, the major reactive metabolite of styrene, was able to induce reverse mutation in *S. typhimurium* TA 1535 and TA 100 in the presence or absence of a metabolic activating system (Milvy and Garro, 1976; Vainio *et al.*, 1976; de Meester *et al.*, 1977; Watabe *et al.*, 1978a,b; Stoltz and Withey, 1977; Busk, 1979; Yoshikawa, 1980; Loprieno *et al.*, 1978) (Table XII). Cytotoxicity was also noted for this substance in bacterial cells (Vainio *et al.*, 1976; de Meester *et al.*, 1977). The mutagenic effect of styrene oxide was reduced when liver homogenate was added to the test, owing to detoxification (Vainio *et al.*, 1976; Watabe *et al.*, 1978a,b; Yoshikawa *et al.*, 1980).

Styrene oxide is detoxified by two major routes; epoxide hydratase and glutathione transferase are implicated in decreased mutagenicity. The addition of trichloropropene oxide increased the S9-mediated mutagenicity of styrene oxide (Watabe *et al.*, 1978a,b), while the addition of microsomes completely abolished this effect (Yoshikawa *et al.*, 1980). On the other hand, the presence of glutathione and of a supernatant liver fraction decreases the mutagenic effect of styrene oxide (Yoshikawa *et al.*, 1980).

Gas chromatographic determinations have shown the disappearance of styrene oxide in the latter conditions (Yoshikawa *et al.*, 1980). The other known metabolites of styrene (styrene glycol, mandelic, phenylglyoxylic, benzoic and hippuric acids) are not mutagenic in *S. typhimurium* (Milvy and Garro, 1976).

Styrene oxide seems thus to be the major mutagenic metabolite of styrene, but is formation cannot completely explain the mutagenic properties of styrene, since other unknown metabolites could also participate in this mutagenic action (Vainio *et al.*, 1976; Watabe *et al.*, 1978b). The arene oxide 1-vinylbenzene 3,4-oxide which is assumed to be a precursor of 4-vinylphenol had a potent killing effect but no mutagenic activity in TA 100 cells (Watabe *et al.*, 1978b).

In a test using yeast, styrene was unable to induce either forward mutations in *S. Pombe* (P₁-strain, ade mutations) or gene conversion in *S. cerevisiae* (D₄-strain-ade locus), although positive results were obtained with styrene oxide (20 mM). In the host mediated assay, both compounds produced gene conversion in *S. cerevisiae*, but did not induce forward mutations in *S. Pombe*. This single positive result obtained for styrene occurred when metabolic activation occured, confirming the results obtained with other tests (Loprieno *et al.*, 1976b).

Further investigations have shown that a loss of monooxygenase activity (due to both enzyme inactivation and inhibition) occurs in the presence of 50 mM styrene. In these conditions, gas chromatographic determinations of styrene oxide in the incubation mixture revealed a styrene oxide concentration too low to act as a mutagen in *S. Pombe*. Positive results have been noted for *S. Pombe* at a concentration of 5 mM styrene oxide (Bauer *et al.*, 1980).

Styrene as well as styrene oxide were able to induce cytogenetic effects on *Allium Cepa*. Styrene caused chromosome breaks, a strong C-mitotic effect, and prolonged, disordered anaphases, indicating an inhibition of the mitotic spindle. After styrene oxide treatment, nuclear bridges and fragments were frequently observed in the anaphases, leading to formation of micronuclei in successive telophases and interphases. Allium cells treated with styrene oxide for 12 h with 0.05% v/v styrene oxide presented a decondensation of the chromatin, suggesting a specific effect of styrene oxide on chromosomal proteins (Linnainmaa *et al.*, 1978). The difference noted between the cytogenetic effects of styrene and styrene oxide suggests that styrene metabolites other than styrene oxide could be formed in the presence of allium cells, causing such effects (Linnainmaa *et al.*, 1978). Styrene oxide, but not styrene, was able to induce forward mutations in Chinese hamster cells (8-Azaguanine resistance) and causes polyploidy in cultured Chinese hamster cells (Loprieno *et al.*, 1976b). The expression curve of mutants induced by styrene oxide decreases after reaching the maximum value, although in general this curve shows a plateau without decrease. This observation seems to be due neither to the instability of a resistant phenotype of clones nor to the selection of stable resistant clones (Bonatti *et al.*, 1978).

Table XI

**Mutagenicity of Styrene**

| | Result | Conditions[a] | References |
|---|---|---|---|
| *Salmonella typhimurium* | + | A,C | Vainio et al., 1976 |
| | | | de Meester et al., 1977 |
| | + | A,D | Watabe et al., 1978a,b,c |
| | − | A,D | de Meester et al., 1981 |
| | | | Stoltz and Withey, 1977 |
| | | | Milvy and Garro, 1976 |
| | | | Busk, 1979 |
| *S. pombe* | − | A,C | Loprieno et al., 1978 |
| *S. cerevisiae* | − | A,C | Loprieno et al., 1976b |
| *S. pombe* | − | Host mediated assay | Loprieno et al., 1976b |
| *S. cerevisiae* | + | Host mediated assay | Loprieno et al., 1976b |
| *Allium cepa* cells chromosomal breaks | + | 0.05% (v/v) | Linnainmaa et al., 1978 |
| *Drosophila melanogaster* | | | |
| Recessive lethal frequency | + | 200 ppm feeding | Donner et al., 1979 |
| Chromosomal non disjunction | − | 500 ppm feeding | Penttilä et al., 1980 |
| Chinese hamster cells (forward mutation) | − | B,C | Loprieno et al., 1976b |

| Test system | Result | Conditions[a] | Reference |
|---|---|---|---|
| Chinese hamster ovary cells (SCE) | − | A,B,C | De Raat, 1979 |
| Chromosomal aberrations | | | |
| Rat | + | Inhalation 300 ppm 2–11 weeks | Meretoja et al., 1978 |
| Mice | − | Oral administration 500 and 1000 mg/kg | Loprieno et al., 1978 |
| Chinese hamster | − | Inhalation 300 ppm | Norppa et al., 1980 |
| | | Ethanol administration | Norppa et al., 1980 |
| | + | Styrene inhalation 300 ppm | |
| Sister chromatid exchanges | | | |
| Alveolar macrophages in mice | | | |
| Bone marrow cells in mice | + | Inhalation 591 to 922 ppm 4 days | Conner et al., 1979 and 1980 |
| Regenerating liver cells in mice | − | 1 g/kg | Penttilä et al., 1980 |
| Micronucleus test: Chinese hamster | + | | Meretoja et al., 1977 |
| Chromosomal aberrations in men | − | | Thiess and Fleig, 1978 |
| Human lymphocytes in culture | + | 0.03% (v/v) | Linnainmaa et al., 1978 |
| EUE Human heteteploid cells | − | A 14.3 mM 28.5 mM 42.8 mM | Loprieno et al., 1976b |
| DNA repair | | | |

[a] A: + S9; B: − S9; C: liquid medium; D: gas phase.

### Table XII
### Mutagenicity of Styrene Oxide

| | Result | Conditions | References |
|---|---|---|---|
| *Salmonella typhimurium* | + | A,B,C | Milvy and Garro, 1976 |
| | | | Vainio *et al.*, 1976 |
| | | | de Meester *et al.*, 1977 |
| | | | Watabe *et al.*, 1978a,b |
| | | | Stoltz and Withey, 1977 |
| | | | Busk, 1979 |
| | | | Yoshikawa, 1980 |
| | | | Loprieno *et al.*, 1978 |
| *S. pombe* | + | A,C | Loprieno *et al.*, 1976b |
| *S. cerevisiae* | + | A,C | Loprieno *et al.*, 1976b |
| *S. pombe* | − | Host mediated assay | Loprieno *et al.*, 1976b |
| *S. cerevisiae* | + | Host mediated assay | Loprieno *et al.*, 1976b |
| *Allium cepa* cells chromosomal aberrations | + | 0.05% (v/v) | Linnainmaa *et al.*, 1978 |
| Chinese hamster cells | + | B,C | Loprieno *et al.*, 1976b |
| Chinese hamster ovary cells | + | A,B,C | de Raat, 1979 |
| *Drosophila melanogaster* Recessive lethal frequency | + | 200 ppm inhalation | Donner *et al.*, 1978 |

| | | | |
|---|---|---|---|
| Chromosomal aberrations | | | |
| Rats | − | 250 mg/kg i.p. | Fabry et al., 1978 |
| Chinese hamsters | − | Inhalation 25–50–75–100 ppm; 2, 4, or 20 days | Norppa et al., 1980 |
| Mice | + | 500 mg/kg, i.p. | Norppa et al., 1980 |
| SCE Bone marrow | + | 50–1,000 mg/kg | Loprieno et al., 1978 |
| Chinese hamster | − | 25–50–75–1000 ppm inhalation; 2, 4, or 20 days | Norppa et al., 1979 |
| | + | 500 mg/kg, i.p. | Norppa et al., 1979 |
| Micronucleus test | | | |
| Chinese hamster | − | 250 mg/kg, i.p. | Penttilä et al., 1980 |
| Micronucleus test | − | 250 mg/kg, i.p. | Fabry et al., 1978 |
| Erythrocytes rats | | | |
| Human lymphocytes in culture | + | 0.5 mM | Fabry et al., 1978 |
| Human lymphocytes in culture | + | 0.003% (v/v) | Linnainmaa et al., 1978 |
| Human EUE cells DNA repair | + | B 4.4 mM 8.7 mM | Loprieno et al., 1978 |

Negative results were noted when Chinese hamster ovary cells were treated with styrene, even in the presence of a metabolic activating system, and a positive result was noted only with the addition of cyclohexene oxide (inhibitor of the epoxide hydratase) to the test. SCEs occurred when Chinese hamster ovary cells were treated with styrene oxide, but the addition of a metabolic activating system decreased this effect (de Raat, 1978).

*Drosophila melanogaster* (white and BASC strains) showed an increase in the recessive lethal frequency after exposure to styrene and styrene oxide.

Phenobarbitone pretreatment caused an increased frequency in both cases, while trichloropropene oxide, only assayed in the presence of styrene oxide, also exacerbated this frequency (Donner *et al.*, 1979).

Styrene, when administered to *Drosophila* by feeding (500 ppm), did not induce chromsomal nondisjunction (Penttila *et al.*, 1980).

Styrene given by inhalation to male rats (300 ppm, 2-11 weeks) significantly increased the rate of chromosomal aberrations in their bone marrow cells (8 to 12%), as compared to the control group (1 to 6%) after 9 weeks of treatment. In addition, polyploid cells were noted only in the exposed animals (Meretoja *et al.* 1978).

No significant increase was observed in the frequency of chromosomal aberrations or gaps in the bone marrow cells of Chinese hamsters after inhalation (300 ppm) (Norppa *et al.*, 1980a) or after i.p. administration (Penttilä *et al.*, 1980). When styrene treatment was combined with ethanol oral administration, no more significant results were noted (Norppa *et al.*, 1980a).

Styrene oxide, when assayed in Chinese hamsters (Norppa *et al.*, 1979; Penttilä *et al.*, 1980), or rats (Fabry *et al.*, 1978), had no effects on chromosomal aberration frequency, but when tested in mice, it increased this frequency, indicating that the latter animal species is more sensitive than rats or Chinese hamsters (Loprieno *et al.*, 1978). The administration to rats of a lethal styrene oxide dose (500 mg/kg, i.p.) provoked an increased frequency of chromsomal aberrations (Norppa *et al.*, 1979). A significant increase in SCE frequencies was observed in harvested alveolar macrophages, bone marrow and regenerating liver cells of mice exposed to styrene at doses ranging from 591 to 922 ppm for 4 days, with a dose–effect relationship. In these conditions, no difference was noted for the different cell types studied, and the effect seems not to be due to the styrene oxide produced by the liver (Conner *et al.*, 1979 and 1980).

Styrene oxide given by inhalation (25 to 100 ppm—2,4 or 20 days) to Chinese hamsters was unable to increase the SCE rate of bone marrow cells, but a significant result was noted when styrene was administered at a lethal concentration (500 mg/kg, i.p.) (Norppa *et al.*, 1979).

Styrene oxide was unable to provoke micronuclei in erythrocytes from treated rats (Fabry *et al.*) 1978). Neither styrene nor styrene oxide was able to provoke loss in the micronucleus test, when injected i.p. to Chinese hamsters (Penttilä et al., 1980).

All tests on germ cells (translocation in premeiotic male germ cells and dominant lethality in post-meiotic ones) gave negative results, when styrene oxide was assayed in male rats (250 mg/kg, i.p.) (Fabry et al., 1978).

Chinese hamster seems to be resistant to the clastogenic effects of styrene and styrene oxide, owing to its favorable activation/inactivation ratio (Norppa et al., 1979; Penttilä et al., 1980).

Two contradictory reports exist on the mutagenic activity of styrene for men: Meretoja et al., (1977) reported that occupationally exposed men showed an increased rate of chromsomal aberrations in cultured blood lymphocytes (11 to 26%), as compared with a control group (3%). Decondensation of chromatin and disturbances similar to premature chromsome condensation were observed. The frequencies of micronuclei and cells connected with nuclear bridges were also increased.

The analysis of Thiess and Fleig (1978) revealed no increase in gap or other chromosomal aberrations in the exposed groups when compared to a control group, probably because of the low styrene concentration in the workplace.

Fabry et al. (1978) reported a significant increase in the total number of anomalies after treatment of human lymphocytes with 0.5 mM styrene oxide (mainly because of an increase in chromatid gaps).

Styrene (0.03% v/v) and styrene oxide (0.008% v/v) induced cytogenetic effects in human cultured lymphocytes. Styrene caused primary chromsome breaks and styrene oxide treatment showed the formation of micronuclei, nuclear bridges, and occasional banded staining (Linainmaa et al., 1978). Only styrene oxide was able to increase the incorporation of thymidine in the DNA of human heteroploid cells in the presence of an inhibitor of semiconservative DNA synthesis. Negative results were noted even when a metabolic activating system was added (Loprieno et al., 1976b).

## 4.4. Carcinogenicity

Styrene has been tested for its carcinogenic potential in 020 and C57B1 mice receiving, on the 17th day of gestation, oral doses of 1350 mg/kg and 300 mg/kg, respectively. Their offspring were treated weekly by gavage, with the same dose of styrene, for their life span. Preweaning mortality is considerbly exacerbated in the 020 mice receiving styrene on the 17th day of gestation, but was comparable to the control group in the C57B1 mice. The mortality of their respective progeny was increased in the 020 mice group but not in the C57B1 mice group.

A significantly increased incidence of lung tumors was observed in the progeny of styrene-treated 020 mice who received styrene for 16 weeks (89%

among the males and 100% among the females). Histologically, the lung tumors were adenomas or adenocarcinomas, and the proportion of malignant and nonmalignant lung tumors did not differ for the different groups. No statistically significant increase or tumors was observed in the C57Bl mice groups (Ponomarkov and Tomatis, 1978). Female BD IV rats were given a single oral dose of styrene (1350 mg/kg) on the 17th day of pregnancy; their progeny received weekly oral administrations of styrene (500 mg/kg). There was a slight increase in preweaning mortality compared to the control groups. A few tumors occurring in the styrene-treated animals claim attention, since they are rarely observed in control animals. Three stomach tumors—adenoma, fibrosarcoma, and carcinosarcoma—with diffuse metastases are observed in styrene-treated animals. A single liver tumor (hepatocellular adenoma) and three neurinomas were found in rats treated weekly with styrene (Ponomarkov and Tomatis, 1978).

Fisher 344 rats (50 males and 50 females per dose) received oral doses of 2000 mg/kg, 1000 mg/kg, and 500 mg/kg for 78 weeks, but the variety of tumors in both control and treated rats was not attributed to styrene dosage.

$B_6C_3F_1$ mice (50 males and 50 females per dose) received oral doses of 300 or 150 mg/kg styrene for 78 weeks. Treated and control animals developed various tumors, suggesting that the tumors were not dose-related, except for lung tumors which occurred in 14% of the low-dosed and 18% of the high-dosed male mice (carcinoma and adenoma of the lung). Owing to the high spontaneous tumor incidence in that animal species (National Cancer Institute, 1979), no firm conclusion on carcinogenicity can be drawn.

When administered orally to Sprague–Dawley rats, styrene oxide (250 and 50 mg/kg) increased the incidence of papillomas *in situ*, carcinomas, and invasive carcinomas of the forestomach. Carcinomas often metastatized to the liver. In the forestomach of treated animals (with or without tumors) precursor lesions were frequently observed. The administration route seemed to play an important role in the determination of the target organ (Maltoni *et al.*, 1979).

Lilis and Nicholson (1976) investigated the mortality of workers in a chemical plant producing styrene monomer. The workers were exposed not only to styrene but also to benzene and butadiene. The observation of three leukemias and two lymphomas, or 104 death, indicates the need for further study (Maltoni *et al.*, 1979).

## 4.5. Teratogenicity and Embryotoxicity

Styrene (46–90 mg/kg egg) injected into the yolk sac of fresh, fertile chicken eggs produced no toxic effects (McLaughlin *et al.*, 1964). Injected on the 4th day of incubation, the $LD_{50}$ was 40 $\mu$mol/embryo. In 20% of the treated embryos, malformations are related to both dose and time of injection (Vainio *et al.*, 1977). The embryotoxicity of styrene (mortality of 29% at a dose of 10 $\mu$mole/egg) and styrene oxide (mortality of 38% at a dose of 0.8 $\mu$mole/egg) was significantly increased (72% and 62% respectively) after injection of trichloropropene oxide to chick embryos. An increased malformation rate was noted for both styrene (15%) and styrene oxide (20%) after trichloropropene oxide treatment (33% and 27%, respectively). The macroscopic anomalies were described as stunting, viscera or brain exteriorization (19/29), and eye defects (8/29) (Vainio et al., 1977).

These results confirm the role of styrene oxide as a potent teratogen which could be formed from styrene in chick embryos, since they have been described as able to transform styrene metabolically into styrene oxide (Kankaanpää et al., 1979b). When rats were exposed to styrene vapors (350–1100 ppm) no embryotoxic effects were described (Ragule, 1974). When the fertilized eggs or embryos of sea urchins were exposed to styrene ($5 \times 10^{-4}$M), the differentiation of the embryos was quite abnormal. Pretreatment of the eggs in $10^{-3}$M styrene induced cytolysis; pretreatment in $10^{-4}$M styrene resulted in pathological embryos. Pretreatment of the sperm at a dose of $10^{-3}$M reduced its fertilizing capacity; no such effects were noted at a dose of $10^{-4}$M but the embryos generated by the treated sperm showed abnormal cleavage (Pagano et al., 1978). After inhalation exposure of rats and rabbits to styrene (300 or 600 ppm) from days 6 to 15 (rats) and from days 6 to 18 (rabbits) of gestation, neither embryotoxicity nor fetotoxicity was noted in either species. The same results were described after oral administration of styrene to rats (90 and 150 mg/kg, twice daily, from days 6 to 15 of gestation), but decreased body weight and food consumption were noted in exposed adults. No teratogenic effect was detected in either rats or rabbits (Murray et al., 1978b).

Styrene inhaled by pregnant mice (250 ppm) or Chinese hamsters (300–500–700 ppm/during the period of organogesesis) did not induce teratogenic effects, but skeletal variations were detected among litters of mice. Embryotoxicity was noted in both animal species (only at the highest dose for Chinese hamsters); maternal toxicity was noted among mice exposed at 500 ppm to styrene, but was low in Chinese hamsters. These results show that the Chinese hamster is very resistant to the effects of styrene (Kankaanpää et al., 1980).

CNS defects have been noted in children whose mothers were exposed to styrene in the plastic industry (Holmberg, 1977).

## 5. VINYLIDENE CHLORIDE

### 5.1. Toxicity

Thyroidectomy, which increases the hepatic amount of glutathione and, to a lesser extent, the administration of antithyroid drugs minimized the parameters of liver injury in fasting rats exposed by inhalation to 2000 ppm vinylidene cholride (VDC) for 4 hours (Szabo *et al.*, 1977b). VDC caused an increase in the level of serum transaminase, but its lipoperoxidative mechanism was dissimilar to $CCl_4$ (Jaeger *et al.*, 1973b).

Metabolites of VDC were more toxic than VDC itself. Acute inhalation toxicity in rats was directly dependent on the amount of metabolite formed and not on the concentration of VDC (Andersen *et al.*, 1979a,b). After treatment with 1000 mg/kg VDC per *os*, liver glutathione in rats decreased to 33% of the control value within 4 hours, but returned to the control level after 24 hours. The depletion was dependent on the dose of VDC (Reichert *et al.*, 1978).

Male rats which were starved for 18 hours and exposed to VDC by inhalation revealed increased susceptibility to the short-term hepatotoxic effect, owing to its dependence on hepatic-reduced glutathione. Vinyl chloride monomer, when administered simultaneously with VDC, prevented the injury associated with VDC inhalation in fasted rats (Jaeger, 1975).

Severe hepatic damage was observed in rats after a single dose of 0.5 g/kg VDC per *os*, as evidenced by high increases in serum enzyme activity and histological examinations. Both diethyldithiocarbamate and (+)-cyanidanol-3 antagonized the hepatotoxic effects of VDC (Sieger *et al.*, 1979). Pretreatment of rats with inducers of the mixed-function-oxidase system minimized the hepatotoxicity of VDC. The inducers appeared to alter the secondary reactions involved in the detoxification of the toxic intermediate (Reynold *et al.*, 1975b).

The inhalation $LD_{50}/4$ hours in fed rats is 10,000–15,000 ppm and 500–2,500 ppm in fasting rats (Jaeger *et al.*, 1973a).

Mice appear to be more sensitive than rats to the lethal, hepatotoxic and renal toxic effects of VDC. Disulfiram, diethyldithiocarbamate, and thiram protected mice from the acute lethal effects of VDC. Disulfiram reduced the levels of covalently bound radioactivity in the liver and kidney after i.p. administration of [14]C VDC (Short *et al.*, 1977a).

In humans, the chemical is highly irritating to the eyes and skin, but is most dangerous when inhaled, producing varying degrees of narcosis. Chronic inhalation of small quantities produced chronic hepatic and renal dysfunction; skin contact caused irritation (Haley, 1975b).

The American Conference of Governmental Industrial Hygienists (ACGIH) has recommended that an employee's exposure to VDC should not exceed an 8-hour time average of 10 ppm (ACGIH, 1976). However, the number of workers engaged in the production of VDC monomer in the U.S. appears to be small, and there is paucity of data concerning worker exposure.

## 5.2. Metabolism

The pharmacokinetics of inhaled VDC in rats is dose-dependent. A significant accumulation of covalently bound VDC metabolites occurred when hepatic glutathione concentrations were depleted by more than 30%. Exposure to vinyl chloride in equivalent concentration resulted in less hepatic glutathione depletion and alkylation of tissue macromolecules than with VDC (McKenna *et al.*, 1977). When male rats were given a single oral dose of 1 mg/kg of $^{14}$C VDC, 78% of the dose was metabolized and excreted in the urine and feces as nonvolatile metabolites; the remainder was exhaled as $^{14}$CO$_2$ (21%) or unchanged $^{14}$C VDC (1–3%) (McKenna *et al.*, 1978a). The exposure of rats to 10 ppm of $^{14}$C VDC vapors for 6 hours revealed that approximately 98% of the acquired body burden of $^{14}$C VDC was metabolized into nonvolatile metabolites. After 200 ppm VDC exposure, a reduced capacity to metabolize VDC was observed. Two metabolites were isolated from rat urine: thiodiglycolic acid and $N$-acetyl-$S$-(2-hydroxyethyl)cystein (McKenna *et al.*, 1978b). The main elimination route for $^{14}$C VDC after intragastric, intravenous, or intraperitoneal administration to rats, was pulmonary; unchanged VDC and VDC related CO$_2$ were excreted by that route; the other metabolites

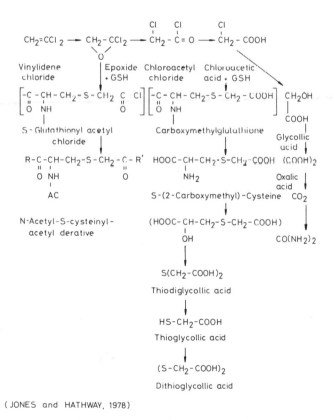

( JONES and HATHWAY, 1978 )

**Figure 4.** Metabolic pathway of vinylidene chloride.

were excreted via the kidneys. Part of the urinary $^{14}C$ was of biliary origin (Jones and Hathway, 1978b).

Due to the strong inhibitory effect of diethyldithiocarbamate on the hepatotoxic effect of VDC, it has been suggested that the action of diethyldithiocarbamate is comparable to that of SKF 525-A (Anderson *et al.*, 1978), an inhibitor of microsomal mixed-function oxidases, which is reported to suppress VDC metabolism. The diminished formation of toxic intermediates of VDC is probably the cause of the reduced GSH depletion.

It should be noted that (+)-cyanidanol-3 also has antihepatotoxic properties against VDC-induced liver injury. No influence of (+)-cyanidanol-3 on VDC metabolism has been detected, but its antihepatotoxic properties are explained by a scavenging activity for free radicals (Sigers *et al.*, 1979). VDC depletion of hepatic glutathione would support a mixed-function-oxidase-dependent conversion into an epoxide (Haley, 1975b). This epoxide, presumed to be formed both by biological and chemical oxidation of VDC (Greim *et al.*, 1975), is extremely reactive and short lived.

Mice metabolized a greater proportion of an oral dose of VDC (50 mg/kg) than rats. Considerably more *N*-acetyl-*S*-cysteinyl acetyl derivative was formed in mice. Chloroacetic acid occupied a key position in the metabolic pathway of VDC (Jones and Hathway, 1978a). It was transformed through the intermediary of glutathione transferae mainly into thiodiglycollic acid and thioglycollic acid (Figure 4).

A specific epoxide-hydrating pathway appears to be of minimal significance in metabolizing the reactive intermediates of VDC. Various epoxides have an exacerbating effect on VDC toxicity that was found to be related to their ability to decrease hepatic GSH (Andersen *et al.*, 1980).

## 5.3. Mutagenicity

When *Salmonella typhimurium* strains TA 1530 and TA 100 were exposed to 0.2, 2, or 20% VDC in air for 4 hours, a reversion increase was observed when S9 (liver, kidney, or lung) from phenobarbitone pretreated mice was added (Bartsch *et al.*, 1975b). The presence of EDTA greatly exacerbated the microsome-mediated mutagenicity of VDC (Malaveille *et al.*, 1977). Low reversion values were observed with S9 from the kidneys or liver of noninduced mice, when strain TA 1535 was incubated in an atmosphere of 5% VDC.

The mutagenic effects recorded were always lower than those of vinyl chloride when tested under the same conditions (Jones and Hathway, 1978c).

The microsome-dependent mutagenicity of VDC on strain TA 100 is in general 20% lower in human liver fractions than in corresponding control experiments with mouse liver. Pretreatment of rats with phenobarbitone and 3-methylcholanthrene has the most exacerbating effects on liver-mediated mutagenicity of VDC. Pretreatment with disulfiram or addition of disulfiram *in vitro* lowered the mutagenic effect. Contrary to vinyl chloride, no 4-(4-nitrobenzyl)pyridine adduct was obtained when vapors of VDC with oxygen were passed through S9 fractions from phenobarbital-treated mice (Bartsch *et al.*, 1979).

VDC was found to be mutagenic in *E. coli* K12 when liver microsomes from phenobarbital-treated mice were added; its mutagenicity was several times lower than that of vinyl chloride (Greim *et al.*, 1975). No germinal mutations were observed in male rats exposed to 55 ppm VDC 6 hours/day for 5 days/week during 11 weeks (Short *et al.*, 1977b).

No mutagenic effects were found in mice exposed by inhalation to 10, 30, and 50 ppm VDC for 6 hours/day for 5 days, as measured by the dominant lethal test (Anderson *et al.*, 1977). The exposure of mice to tumorigenic doses of VDC resulted in massive tissue damage but induced only minimal DNA alkylation or DNA repair synthesis (Reitz *et al.*, 1980).

## 5.4. Carcinogenicity

Comparative investigation of the biological fate of VDC has revealed an agent of low oncogenic potential, likely to be damaging only under special circumstances (Hathway, 1977). When rats inhaled 75 and 100 ppm VDC, no grossly observable interrelation between tumor production and VDC exposure was detected (Viola and Caputo, 1977). The oral administration of VDC to rats did not produce a statistically significant increase in the total number of tumor-bearing animals. The incidence of liver tumors was, however, increased in both sexes, as was that of meningiomas in males (Ponomarkov and Tomatis, 1980).

Vinyl chloride has been demonstrated to be somewhat more carcinogenic in rats and mice than VDC (Lee *et al.*, 1978). Kidney adenocarcinomas have been observed in mice inhaling 50 and 25 ppm VDC, but not at the 10 ppm level. Male mice appear to be more responsive than females (Maltoni *et al.*, 1977c). Certain aspects of the reported carcinogenicity of VDC appear to be conflicting and indicate sex, species, and strain specificity. Exposure of mice to 55 ppm of VDC (6 hours/day and 5 days/week) caused a few acute deaths and a few hepatic hemangiosarcomas (Lee *et al.*, 1977); but investigation of the cancer risk among 138 workers exposed to VDC (where VCM was not used) revealed no finding statistically related or individually attributable to VDC exposure (Ott *et al.*, 1976).

## 5.5. Teratogenicity and Embryotoxicity

Teratogenic effects were not seen in rats or rabbits inhaling concentrations up to 160 ppm VDC for 7 hours/day or in rats given drinking water containing

200 ppm VDC. Some evidence of embryotoxicity and fetotoxicity was, however, noted in both rats and rabbits exposed to VDC by inhalation; these effects were associated with maternal toxicity (Murray *et al.*, 1979).

## 6. BUTADIENE

### 6.1. Toxicity

Sprague–Dawley rats were unaffected when exposed to butadiene (BUT) atmospheres at concentrations of 8000 ppm (v/v) 6 hours/day, 5 days/week for 13 weeks (Crouch *et al.*, 1979); examination of workers chronically exposed to BUT concentrations of 5000 ppm (v/v) revealed no adverse effects (Wilson and McCormich, 1954).

### 6.2. Metabolism

The cytochrome-$P_{450}$-dependent metabolism of 1,3-butadiene has been demonstrated; 1,2-epoxybutene-3 was detected as the first metabolite, which was further converted into 1,2,3,4-diepoxybutane (Malvoisin *et al.*, 1979).

### 6.3. Mutagenicity

BUT induced reverse mutations in *Salmonella typhimurium* strains TA 1530 and TA 1535 when the incubation mixture was supplemented with NADPH-fortified rat liver S9 (de Meester *et al.*, 1978b,c,d; 1979b). This mutagenic activity was only detected in the presence of gaseous BUT. Assays in the classical plate incorporation method with ethanolic solutions of BUT failed to reveal any activity. The mutagenic activity of BUT on TA 1530 was strongly influenced by pretreatment of the animals from which the liver S9 was prepared (de Meester *et al.*, 1980b).

Both 1,2-epoxybutene-3 and 1,2,3,4-diepoxybutane, two possible metabolites of BUT, appeared to be direct mutagens in several test systems: in *Salmonella typhimurium* (McCann *et al.*, 1975b), (Clarke and Loprieno, 1965), *Escherichia coli* (Glover, 1956), *Neurospora crassa* (Kolmark and Westergaard, 1953), *Saccharomyces cerevisiae* (Zimmerman and Vig, 1975), *Drosophila melanogaster* (Watson, 1972), and induced prophage in *Escherichia coli* K-12 (Heineman and Howard, 1964).

### 6.4. Carcinogenicity

No data are available on the carcinogenic properties of BUT in humans. Two possible oxidative metabolites, 1,2-epoxybutene-3, as well as D, L, and meso-1,2,3,4-diepoxybutane, produced squamous cell skin carcinomas when applied to mouse skin (Van Duuren *et al.*, 1963). Local fibrosarcomas were observed in mice and rats after subcutaneous injection of D, L-1,2,3,4-diepoxybutane (Van Duuren et al., 1966), and lung tumors were detected in mice when injected i.p. (Skimkim et al., 1966).

### 6.5. Teratogenicity and Embryotoxicity

No data are available on embryotoxic or teratogenic studies with BUT.

## 7. CHLOROBUTADIENE

### 7.1. Toxicity

Animal experiments have shown that a concentration of 250 ppm chlorobutadiene (CBD) in air is an irritant to the respiratory tract. The vapor was a CNS depressant, caused degenerative changes in the liver and kidney, lowered the blood pressure, and provoked lung changes (Sax, 1968). It decreased the number of lymphocytes in rats (Agakhanyan et al., 1973) and affected male reproductive organs (Von Oettingen et al., 1936).

The threshold dose for hepatic toxicity due to CBD inhalation in fasting rats was 160 ppm for 5 hours; Aroclor 1254 pretreatment exerted a protective effect (Plugge and Jaeger, 1979). The fasting of male rats increased their susceptibility to the short-term hepatotoxic effects of CBD (Jaeger et al., 1975b). The oral $LD_{50}$ of CBD in rats and mice were 251 mg/kg and 260 mg/kg, respectively, (IARC, 1979). Repeated exposures by inhalation of rats and hamsters for 4 weeks, 6 hours/day, 5 days/week demonstrated the cumulative toxicity of CBD. The lower exposure level (39 ppm) was irritating in both species. The chemical stability of CBD is important in toxicological studies; oxidized CBD was four times as acutely toxic in rats as the nonoxidized form (Clary et al., 1978).

The primary response of human exposure to CBD is CNS depression and injury to the lungs, liver, and kidneys (Patty, 1963). Functional disturbances in spermatogenesis have been observed in workers, and the frequency of spontaneous abortions in the wives of CBD workers was 3 times higher than in those of the controls (Sanotskii, 1976). Approximately 2500 workers are estimated to be exposed to CBD in the U.S. (Lloyd et al., 1975). The ACGIH has established a threshold limit for chloroprene exposure of 25 ppm (IARC, 1979). A maximum occupational exposure of 1 ppm has been recommended, as a ceiling concentration for a 15 minute period during a 40 hour working week (Niosh, 1977).

### 7.2. Metabolism

The biochemical effects of chloroprene (CBD) on various metabolic processes have been reviewed (Haley, 1978) (Figure 5). The main effects were

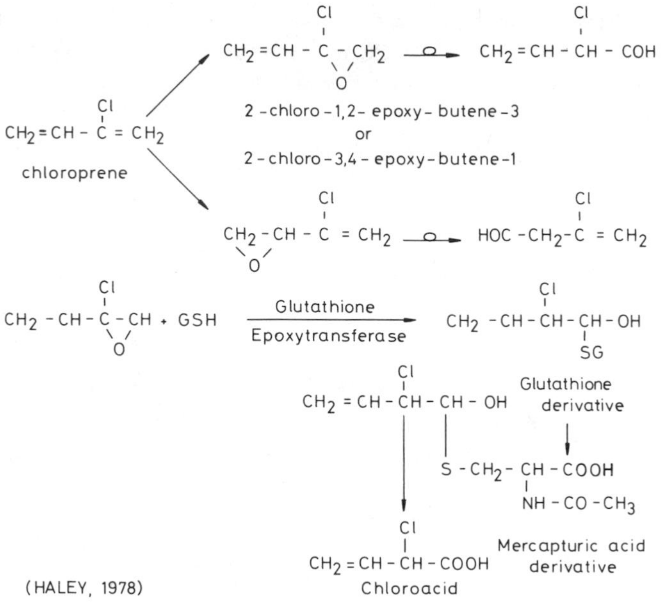

**Figure 5.** Metabolic pathway of chlorobutadiene.

inhibition of liver detoxification mechanisms, decreased activity of hepatic enzymes, and decreased liver glycogen content. It has been postulated that CBD is probably handled in the body similarly to vinyl chloride and vinylidene chloride (Haley, 1978).

The adduct obtained between CBD and 4-(4-nitrobenzyl)pyridine was increased when co-factors were added to the mouse-liver microsomes; this suggests that the formation of a reactive intermediate (probably an epoxide) is a 1 enzymatic process (Bartsch *et al.*, 1979).

### 7.3. Mutagenicity

A direct mutagenic action of CBD was described when *Salmonella typhimurium* TA 100 was exposed to 0.5–8% vapors. An increased mutagenic response was observed when a fortified 9000 × g liver supernatant from either phenobarbital-treated or untreated mice was added. Likewise, liver supernatant from human biopsies exacerbated the mutagenicity of CBD (Bartsch *et al.*, 1975b). CBD dimers also caused a small increase in the reversion rate in *Salmonella typhimurium* strains TA 1535 and TA 100 in the presence of a mouse-liver S9 fraction (Bartsch *et al.*, 1979).

CBD induced recessive lethal mutations in *Drosophila melanogaster* by feeding males with 5.7 to 34.3 mM CBD for 3 days (Vogel, 1979). No mutagenicity was detected in 8-azaguanine and ouabain-resistant $V_{79}$ Chinese hamster cells, exposed for 5 hours to up to 10% (v/v) CBD vapors in the presence of microsomes (Drevon and Kuroki, 1979). Malignant transformation of hamster lung cells was observed *in vitro* with 1 $\mu$g/ml CBD, 14 weeks after treatment (Menezes *et al.*, 1979).

Spermatogenesis in mice was affected after 2 months exposure to 0.32 ppm CBD. Dominant lethal mutations were induced in germ cells exposed to 1 ppm CBD. Chromosome aberrations at a highly significant level appeared in mouse bone marrow after 2 months exposure. An increased number of chromosomal aberrations has also been reported in lymphocyte cultures from workers occupationally exposed to CBD (Sanotskii, 1976).

## 7.4. Carcinogenicity

When CBD was given orally to pregnant female rats (100 mg/kg body weight) and to their offspring (50 mg/kg body weight weekly from the time of weaning for the entire life span), the total incidence of tumors was similar in treated and untreated animals (Ponomarkov and Tomatis, 1980). No carcinogenic effect of CBD has been noted in mice or rats after oral, intratracheal, dermal, or subcutaneous administration (Zil'Fyan *et al.*, 1977).

CBD exposure has been associated with an increased incidence of skin and lung cancer in industrial workers in the Yerevan region of the USSR. Epidemiological studies revealed 137 cases of skin cancer among approximately 25,000 workers. During the same period 87 cases of lung cancer were identified among 19,979 workers in the same region. Persons exposed only to chloroprene derivatives showed an increased incidence of skin cancer (Khachatryan, 1972).

Another study of lung cancer mortality in a high-exposure occupational group indicates that CBD does not increase the risk of lung cancer, but enhances the risks of digestive cancer (19 vs. 13.3) and of lymphatic and hematopoietic cancer (7 vs. 4.5) (Pell, 1978).

## 7.5. Teratogenicity and Embryotoxicity

In rats and mice CBD caused an increase in the total embryonic mortality and lower fetal weight of the offspring of females exposed during pregnancy (Salnikova and Fomenko, 1973). In a reproduction study, where rats were exposed by inhalation to 25 ppm CBD, 4 hours daily for 22 days, no embryotoxic or teratogenic effects were found, and the reproductive capacity of male rats was unimpaired (Culik *et al.*, 1978).

## 8. HEXACHLOROBUTADIENE

### 8.1. Toxicity

Toxic effects have been observed in rats after ingestion of hexachloro-butadiene (HCBD) (Gudumak, 1968). Accumulation in fatty tissue was noted (Jacobs *et al.*, 1974). Lesions were observed in the kidneys (Dmitrienko and Vasilos, 1972; Lock and Ishmael, 1979) and CNS (Murzakaev, 1967). HCBD was moderately toxic to the rat; the oral $LD_{50}$ was in the range of 250–350 mg/kg and the intraperitoneal $LD_{50}$ about 200 mg/kg (Gradiski *et al.*, 1975). The $LD_{50}$ for rabbits, exposed epicutaneously to HCBD is reported to be 0.72 mg/kg (Duprat and Gradiski, 1978). Acute and chronic effects have been detected in fish (Laska *et al.*, 1976). Several disturbances have also been found in Russian farm workers as a result of exposure to HCBD fumigation (Krasmyuk *et al.*, 1969).

### 8.2. Metabolism

No data are available on the possible metabolites of hexachloro-1,3-butadiene (HCBD), which is highly resistant to physicochemical and biological degradation processes.

### 8.3. Mutagenicity

A direct mutagenic effect of HCBD has been described in *Salmonella typhimurium* strains TA 1535 and TA 100 (Simon, 1977). However, no such effects could be observed in the same strains, with or without fortified liver S9 from Aroclor 1254-pretreated rats in the classical plate incorporation assay, with HCBD concentrations reaching 250 $\mu$moles/plate (de Meester *et al.*, 1981a).

### 8.4. Carcinogenicity

Neoplasms in rats have occurred only at a dose level that caused significant tissue injury. The ingestion of 20 mg/kg/day of HCBD for up to 2 years caused renal tubular adenomas and adenocarcinomas, some of which metastasized to the lungs. The ingestion of 2 mg/kg/day of HCBD for up to 2 years caused lesser degrees of toxicity; no neoplasms were attributable to ingestion at this dose level (Kociba *et al.*, 1977).

### 8.5. Teratogenicity and Embryotoxicity

The death of newborn rats from mothers given a single subcutaneous dose of 20 mg HCBD/day, 3 months previously, has been reported

(Poteryayeva, 1966). When female rats were fed diets containing 150 ppm HCBD, the progeny were found to have a decreased body weight but no manifest malformations (Harleman and Seinen, 1979). With diets containing 0.2 or 2.0 mg/kg/day, no effects on pregnancy or on neonatal survival and development were observed (Schwetz *et al.*, 1977).

## 9. GENERAL DISCUSSION AND CONCLUSION

The toxicity of the monomers described here seems to be highly related to their metabolic activation. Metabolism occurs essentially in the liver, via the mixed-function-oxidase system; however, radicalar activation has been suggested for several of these monomers. The formation of highly electrophilic, reactive intermediates (oxiranes, aldehydes) has been directly or indirectly proved by trapping with nucleophilic sites, leading to the formation of glutathione conjugates or to nucleic acid alkylation products. The main detoxification routes involve epoxide hydratase, glutathione-S-transferases, and dehydrogenases; the role of each compound varies. Extensive urinary excretion of metabolites might explain the toxic renal effects observed for some of them. VCM is known to induce several types of tumors in experimental animals as well as in exposed workers. VDC, ACN, and STY are said to increase the incidence of cancer in experimental animals, while for STY and ACN, human data are also available. These six monomers are able to induce base pair substitutions in *Salmonella typhimurium*; VCM, VDC, and ACN produce reverse mutations in *E. coli*; VCM is able to produce forward mutations in *Schizosaccharomyces pombe* in the presence of S9 mix as well as in the host-mediated assay. An increase in gene conversion frequency is noted in *Saccharomyces cerevisiae* for VCM when tested *in vitro* in the presence of S9 mix, and for styrene when using the host-mediated assay.

Chromosome aberrations occur in the cells of animals exposed to VCM and STY vapors. An increased incidence of chromosomal aberrations has been noted among workers exposed to VCM, STY, and chlorobutadiene. Among the six monomers reveiwed, VCM along is classified as a human carcinogen; a good correlation exists between its mutagenic properties and its carcinogenicity. The results of mutagenicity studies reported for the other substances need further investigations to evaluate more adequately their toxicogenetic potential.

## REFERENCES

Abreu, M. E., and Ahmed, A. E., 1980, Metabolism of acrylonitrile to cyanide, *Drug Met. and Disp.* **8**:376–379.

Agakhanyan, A. G., Fridenshtein, A. Y., Allverdyan, A. G., 1973, Immunomorphology of chloroprene toxicosis, *Zh. Eksp. Klin. Med.*: **13**:3–7.

American Conference of Governmental Industrial Hygienists, 1976, TLVs[R], Threshold limit values for chemical substances in workroom air adopted by ACGIH for 1976, Cincinnati, Ohio, p. 30.

Andersen, M. E., Jones, R. A. and Jenkins, L., 1978, The acute toxicity of vinyle, oral doses of 1,1-dichloroethylene in the fasted, male rat: Effect of induction and inhibition of microsomal enzyme activities on mortality, *Toxicol. Appl. Pharmacol.* **46**:227–234.

Andersen, M. E., Gargas, M. L., Jones, R. A. and Jenkins, L. J., 1979a, The use of inhalation techniques to assess the kinetic constants of 1,1-dichloroethylene metabolism, *Toxicol. Appl. Pharmacol.* **47**:395–409.

Andersen, M. E., French, J. E., Gargas, M. L., Jones, R. A., and Jenkins, L. J., 1979b, Saturable metabolism and acute toxicity of 1,1-dichloroethylene, *Toxicol. Appl. Pharmacol.* **47**:385–393.

Andersen, M. E., Thomas, O. E., Gargas, M. L., Jones, R. A. and Jenkins, L. J., 1980, The significance of multiple detoxification pathways for reactive metabolites in the toxicity of 1,1-dichloroethylene, *Toxicol. Appl. Pharmacol.* **52**:422–432.

Anderson, D., Hodge, M. C. E. and Purchase, I. F. H., 1977, Dominant lethal studies with the halogenated olefins vinyl chloride and vinylidene dichloride in male CD-1 mice, *Environ. Health Persp.* **21**:71–78.

Anderson, D., Hodge, M. C. E. & Purchase, I. F. H., 1976, Vinyl chloride: Dominant lethal studies in male CD-1 mice, *Mutat. Res.* **40**:359–370.

Andrews, A. W., Zawistowski, E. S., and Valentine, C. R., 1976, A comparison of the mutagenic properties of vinyl chloride and methyl chloride, *Mutat. Res.* **40**:273–276.

Anonymous, 1980, ACN testing shows tumors at all levels, *Food and Drug Packaging*, March 20, 1980, 43–44.

Antweiler, H., 1976, Studies on the metabolism of vinyl chloride, *Environ. Health Perspect.* **17**:217–219.

Baggett, M. S., Morie, G. P., Simmons, M. W. and Lewis, J. S., 1974, Quantitative determination of semivolatile compounds in cigarette smoke, *J. Chromatogr.* **97**:79–82.

Bakke, O. N., and Sheline, R. R., 1970, Hydroxylation of aromatic hydrocarbons in the rat, *Toxicol. Appl. Pharmacol.* **16**:691–700.

Barbin, A., Brésil, H., Croisy, A., Jacquignon, P., Malaveille, C., Montesano, R., and Bartsch, H., 1975, Liver-microsome-mediated formation of alkylating agents from vinyl bromide and vinyl chloride, *Biochem. Biophys. Res. Commun.*, **67**:596–603.

Bardodej, Z., and Bardodejova, E., 1970, Biotransformation of ethylbenzene, styrene, and alpha-methylstyrene in man, *Am. Ind. Hyg. Assoc. J.* **31**:206–209.

Barrio, J. R., Secrist, J. A., and Léonard, N. J., 1972, Fluorescent adenosine and cytidine derivatives, *Biochem. Biophys. Res. Commun.* **46**:597–604.

Bartsch, H., and Montesano, R., 1975, Mutagenic and carcinogenic effects of vinyl chloride, *Mutat. Res.* **32**:93–114.

Bartsch, H., Malaveille, C., Montesano, R., 1975a, Human rat and mouse liver-mediated mutagenicity of vinyl chloride in *S. typhimurium* strains, *Int. J. Cancer* **15**:429–437.

Bartsch, H., Malaveille, C., Montesano, R. and Tomatis, L., 1975b), Tissue-mediated mutagenicity of vinylidene chloride and 2-chlorobutadiene in *Salmonella typhimurium*, *Nature* **255**:641–643.

Bartsch, H., Malaveille, C., Barbin, A., Brésil, H., Tomatis, L., and Montesano, R., 1976, Mutagenicity and metabolism of vinyl chloride and related compounds, *Environ. Health Perspect.* **17**:193–198.

Bartsch, H., Malaveille, C., Barbin, A. and Planche, G., 1979, Mutagenic and alkylating metabolites of halo-ethylenes, chlorobutadienes and dichlorobutenes produced by rodent or human liver tissues. Evidence for oxirane formation by $P_{450}$-linked microsomal mono-oxygenases, *Arch. Toxicol.* **41**:249–277.

Basler, A., and Röhrborn, G., 1980, Vinyl chloride: An example for evaluating mutagenic effects in mammals *in vivo* after exposure to inhalation, *Arch. Toxicol.* **45**:1–7.

Bauer, C., Leporini, C., Bronzetti, G., Corsi, C., Nieri, R., Del Carratore, R., Tonarelli, S., 1980, The problem of negative results for styrene in the *in vitro* mutagenesis test with metabolic activation, *Boll. Soc. It. Biol. Sper.* **56**:203–207.

Baxter, P. J., Anthony, P. P., McSween, R. N. M., and Scheuer, P. J., 1977, Angiosarcoma of the liver in Great Britain, 1963–1973. *Brit. Med. J.*:919–921.

Belvedere, G., Cantoni, L., Tacchinetti, T., and Salmona, M., 1977, Kinetic behaviour of microsomal styrene monooxygenase and styrene epoxide hydratase in different animal species, *Experientia* **33**:708–709.

Biersack, H. J., Sanluis, T. Jr., Lange, C. E., Thelen, M., Veltman, G., Winkler, C., 1977, Scintigraphy of liver and spleen in vinyl chloride workers, *Acta Hepato-Gastroenterol.* **24**:357–361.

Binns, C. H. B., 1979, Vinyl chloride: a review, *J. Soc. Occup. Med.* **29**:134–141.

Block, J. B., 1974, Angiosarcoma of the liver following vinyl chloride exposure, *J. Am. Med. Assoc.* **229**:53–54.

Bolt, H. M., Kappus, H., Buchter, A., and Bolt, W., 1976, Disposition of (1,2-$^{14}$C) vinyl chloride in the rat, *Arch. Toxicol.*, **35**:153–162.

Bolt, H. M., and Filser, J. G., 1977, Irreversible binding of chlorinated ethylenes to macromolecules, *Environ. Health Perspect.* **21**:107–112.

Bonatti, S., Abbondandolo, A., Corti, G., Fiorio, R., and Mazzaccaro, A., 1978, The expression curve of mutants induced by styrene oxide at the HGPRT locus in V 79 cells, *Mutation Res.* **52**:295–300.

Border, E. A., and Webster, I., 1977, The effect of vinyl chloride monomer, chloroethylene oxide and chloroacetaldehyde on DNA synthesis in regenerating rat liver, *Chem. Biol. Interact.* **17**:239–247.

Bos, R., Guicherit, R. and Hoogeveen, A., 1977, Distribution of some hydrocarbons in ambient air near Delft and the influence of the formation of secondary air pollutants, *Sci. Total Environ.* **7**:269–281.

Boyland, F., and Williams, K., 1965, An enzyme catalysing the conjugation of epoxides with glutathione, *Biochem. J.* **94**:190–197.

Brady, J, Liberatore, F., Harper, Ph., Greenwald, P., Burnett, W., Davies, J. N. P., Bishop, M., Polan, A., and Vianna, N., 1977, Angiosarcoma of the liver: an epidemiologic study, *J. Nat'l Cancer Inst.* **59**:1383–1385.

Brand, K. G., Buoen, L. C., and Brand, I., 1975, Foreign-body tumorigenesis by vinyl chloride vinyl acetate copolymer: No evidence for chemical cocarcinogenesis, *J. Nat'l Cancer Inst.* **54**:1259–1262.

Buffler, P. A., Wood, S., Eifler, C., Suarez, L., Kilian, D. J., 1979, Mortality experience of workers in a vinyl chloride monomer production plant, *J. Occup. Medicine* **21**:195–203.

Busk, L., 1979, Mutagenic effects of styrene and styrene oxide, *Mutat. Res.* **67**:201–208.

Byrén, D., and Holmberg, B., 1975, Two possible cases of angiosarcoma of the liver in a group of Swedish vinyl chloride–polyvinyl chloride workers, *Ann. N.Y. Acad. Sci.* **246**:249–250.

Byrén, D., Engholm, G., Englund, A., and Westerholm, P., 1976, Mortality and cancer morbidity in a group of Swedish VCM and PVC production workers, *Environ. Health Perspect.* **17**:167–170.

Cantoni, L., Salmona, M. Facchinetti, T., Pantarotto, C., and Belvedere, G., 1978, Hepatic and extrahepatic formation and hydration of styrene oxide *in vitro*, in animals of different species and sexes, *Tox. Letters* **2**:179–186.

Caperos, J. R., Humbert, B. and Droz, P. O., 1979, Exposition au Styrène. II. Bilan de l'absorption, de l'excrétion et du métabolisme sur des sujets humains, *Int. Arch. Occup. Environ. Health* **42**:223–230.

Caputo, A., Viola, P. L., and Bigotti, A., 1974, Oncogenicity of vinyl chloride at low concentrations in rats and rabbits, *Int. Res. Commun.* **2**:1582.

Chiazze, L., Jr., Nichols, W. E., and Wong, O., 1977, Mortality among employees of PVC fibricators, *J. Occup. Med.* **19**:623–628.

Chmielewski, J., and Renke, W., 1976, Clinical and experimental research into the pathogenesis of toxic effect of styrene, *Bull. Inst. Mar. Trop. Med. Gdynia* **27**:63–68.

Chmielewski, J., and Hac, E., 1976, Clinical and experimental research into the pathogenesis of toxic effects of styrene. IV. Estimation of liver functions in persons exposed to the action of styrene during their work, *Bull. Inst. Mar. Trop. Med. Gdynia* **27**:69–74.

Chmielewski, J., 1976, Clinical and experimental research into the pathogenesis of toxic effects of styrene. V. Impact of styrene on carbohydrate balance in people in the course of their work, *Bull. Inst. Mar. Trop. Med. Gdynia* **27**:177–184.

Clarke, C. H., and Loprieno, N., 1965, The influence of genetic background on the induction of methionine reversions by diepoxybutane in *Schizosaccharomyces pombe*, *Microb. Genet. Bull.* **22**:11–12.

Clary, J. J., Feron, V. J., and Reuzel, P. G. J., 1978, Toxicity of $\beta$-chloroprene (2-chlorobutadiene-1,3): Acute and subacute toxicity, *Toxicol. Appl. Pharmacol.* **46**:375–384.

Conner, M. K., Alarie, Y. and Dombroske, R. L., 1979, Sister chromatid exchange in regenerating liver and bone marrow cells of mice exposed to styrene, *Toxicol. Appl. Pharmacol.* **50**:365–367.

Conner, M. K., Alarie, Y., and Dombroske, R. L., 1980, Sister chromatid exchange in murine alveolar macrophages, bone marrow and regenerating liver cells induced by styrene inhalation, *Toxicol. Appl. Pharmacol.* **55**:37–42.

Conolly, R. B., Jaeger, R. J., and Szabo, S., 1978, Acute hepatotoxicity of ethylene, vinyl fluoride, vinyl chloride and vinyl bromide after Aroclor 1254 pretreatment, *Exper. Molec. Pathol.* **28**:25–33.

Conolly, R. B., and Jaeger, R. J., 1979, Acute hepatotoxicity of vinyl chloride and ethylene: Modification by trichfloropropene oxide, diethylmaleate, and cysteine, *Toxicol. Appl. Pharmacol.* **50**:523–531.

Couderc, P., Panh, M.-H., Pasquier, B., Pasquier, D., N'Golet, A., and Faure, H., 1976, Angiosarcoma of the bone indicating a hepatic tumor in a worker exposed to vinyl chloride (Fr.), *Semin. Hop. Paris* **52**:1721–1722.

Creech, J. L., Jr., and Johnson, M. N., 1974, Angiosarcoma of liver in the manufacture of polyvinyl chloride, *J. occup. Med.* **16**:150–151.

Crouch, C. N., Pullinger, D. H., and Gaunt, J. F., 1979, Inhalation toxicity studies with 1,3-butadiene-2. 3 month toxicity study in rats, *Am. Ind. Hyg. Assoc. J.* **40**:796–802.

Culik, R., Kelly, D. P., and Clary, J. J., 1978, Inhalation studies to evaluate the teratogenic and embryotoxic potential of $\beta$-chloroprene(2-chlorobutadiene-1,3), *Toxicol. Appl. Pharmacol.* **44**:81–88.

Danishefsky, I., and Willhite, M., 1954, The metabolism of styrene in the rat, *J. Biol. Chem.* **211**:549–553.

Delorme, F., and Thériault, G., 1978, Ten cases of angiosarcoma of the liver in Shawinigan, Quebec, *J. Occup. Med.* **20**:338–340.

Delorme, F., 1978, Association d'un angiosarcome du foie et d'un hépatome chez un ouvrier du chlorure de vinyle, *Ann. Anat. Pathol.* **23**:105–114.

de Meester, C., Poncelet, F., Roberfroid, M., Rondelet, J., and Mercier, M., 1977, Mutagenicity of styrene and styrene oxide, *Mutat. Res.* **56**:147–152.

de Meester, C., Poncelet, F., Roberfroid, M., Mercier, M., 1978a, Mutagenicity of acrylonitrile, *Toxicology* **11(1)**:19–27.

de Meester, C., Poncelet, F., Roberfroid, M., and Mercier, M., 1978b, Etude de l'activite mutagene du butadiene, de l'acrylonitrile de du styrene. Presented at the National Congres of the Belgian Society for Pharmaceutical Science. Liege, Belgium, March 16–17, Abst., p. 47.

de Meester, C., Poncelet, F., Roberfroid, M., and Mercier, M., 1978c, Impact of microsomal enzymes on the mutagenicity of acrylonitrile, butadiene and styrene. Presented at the Eighth Annual Meeting of the European Environmental Mutagen Society. Dublin, July 11–13, Abst. p. 63.

de Meester, C., Poncelet, F., Roberfroid, M., and Mercier, M., 1978d. Mutagenicity of butadiene and butadiene monoxide, *Biochem. Biophys. Res. Commun.* **80:**298–305.

de Meester, C., Duverger-van Bogaert, M., Lambotte-Vandepaer, M., Roberfroid M., Poncelet, F., Mercier, M., 1979a, Liver extract mediated mutagenicity of acrylonitrile, *Toxicology* **13(1):**7–15.

de Meester, C., Poncelet, F., Roberfroid, M., and Mercier, M., 1979b, Mutagenic activity of butadiene and related compounds. Presented at the Ninth Annual Meeting of the European Environmental Mutagen Society. Makarska, September 30–October 5, 1979, Abst. p. 94.

de Meester, C., Duverger-van Bogaert, M., Lambotte-Vandepar, M., Roberfroid, M., Poncelet, F., and Mercier, M., 1980a, Mutagenicity of vinyl chloride in the Ames test: Possible artifacts related to experimental conditions, *Mutat. Res.* **77:**175–179.

de Meester, C., Poncelet, F., Roberfroid, M., and Mercier, M., 1980b, The mutagenicity of buradiene towards *Salmonella typhimurium. Tox. Letters* **6:**125–130.

de Meester, C., Duverger-van Bogaert, M., Lombotte-Vandepaer, M., Mercier, M., and Poncelet, F., 1981, Mutagenicity of styrene in the *Salmonella typhimurium* test system, *Mutat. Res.*, **90:**443–450.

de Meester, C., Mercier, M., and Poncelet, F., Mutagenic activity of butadiene, hexachloro-butadiene, and isoprene (to be published).

de Raat, W. K., 1978, Induction of sister chromatic exchanges by styrene and its presumed metabolite styrene oxide in the presence of rat liver homogenate, *Chem.-biol. Interact.* **20:**163–170.

Dinu, V., 1975, Activity of GSH peroxidase and catalase and the concentration of lipid peroxides in acute intoxication with Acrylonitrile, *Rev. Roum. Biochim. 12(1):*11–14.

Dinu, V., and Klein, R., 1976, Activité catalasique et concentration de glutathion et d'acide lactique dans l'intoxication aiguë par l'acrylonitrile chez le rat, *J. Pharmacol. (Paris)* 7:2, 223–226.

Dmitrienko, V. D., and Vasilos, A. F., 1972, Kidney damage during the experimental acute poisoning with hexachlorobutadiene, *Zdravookhranenie (Kishinev)* **15:**11–12. Abstructed in *Chem. Abstr.* 77, 44061.

Dolmierski, R., Kwaiktowski, S. R., and Nitka, J., 1976, Clinical and experimental research into the pathogenesis of toxic effects of styrene: VII. Appraisal of the nervous system in the workers exposed to styrene, *Bull. Inst. Mar. Trop. Med. Gdynia* 27:193–196.

Donner, M., Sorsa, M., and Vainio, H., 1979, Recessive lethals induced by styrene and styrene oxide in *Drosophila melanogaster. Mutat. Res.* **67:**373–376.

Drevon, C., and Kuroki, T., 1979, Mutagenicity of vinyl chloride, vinylidene chloride, and chloroprene in V 79 Chinese hamster cells, *Mutat. Res.* **67:**173–182.

Drew, R. T., Harper, C., Gupta, B. N., Talley, F. A., 1975, Effects of vinyl chloride exposures to rats pretreated with phenobarbital, *Environ. Health Persp.* **11:**235–242.

Drozdowicz, B. Z., and Huang, P. C., 1977, Lack of mutagenicity of vinyl chloride in two strains of *Neurospora crassa*, *Mutat. Res.* **48:**43–50.

Du, J. T., Sandoz, J. P., Tseng, M. T., and Tamburro, C. H., 1979, Biochemical alterations in livers of rats exposed to vinyl chloride, *J. Toxicol. Environm. Health* **5:**1119–1132.

Ducatman, A., Hirschhorn, K., and Selikoff, I. J., 1975, Vinyl chloride exposure and human chromsome aberrations, *Mutat. Res.* **31:**163–168.

Duck, B. W., and Carter, J. T., 1976, Vinyl chloride and mortality? *Lancet* **ii:**195.

Duprat, P., and Gradiski, O., 1978, Percutaneous toxicity of hexachlorobutadiene, *Acta Pharmacol. Toxicol.* **43:**346–353.

Duverger–van Bogaert, M., Lambotte–Vandepaer, M., Noël, G., Roberfroid, M., and Mercier, M., 1978a, Biochemical effects of acrylonitrile on the rat liver, as influenced by various pretreatments of the animals, *Biochem. Biophys. Res. Commun.* **83:**3, 1117–1124.

Duverger–van Bogaert, M., Noël, G., Rollmann, B., Cumps, J., Roberfroid, M., and Mercier, M., 1978b, Determination of oxide synthetase and hydratase activities by a new highly sensitive gas chromatographic method using styrene and styrene oxide as substrates, *Biochim. Biophys. Acta* **526:**77–84.

Duverger–van Bogaert, M., Lambotte–Vandepaer, M., de Meester, C. Mercier, M., and Poncelet, F., Vinyl chloride and acrylonitrile: activation mechanism and mutagenicity, *Tox. Eur. Res.* (in press).

Duverger–van Bogaert, M., Lambotte–Vandepaer, M., de Meester, C., Rollmann, b., Poncelet, F., and Mercier, M., 1981b, Effect of several factors on the liver extract mediated mutagenicity of acrylonitrile and identification of four new *in vitro* metabolites. *Tox. Lett.* **7:**311–318.

Edmonds, L. D., Anderson, C. E., Flynt, J. W., Jr., and James, L. M., 1978, Congenital central nervous system malformations and vinyl chloride monomer exposure: A community study, *Teratology* **17:**137–142.

El Masri, A. M., Smith, J. N., and Williams, R. T., 1958, Studies in detoxications 73. The metabolism of alkylbenzenes: phenyl acetylene and phenylethylene, *Biochem. J.* **68:**199–204.

Elmore, J. D., Wong, J. L., Laumback, A. D., and Streips, U. N., 1976, Vinyl chloride mutagenicity via the metabolites chlorooxirane and chloroacetaldehyde monomer hydrate, *Biochim. Biophys. Acta* **442:**405–419.

Engström, J., Bjurström, R., Astrand, I., and Övrum, B., 1978, Uptake, distribution and elimination of styrene in man, *Scand. J. Work. Environ. Health* **4:**315–323.

Eurocop-Cost, 1976, A comprehensive list of polluting substances which have been identified in various fresh waters, effluent discharges, aquatic animals and plants, and bottom sediments, EUCO/MDU/73/76, XII/476/76, 2nd ed., Luxembourg, Commission of the European Communities, p. 19.

Fabry, L., Leonard, A. and Roberfroid, M., 1978, Mutagenicity tests with styrene oxide in mammals, *Mutat. Res.* **51:**377–381.

Falk, H., Creech, J. L., Jr., Heath, C. W., Jr., Johnson, M. N., & Key, M. M., 1974, Hepatic disease among workers at a vinyl chloride polymerization plant, *J. Am. Med. Assoc.* **230:**59–63.

Fasset, D. W., 1963, Cyanides and nitriles, in Industrial Hygiene and Toxicology (edited by F. A. Patty) 2nd Revised edition, New York, Interscience, Vol. II, pp. 2009–2012.

Feron, V. J., Kruysse, A., and Til, H. P., 1979a, One-year time sequence inhalation toxicity study of vinyl chloride in rats. I. Growth, mortality, haematology, clinical chemistry and organ weights, *Toxicology* **13:**25–28.

Feron, V. J., Spit, B. J., Immel, H. R., and Kross, R., 1979b, One year time sequence inhalation toxicity study of vinyl chloride in rats. III. Morphological changes in the liver. *Toxicology* **13:**143–154.

Filatova, V. S., and Gronsberg, E. S., 1957, Sanitary-hygienic conditions of work in the production of polychlorvinylic tar and measures of improvement (Russ.) *Gig. i Sanit.* **22:**38–42.

Fishbein, L., 1979, *Potential Industrial Carcinogens and Mutagens*, Elsevier, Amsterdam, pp. 165, 178, 189, 193–194, 495.

Fleig, I., and Thiess, A. M., 1978, Mutagenicity of vinyl chloride. External chromosome studies on persons with and without illness and on VC exposed animals. *J. Occup. Med.* **20:**557–560.

Fox, A. J., and Collier, P. F., 1976, Low mortality rates in industrial cohort studies due to selection for work and survival in the industry, *Br. J. Prev. Soc. Med.* **30**:225–230.

Fox, A. J., and Collier, P. F., 1977, Mortality experience of workers exposed to vinyl chloride monomer in the manufacture of polyvinyl chloride in Great Britain, *Br. J. Ind. Med.* **34**:1–10.

Fuchs, G., Gawell, B. M., Albanus, L., and Slorach, S., 1975, Vinyl chloride monomer levels in edible fats (Swed.), *Var Foeda* **27**:134–145. *Chem. Abstr.* **83**:145870g.

Funes–Cravioto, F., Lambert, B., Lindsten, J., Ehrenberg, L., Natarajan, A. I., and Osterman–Golkar, S., 1975, Chromsome aberrations in workers exposed to vinyl chloride, *Lancet* i:459.

Gadzhiev, F. M., and Aliev, T. V., 1974, New method of studying free amino acids and their metabolism in brain tissues under the prolonged effects of gasoline and styrene vapors, *Izv. Akad. Nauk. Az. SSR Ser. Biol. Nauk.* **4**:112–118.

Garro, A. J., Guttenplan, J. B., and Milvy, P., 1976, Vinyl chloride dependent mutagenesis: Effects of liver extracts and free radicals, *Mutat. Res.* **38**:81–88.

Gazzotti, G., Garatti, E., and Salmona, M., 1980, Nuclear metabolism. I. Determination of styrene monooxygenase activity in rat liver nuclei, *Chem.-Biol. Interact.* **29**:189–195.

Gehring, P. J., Watanabe, P. g., and Park, C. N., 1978, Resolution of dose-response toxicity data for chemicals requiring metabolic activation: example—Vinyl chloride, *Toxicol. Appl. Pharmacol.* **44**:581–591.

Glover, S. W., 1956, A comparative study of induced reversions in *Escherichia coli*, in Genetic studies with bacteria, Carnegie Institution of Washington, Publication G12, Washington D.C., p. 121–136.

Gotell, P., Axelson, O., and Lindelof, B., 1972, Field studies on human styrene exposure, *Work Environ. Health* **9**:76–83.

Göthe, R., Calleman, C. J., Ehrenberg, L., and Wachtmeister, C. A., 1974, Trapping with 3,4-dichlorobenzenethiol of reactive metabolites formed *in vitro* from the carcinogen vinyl chloride, *Ambio* **3**:234–236.

Gradiski, D., Duprat, P., Magadur, J. L., Fayein, E., 1975, Etude toxicologique expérimentale de l'hexachlorobutadiène, *Eur. J. Toxicol.* **8**:180–187.

Green, T., and Hathway, D. E., 1975, The biological fate in rats of vinyl chloride in relation to its oncogenicity, *Chem. Biol. Interact.* **11**:545–562.

Green, T., and Hathway, D. E., 1977, The chemistry and biogenesis of the S-containing metabolites of vinyl chloride in rats, *Chem. Biol. Interact.* **17**:137–150.

Green, T., and Hathway, D. E., 1978, Interactions of vinyl chloride with rat liver DNA *in vivo*, *Chem. Biol. Interact.* **22**:211–224.

Greim, H., Bonse, G., Radwan, Z., Reichert, D., and Henschler, D., 1975, Mutagenicity *in vitro* and potential carcinogenicity of chlorinated ethylenes as a function of metabolic oxirane formation, *Biochem. Pharmacol.* **24**:2013–2017.

Grigorescu, I., and Toba, G., 1966, Chlorura di vino. Aspects de toxicologie industrielle, *Rev. Chim. Rom.* **17**:499–501.

Gross, H., and Freiberg, J. 1969, Zür existenz von chloroâthylenoxid, *J. Prak. Chem.* **311**:506–510.

Gudumak, V. S., 1968, The change in activity of the oxidative enzymes in the organs of white rats given hexachlorobutadiene in acute experiments, *Zdravookyr (Kishinev)* **3**:47–50. Abstracted in *Ref. Zh. Otd. Vyp. Farmakol. Khimioter. Sredstva. Toksikol.* 4.54.828 (1969).

Guengerich, F. P., Grawford, W. M., Watanabe, P. G., Jr., 1979, Activation of vinyl chloride to covalently bound metabolites: Roles of 2-chloroethylene oxide and 2-chloroacetaldehyde, *Biochemistry* **18**:5177–5182.

Guerin, M. R., Olerich, G., and Horton, A. D., 1974, Routine gas chromatographic component profiling of cigarette smoke for the identification of biologically significant constituents, *J. Chromatogr. Sci.* **12**:385–391.

Guillemin, M. P., and Bauer, D., 1979, Human exposure to styrene. Elimination kinetic of urinary mandelic and phenylglyoxylic acids after single experimental exposures, *Int. Arch. Occup. Environ. Health* **44**:249–263.

Gut, I., Nerudova, J., Kopecky, J., and Holecek, V., 1975, Acrylonitrile biotransformation in rats, mice and Chinese hamsters as influenced by the route of administration and by phenobarbital, SKF 525-A, cysteine, dimercaprol or thiosulfate, *Arch. Toxico.* **33**:151–161.

Gut, I., Kopecky, J., and Filip, J., 1981, Acrylonitrile [14]C metabolism in rats: Effect of the route of administration on the elimination of thiocyanate and other radioactive metabolites in urine and faeces, *J. Hyg. Epid. Microbiol. and Immunol.* **25**:12–16.

Haley, T. J., 1975a, Vinyl chloride: How many unknown problems, *J. Toxicol. Environm. Health* **1**:47–73.

Haley, T. J., 1975b, Vinylidene chloride: A review of the literature, *Clin. Toxicol.* **8**:633–643.

Haley, T. J., 1978, Chloroprene (2-chloro-1,3-butadiene). What is the evidence for its carcinogenicity? *Clin. Toxicol.* **13**:153–170.

Hansteen, I. L., Hillestad, L., Thiis–Evensen, E., and Heldaas, S. S., 1978, Effects of vinyl chloride in man, a cytogenetic follow up study, *Mutat. Res.* **51**:271–278.

Harleman, J. H., and Seinen, W., 1979, Short-term toxicity and reproduction studies in rats with hexachloro-(1,3)-butadiene, *Toxicol. Appl. Pharmacol.* **47**:1–14.

Härkönen, H., 1978, Styrene: Its experimental and clinical toxicology, *Scand. J. Work Environ. Health* **4(2)**:104–113.

Härkönen, H., Lindström, H., Sepäläinen, A. M., Asp. S., and Hernberg, S., 1978, Exposure relationship between styrene exposure and central nervous functions, *Scand. J. Work. Environ. Health* **4(2)**:53–59.

Hashimoto, K., and Kanai, R., 1965, Studies on the toxicology of acrylonitrile. Metabolism, mode of action and therapy, *Ind. Health* **3**:30–46.

Hashimoto, K., and Kanai, R., 1972, Effect of acrylonitrile on sulfhydryls and pyruvate metabolism in tissues, *Biochem. Pharmacol.* **21**:635–640.

Hathway, D. E., 1977, Comparative mammalian metabolism of vinyl chloride and vinylidene chloride in relation to oncogenic potential, *Environ. Health Persp.* **21**:55–59.

Hawley, G. G., Ed., 1971, *The Condensed Chemical Dictionary*, 8th ed., Van Nostrand–Reinhold, New York, p. 206.

Heath, C. W., Jr., Dumont, C. R., Gamble, J., and Waxweiler, R. J., 1977, Chromosomal damage in men occupationally exposed to vinyl chloride monomer and other chemicals, *Environ. Res.* **14**:68–72.

Hedley, W. H., Cheng, J. T., McCormick, R. J., and Lewis, W. A., 1976, Sampling of automobile interiors for vinyl chloride monomer, EPA-600/2-76-124, Springfield, Va., National Technical Information Service.

Hefner, R. E., Jr., Watanabe, P. G., and Gehring, P. J., 1975, Preliminary studies on the fate of inhaled vinyl chloride monomer (VCM) in rats, *Environ. Health Perspect.* **11**:85–95.

Heineman, B., and Howard, A. J., 1964, Induction of lambda-bacteriophage in *Escherichia coli* as a screening test for potential antitumor agents, *Appl. Microbiol.* **12**:234–239.

Hoffmann, D., Patrianakos, C., Brunnemann, K. D., and Gori, G. B., 1976, Chromatographic determination of vinyl chloride in tobacco smoke, *Anal. Chem.* **48**:47–50.

Holmberg, B., Kronevi, T., and Winell, M., 1976, The pathology of vinyl chloride exposed mice, *Acta Vet. Scand.* **17**:328–342.

Holmberg, P. C., 1977, Central nervous defects in two children of mothers exposed to chemicals in the reinforced plastic industry: Chance or a causal relation? *Scand. J. Work Environ. Health* **3**:212–214.

Hopkins, J., 1980, Vinyl chloride. V. Mutagenicity in man, *Food Cosmet. Toxicol.* **18**:200–201.

Huberman, E., Bartsch, H., and Sachs, L., 1975, Mutation induction in Chinese hamster V79 cells by two vinyl chloride metabolites, chloroethylene oxide and 2-chloroacetaldehyde, *Int. J. Cancer* **16**:639–644.

Hushon, J., and Kornreich, M., 1976, Air pollution assessment of vinylidene chloride, Springfield, Va., U.S. National Technical Information Service, PB 256, 738, p. 40.

IARC, 1979, IARC monographs on the evaluation of the carcinogenic risk of chemicals to human, 19, some monomers, plastics and synthetic elastomers and acrolein, pp. 73–86; pp. 131–156; pp. 231–244; pp. 377–401; pp. 439–459.

Ikeda, M., Ohtsuji, H., and Imamura, I., 1972, *In vivo* suppression of benzene and styrene oxidation by co-administration of toluene in rats and effects of phenobarbital, *Xenobiotica* **2**:101–106.

Infante, P. F., Wagoner, J. K., and Waxweiller, R. J., 1976, Carcinogenic, mutagenic and teratogenic risks associated with vinyl chloride, *Mutat. Res.* **41**:131–142.

Infante, P. F., Wagoner, J. K., and Young, R. J., 1977, Chloroprene: Observations of carcinogenesis and mutagenesis, in *Origins of Human Cancer*, Book A, (edited by H. H. Hiatt, J. D. Watson, and J. A. Winsten), Cold Spring Harbor Laboratory, Cold Spring Harbor, New York, pp. 205–217.

Ivanov, V. V., Kutznetsova, G. P., Archakov, A. I., 1978, Stimulation of lipid peroxidation by acrylonitrile in rat liver tissue, *Vopr. Med. Khim.* **24**(6):816–818.

Ivanetich, K. M., Aronson, I., and Katz, I. D., 1977, The interaction of vinyl chloride with rat hepatic microsomal cytochrome $P_{450}$ *in vitro*, *Biochem. Biophys. Res. Comm.* **74**:1411–1418.

Jacobs, A., Blangetti, M., and Hellmond, F., 1974, Accumulation of noxious chlorinated substances from Rhine River water in the fatty tissue of rats, *Vom. Wasser* **43**:259–274, Abstracted in *Chem. Abstr.* **82**:165547.

Jaeger, R. J., Trabulus, M. J., and Murphy, S. D., 1973a, The interaction of adrenalectomy partial adrenal replacement therapy, and starvation with hepatotoxicity and lethality of 1,1-dichloroethylene intoxication, *Toxicol. Appl. Pharmacol.* **25**:491.

Jaeger, R. J., Trabulus, M. J., and Murphy, S. D., 1973b, Biochemical effects of 1,1-dichloroethylene in rats: Dissociation of its hepatotoxicity from a lipoperoxidative mechanism, *Toxicol. Appl. Pharmacol.* **24**:457–467.

Jaeger, R. J., Reynolds, E. S., Conolly, R. B., Moslen, M. T., Szabo, S., and Murphy, S. D., 1974, Acute hepatic injury by vinyl chloride in rats pretreated with phenobarbital, *Nature* **252**:724–725.

Jaeger, R. J., Conolly, R. B., Reynolds, E. S., and Murphy, S. D., 1975a, Biochemical toxicology of unsaturated halogenated monomers, *Environ. Health Persp.* **11**:121–128.

Jaeger, R. J., Conolly, R. B., and Murphy, S. D., 1975b, Short-term inhalation toxicity of halogenated hydrocarbons, *Arch. Environm. Health.* **30**:26–31.

Jaeger, R. J., 1975, Vinyl chloride monomer: Comments on its hepatotoxicity and interaction with 1,1-dichloroethylene, *Ann. N.Y. Acad. Sci.* **246**:150–151.

Jaeger, R. J., Murphy, S. D., Reynolds, E. S., Szabo, S., and Moslen, M. T., 1977, Chemical modification of acute hepatotoxicity of vinyl chloride monomer in rats, *Toxicol. Appl. Pharmacol.* **41**:597–607.

James, S. P., and White, D. A., 1967, The metabolism of phenethyl bromide, styrene, and styrene oxide in the rabbit and rat, *Biochem. J.* **104**:914–921.

James, M. O., Fouts, J. R., and Bend, J. R., 1975, Hepatic and extrahepatic metabolism *in vitro* of an epoxide (8-$^{14}$C styrene oxide) in the rabbit, *Biochem. Pharmacol.* **25**:187–193.

John, J. A., Smith, F. A., Leong, B. K. J., and Schwetz, B. A., 1977, The effects of maternally inhaled vinyl chloride on embryonal and foetal development in mice, rats and rabbits, *Toxicol. Appl. Pharmacol.* **39**:497–513.

Jones, B. K., and Hathway, D. E., 1978a, Differences in metabolism of vinylidene chloride between mice and rats, *Br. J. Cancer* **37**:411–417.

Jones, B. K., and Hathway, D. E., 1978b, The biological fate of vinylidene chloride in rats, *Chem. Biol. Interact.* **20**:27–41.

Jones, B. K., and Hathway, D. E., 1978c, Tissue-mediated mutagenicity of vinylidene chloride in *Salmonella typhimurium* TA 1535. *Cancer Lett.* **5**:1–6.

Kankaanpää, J., Elovaara, E., Hemminki, K., and Vainio, H., 1979a, Embryotoxicity of acrolein, acrylonitrile and acrylamide, in developing chick embryos, *Tox. Lett.* **4**:93–96.

Kankaanpää, J. T., Hemminki, K., and Vainio, H., 1979b, Embryotoxicity and teratogenicity of styrene and styrene oxide on chick embryos enhanced by trichloropropene oxide, *Acta Pharmacol. Toxicol.* **45**:399–402.

Kankaanpää, J. T., Elovaara, E., Hemminki, K., and Vainio, H., 1980, The effects of maternally inhaled styrene on embryonal and foetal development in mice and Chinese hamsters, *Acta Pharmacol. Toxicol.* **47**:127–129.

Kappus, H., Bolt, H. M., Buchter, A., and Bolt, W., 1976, Liver microsomal uptake of $^{14}$C vinyl chloride and transformation to protein alkylating metabolites *in vitro*, *Toxicol. Appl. Pharmacol.* **37**:461–471.

Keplinger, M. L., Goode, J. W., Gordon, D. E., and Calandra, J. C., 1975, Interim results of exposure of rats, hamsters, and mice to vinyl chloride, *Ann. N.Y. Acad. Sci.* **246**:219–224.

Khachatryan, E. A., 1972, The occurrence of lung cancer among people working with chloroprene, *Probl. Oncol.* **18**:85.

Klimkova–Deutschova, E., Jandova, D., Salcmanova, Z., Schwartzova, K., and Titman, O., 1973, Recent advances concerning the clinical picture of professional styrene exposure (Czech.), *Cesk. Neurol. Neurochir.* **36**:20–25.

Kociba, R. J., Keyes, D. G., Jersey, G. C., Ballard, J. J., Dittenber, D. A., Quast, J. F., Wade, C. E., Humiston, C. G., and Schwetz, B. A., 1977, Results of a two year chronic toxicity study with hexachlorobutadiene in rats, *Ann. Ind. Hyg. Assoc. J.* **38**:589–602.

Kølmark, G., and Westergaard, M., 1953, Further studies on chemically induced reversions at the adenine locus of *Neurospora Hereditas* **39**:209–224.

Kopecky, J., Gut, I., Nerudova, J., Zachardova, D., Holecek, V., Filip, J., 1980, Acrylonitrile metabolism in the rat, *Arch. Toxicol. Suppl.* **4**:322–324.

Kopecky, J., Gut, I., Nerudova, J., Zachardova, D., Holecek, V. 1980a, Two routes of acrylonitrile metabolism, *J. Hyg. Epid. Microbiol. Immunol.* **24**:356–362.

Kramer, C. G., and Mutchler, J. E., 1972, The correlation of clinical and environmental measurements for workers exposed to vinyl chloride, *Am. Ind. Hyg. Assoc. J.* **33**:19–30.

Krasmyuk, E. P., Zaritskaya, L. A., Bioko, V. G., Viotenko, G. A., and Matokhmyuk, L. A., 1969, Health of vineyard workers having contact with the fumigants hexachlorobutadiene and polychlorobutane, 80, *Vrach. Delo.* **7**:111–115.

Kucerova, M., Polivkova, Z., and Batora, J., 1979, Comparative evaluations of the frequency of chromosomal aberrations and the SCE numbers in peripheral lymphocytes of workers occupationally exposed to vinyl chloride monomer, *Mutat. Res.* **67**:97–100.

Laib, R. J., and Bolt, H. M., 1978, Formation of 3, $N^4$-ethenocytidine moietis in RNA by vinyl chloride metabolites *in vitro* and *in vivo*, *Arch. Toxicol.* **39**:235–240.

Lambotte–Vandepaer, M., Duverger–van Bogaert, M., de Meester, C., Noël, G., Poncelet, F., Roberfroid, M., and Mercier, M., 1979, Styrene induced modification of some rat liver enzymes involved in the activation and inactivation of xenobiotics, *Biochem. Pharmacol.* **28**:1653–1659.

Lambotte–Vandepaer, M., Duverger–van Bogaert, M., de Mecster, C., Poncelet, F., and Mercier, M., 1980, Mutagenicity of urine from rats and mice treated with Acrylonitrile, *Toxiciology* **16**:67–71.

Lambotte–Vandepaer, M., Duverger–van Bogaert, M., de Meester, C., Rollmann, B., Poncelet, F., and Mercier, M., 1981, Identification of two urinary metabolites of rats treated with acrylonitrile: Influence of several inhibitors on the mutagenicity of those urine, *Tox. Lett.* **7**:321–328.

Lange, C. E., Jühe, S., Stein, G., and Veltman, G. 1975, Further results in polyvinyl chloride production workers, *Ann. N. Y. Acad. Sci.* **246**:18–21.

Langvardt, P. W., Putzig, C. L., Braun, W. H., and Young, J. D., 1980, Identification of the major urinary metabolites of acrylonitrile in the rat, *J. Toxicol. Environ. Health* **6**:273–282.

Laska, A. L., Bartell, C. K., Condie, D. B., Brown, J. W., Evans, R. L., and Laseter, J. L., 1978, Acute and chronic effects of hexachlorobenzene and hexachlorobutadiene in red swamp crayfish (*Procambarus clarki*) and selected fish species, *Toxicol. Appl. Pharmacol.* **43**:1–12.

Lee, F. I., and Harry, D. S., 1974, Angiosarcoma of the liver in a vinyl chloride worker, *Lancet.* **i**:1316–1318.

Lee, C. C., Bhandari, J. C., Winston, J. M., House, W. B., Peters, P. J., Dixon, R. L., and Woods, J. S., 1977, Inhalation toxicity of vinyl chloride and vinylidene chloride, *Environ. Health Perspect.* **21**:25–32.

Lee, C. C., Bhandari, J. C., Winston, J. M., House, W. B., Dixon, R. L., and Woods, J. S., 1978, Carcinogenicity of vinyl chloride and vinylidene chloride, *J. Toxicol. Environ. Health* **4**:15–30.

Leibman, K. C., and Ortiz, E., 1969, Oxidation of styrene in liver microsome, *Biochem. Pharmacol.* **18**:552–554.

Leibman, K. C., 1975, Metabolism and toxicity of styrene, *Environ. Health Perspect.* **11**:115–119.

Léonard, A., Decat, G., Léonard, E. D., Lefèvre, M. J., Decuyper, I. I., and Nicaise, C., 1977, Cytogenetic investigations on lymphocytes from workers exposed to vinyl chloride, *J. Toxicol. Environ. Health* **2**:1135–1141.

Léonard, A., Garny, V., Poncelet, F., and Mercier, M., 1981, Mutagenicity of acrylonitrile in mouse, *Tox. Lett.* **7**:329–334.

Lilis, R., and Nicholson, W. J., 1976, Cancer experience among workers in a chemical plant producing styrene monomers, in *Proceedings of NIOSH Styrene-Butadiene briefing*, Covington, Kentucky, 1976, (edited by L. Ede), HEW Publ. No. (NIOSH) 77-129, Cincinnati, Ohio, U.S. Department of Health, Education, and Welfare, pp. 22–27.

Lilis, R., Lorimer, W. V., Diamond, S., and Selikoff, I. J., 1978, Neurotoxicity of styrene in production and polymerization workers, *Environ. Res.* **15**:133–138.

Lindström, K., Härkönen, H., and Hernberg, S., 1976, Disturbances in psychological functions of workers occupationally exposed to styrene, *Scand. J. Work. Environ. Health* **3**:129–139.

Lingeman, C. H., 1976, The vinyl chloride story, *The Bulletin of SPEP* **IV**:9–15.

Linnainmaa, K., Meretoja, T., Sorsa, M., and Vainio, H., 1978, Cytogenetic effects of styrene and styrene oxide on human lymphocytes and "*Allium Cepa.*" *Scand. J. Work. Environ. Health* **4**(2):156–162.

Lloyd, J. W., 1975, Angiosarcoma of the liver in vinyl chloride/polyvinyl chloride workers, *J. Occup. Med.* **17**:333–334.

Lloyd, J. W., Decoufle, P., Moore, R. M., 1975, Background information on chloroprene, *J. Occup. Med.* **17**:263–264.

Lock, E. A., and Ishmael, J., 1979, The acute toxic effects of hexachloro-1,3-butadiene on the rat kidney, *Arch. Toxicol.* **43**:47–57.

Locker, G. Y., Doroshow, J. H., Zwelling, L. A., and Chabner, B. A., 1979, The clinical features of hepatic angiosarcomas. A report of four cases and a review of the English literature, *Medicine* **58**:48–64.

Loprieno, N., Barale, R., Baroncelli, S., Bauer, C., Bronzetti, G., Cammellini, A., Cercignani, G., Corsi, C., Gervasi, G., Leporini, C., Nieri, R., Rossi, A. M., Stretti, G., and Turchi, G., 1976a, Evaluation of the genetic effects induced by vinyl chloride monomer (VCM) under mammalian metabolic activation: Studies *in vitro* and *in vivo*, *Mutat. Res.* **40**:85–96.

Loprieno, N., Abbondandolo, A., Barale, R., Baroncelli, S., Bonatti, S., Bronzetti, G., Cammellini, A., Corsi, C., Corti, G., Frezza, D., Leporini, C., Mazzaccaro, A., Nieri, R.,

Rosellini, D., and Rossi, A. M., 1976b, Mutagenicity of industrial compounds; Styrene and its possible metabolite styrene oxide, *Mutat. Res.* **40**:317–324.

Loprieno, N., Barale, R., Baroncelli, S., Bartsch, H., Bronzetti, G., Cammellini, A., Corsi, C., Frozza, D., Nieri, R., Leporini, C., Rosellini, D., and Rossi, A. M., 1977, Induction of gene mutations and gene conversions by vinyl chloride metabolites in yeast, *Cancer Res.* **36**:253–257.

Loprieno, N., Presciuttini, S., Sbrana, I., Stretti, G., Zaccaro, L., Abbondandolo, A., Bonatti, S., Fiorio, R., and Mazzaccaro, A., 1978, Mutagenicity of industrial compounds VII: Styrene and styrene oxide. II. Point mutations, chromosome aberrations and DNA repair induction analyses, *Scand. J. Work. Environ. Health.* **4**:(suppl. 2):169–178.

Lorimer, W. V., Lilis, R., Nicholson, W. J., Anderson, H., Fischbein, A., Daum, S., Rom, W., Rice, C., and Selikoff, I. J., 1976, Clinical studies of styrene workers: Initial findings, *Environ. Health Perspect.* **17**:171–181.

Lukoshkima, L. P., and Alekperov, I. I., 1973, Lipid protein metabolism in workers handling divinylbenzene and styrene, *Gig. Tr. Prof. Zabol.* **17**:42–44.

Magnusson, J., and Ramel, C., 1978, Mutagenic effect of vinyl chloride on *Drosophila melanogaster* with and without pretreatment with sodium phenobarbitone, *Mutat. Res.* **57**:307–312.

Magnusson, J., Hällström, I., and Ramel, C., 1979, Studies on metabolic activation of vinyl chloride in *Drosophila melanogaster* after pretreatment with phenobarbital and polychlorinated biphenyls, *Chem. Biol. Interact.* **24**:287–298.

Magos, L., 1962, A study of acrylonitrile poisoning in relation to methaemoglobin-CN complex formation, *Brit. J. Ind. Med.* **19**:283–286.

Makk, L., Creech, J. L., Whelan, J. G., Jr., and Johnson, M. N., 1974, Liver damage and angiosarcoma in vinyl chloride workers. A systematic detection program, *J. Am. Med. Assoc.* **230**:64–68.

Malaveille, C., Bartsch, H., Barbin, A., Camus, A. M., Montesano, R., Croisy, A., and Jacquignon, P., 1975, Mutagenicity of vinyl chloride, chloroethyleneoxide, chloroacetaldehyde, and chloroethanol, *Biochem. Biophys. Res. Commun.* **63**:363–370.

Malaveille, C., Planche, G., and Bartsch, H., 1977, Factors for efficiency of the *Salmonella*/microsome mutagenicity assay, *Chem. Biol. Interact.* **17**:129–136.

Maltoni, C., 1974, Angiosarcoma of the liver in workers exposed to vinyl chloride. First two cases found in Italy (Ital.), *Med. Lav.* **65**:445–450.

Maltoni, C., Lefemine, G., Chicco, P., and Carreti, D., 1974, Vinyl chloride carcinogenesis: Current results and perspectives, *Med. Lav.* **65**:421–444.

Maltoni, C., 1976a, Vinyl chloride pathology, *Med. Biol. Environ.* **4**:267–278.

Maltoni, C., 1976b, Occupational chemical carcinogenesis New facts, priorities and perspectives, *Colloq. Inst. Natl. Scint. Rech. Med.* **52**:127–150.

Maltoni, C., 1977a, Vinyl chloride carcinogenecity: An experimental model for carcinogenesis studies, in *Origins of Human Cancer*, (edited by H. H. Hiatt, J. D. Watson, and J. A. Winsten), Cold Spring Harbor Laboratory, Cold Spring Harbor, N.Y., pp. 119–146.

Maltoni, C., Ciliberti, A., and DiMaio, V., 1977b, Carcinogenicity bioassays on rats of acrylonitrile administered by inhalation and by ingestion, *Med. Lav.* **68**:401–411.

Maltoni, C., Cotti, G., Morisi, L., and Chieco, P. 1977c, Carcinogenicity bioassays of vinylidene chloride, Research plan and early results, *Med. Lav.* **68**:241–262.

Maltoni, C., Failla, G., and Kassapidis, G., 1979, First experimental demonstration of the carcinogenic effects of styrene oxide, *Med. Lav.* **5**:358–362.

Malvoisin, E., Lhoest, G., Poncelet, F., Roberfroid, M., and Mercier, M., 1979, Identification and quantitation of 1,2-epoxybutene-3 as the primary metabolite of 1,3-butadiene. *J. Chrom.* **178**:419–425.

Maricq, H. R., Johnson, M. N., Whetstone, C. L., and Carwille, E., 1976, Capillary abnormalities in polyvinyl chloride production workers. Examination by *in vivo* microscopy, *Jama* **236:**1368–1371.

Marniemi, J., Suolinna, E. M., Kaartinen, N., and Vainio, H., 1976, Covalent binding of styrene oxide to rat liver macromolecules *in vivo* and *in vitro*. Hoppe Seyler's, *Z. Physiol. Chem.* **357:**140.

Martynenko, D. N., 1973, Hygienic characteristics of working conditions during production of articles from polymeric materials used in machine construction (Russ.), *Cig. Tr.* **9:**57–61. *Chem. Abstr.* **85:**148321f.

Mattern, I. E., Van der Zwaan, W. B., and Willems, M. J., 1977, Mutagenicity testing of urine from vinyl chloride treated rats using the *Salmonella* test system, *Mutat. Res.* **46:**230–231.

McCann, J., Simmon, V., Streitwieser, D., and Ames, B. N., 1975a, Mutagenicity of chloroacetaldehyde, a possible metabolic product of 1,2-dichloroethane (ethylene dichloride), chloroethanol (ethylene chlorohydrin), vinyl chloride, and cyclophosphamide, *Proc. Natl. Acad. Sci. (Wash.)* **72:**3190–3193.

McCann, J., Choi, E., Yamasaki, E., and Ames, B. N., 1975b, Detection of carcinogens as mutagens in the *Salmonella*/microsome test: Assay of 300 chemicals, *Proc. Natl. Acad. Sci. U.S.A.* **72:**5135–5139.

McKenna, M. J., Watanabe, P. G., and Gehring, P. J., 1977, Pharmacokinetics of vinylidene chloride in the rat, *Environm. Health Perspect.* **21:**99–105.

McKenna, M. J., Zempel, J. A., Madrid, E. O., Braun, W. H., and Gehring, P. J., 1978a, Metabolism and pharmacokinetic profile of vinylidene chloride in rats following oral administration, *Toxicol. Appl. Pharmacol.* **45:**821–835.

McKenna, M. J., Zempel, J. A., Madrid, E. O., and Gehring, P. J., 1978b, The pharmacokinetics of $^{14}$C vinylidene chloride in rats following inhalation exposure, *Toxicol. Appl. Pharmacol.* **45:**599–610.

McLaughlin, J., Jr., Marliac, J.-P., Verrett, M. J., Mutchler, M. K., and Fitzhugh, O. G., 1964, Toxicity of fourteen volatile chemicals as measured by the chick embryo method, *Am. Ind. Hyg. Assoc. J.* **25:**282–284.

Menezes, S., Papadopoulo, D., Levry, S., and Markovits, P., 1979, Transformation *in vitro* de cellules de poumons de jeunes hamsters par le chloro-2-butadiène, *C. R. Acad. Sci. Paris* **288:**923–926.

Meretoja, T., Vainio, H., Sorsa, M., and Härkönen, H., 1977, Occupational styrene exposure and chromosomal aberrations, *Mutat. Res.* **56:**193–197.

Meretoja, T., Vainio, H., and Järventaus, H., 1978, Clastogenic effects of styrene exposure on bone marrow cells of rats, *Tox. Lett.* **1:**315–318.

Miller, A., Teirstein, A. S., Chuang, M., and Selikoff, I. J., 1975, Changes in pulmonary function in workers exposed to vinyl chloride and polyvinyl chloride, *Ann. N. Y. Acad. Sci.* **246:**42–52.

Milvy, P., and Garro, A. J., 1976, Mutagenic activity of styrene oxide (1,2-epoxyethylbenzene), a presumed styrene metabolite, *Mutat. Res.* **40:**15–18.

Milvy, P., and Wolff, M., 1977, Mutagenic studies with acrylonitrile, *Mutat. Res.* **48(3–4):**271–278.

Monson, R. R., Peters, J. M., and Johnson, M. N., 1974, Proportional mortality among vinyl-chloride workers, *Lancet* **ii:**397–398.

Morris, G. E., 1953, Vinyl plastics. Their dermatological and chemical aspects, *Arch. Ind. Occup. Med.* **3:**535.

Morisset, Y., P'an, A., and Jegier, Z., 1979, Effect of styrene and fiber glass on small airways of mice, *J. Toxicol. Environ. Health* **5:**943–956.

Müller, G. Norpoth, K., and Eckard, R., 1976, Identification of two urine metabolites of vinyl chloride by GC-MS investigations, *Int. Arch. Occup. Environ. Health* **38:**69–75.

Muller, G., Norpoth, C. K., and Owzarski, W., 1978, *In vivo* trapping of a vinyl chloride metabolite by means of 3,4-dichlorobenzenethiol, *Int. Arch. Occup. Environ. Health* **42**:137–139.

Muratov, M. M., and Gus'Kova, S. I., 1978, The question of the mutagenic activity of vinyl chloride, *Hyg. Sanit.* **7**:111–112.

Murdoch, I. A., and Hammond, A. R., 1977, A practical method for the measurement of vinyl chloride monomer (VCM) in air, *Ann. Occup. Hyg.* **20**:55–61.

Murray, F. J., Schwetz, B. A., Nitschke, K. D., John, J. A., Norris, J. M., and Gehring, P. J., 1978a, Teratogenicity of acrylonitrile given to rats by gavage or by inhalation, *Food Cosmet. Toxicol.* **16**:547–551.

Murray, F. J., John, J. A., Balmer, M. F., and Schwetz, B. A., 1978b, Teratologic evaluation of styrene given to rats and rabbits by inhalation or by gavage, *Toxicology* **11**:335–343.

Murray, F. J., Mitschke, K. D., Rampy, L. W., and Schwetz, B. A., 1979, Embryotoxicity of fetotoxicity of inhaled or ingested vinylidene chloride in rats and rabbits, *Toxicol. Appl. Pharmacol.* **49**:189–202.

Murzakaev, F. G., 1967, Action exerted by low hexachlorobutadiene doses on the activity of the central nervous system and morphological changes in animals so poisoned, *Gig. Tr. Prof. Zabol.* **11**:23–28. Abstracted in *Chem. Abstr.* **67**:31040.

National Cancer Institute, 1979, Bioassay of styrene for possible carcinogenicity. Technical report series No. 185, case No. 100-42-5, U.S. Department of Health, Education, and Welfare. Public Health Service, National Institute of Health.

National Institute for Occupational Safety and Health, 1977, Criteria for a Recommended Standard—Occupational Exposure to Chloroprene, DHEW (NIOSH) Publ. No. 77-210. Washington, D.C., U.S. Government Printing Office.

Nerudova, J., Kopecky, J., Hatle, K., 1978, Acrylonitrile biotransformation in microsomes, isolated perfused liver, and in living rats, *Int. Congr. Ser. Exc. Med.* **440**:121–123.

Nicholson, W. J., Hammond, E. C., Seidman, H., and Selikoff, I. J., 1975, Mortality experience of a cohort of vinyl chloride–polyvinyl chloride workers, *Ann. N. Y. Acad. Sci.* **246**:225–230.

Nilsen, O. G., Toftgard, R., Eneroth, P., 1980, Effects of acrylonitrile on rat liver cytochrome $P_{450}$, benzo(a)pyrene metabolism and serum hormone levels, *Tox. Lett.* **6(6)**:399–404.

Noria, D. F., Ritchie, S., and Silver, M. D., 1976, Angiosarcoma of the liver after vinyl chloride exposure: Report of a case and review of the literature (abstract), *Lab. Invest.* **34**:346.

Norpoth, K., Gottschalk, D., Gottschalk, I., Witting, U., Thomas, H., Fichner, D., and Schmidt, E. H., 1980, Influence of vinyl chloride monomer and $As_2O_3$ on rat liver cell proliferation after partial hepatectomy, *J. Cancer Res. Clin. Oncol.* **97**:41–50.

Norppa, H., Elovaara, E., Husgafvel-Pursainen, H., Sorsa, M., and Vainio, H., 1979, Effects of styrene oxide on chromosome aberrations, sister chromatid exchanges and hepatic drug biotransformation in Chinese hamsters *in vivo*, *Chem. Biol. Interact.* **26**:305–315.

Norppa, H., Sorsa, M., and Vainio, H., 1980a, Chromosomal aberrations in bone marrow of Chinese hamsters exposed to styrene and ethanol, *Tox. Lett.* **5**:241–244.

Norppa, H., Sorsa, M., Pfäffli, P., and Vainio, H., 1980b, Styrene and styrene oxide induce SCEs and are metabolized in human lymphocytes cultures, *Carcinogenesis* **1**:357–361.

Oesch, F., Jerina, D. M., and Daly, J. W., 1971, A radiometric assay for hepatic epoxide hydrase activity with (7-$^{3H}$) styrene oxide, *Biochim. Biophys. Acta.* **227**:685–691.

Ogata, M., and Sugishara, R., 1978, HPLC procedure for quantitative determination of urinary phenyl glyoxylic, mandelic, and hippuric acids as indices of styrene exposure, *Int. Arch. Occup. Environ. Health.* **42**:11–19.

Ohtsuji, H., and Ikeda, M., 1971, The metabolism of styrene in the rat and the stimulatory effect of phenobarbital, *Toxicol. Appl. Pharmacol.* **18**:321–328.

O'Mara, M. M., Crider, L. B., and Daniel, R. L., 1971, Combustion products from vinyl chloride monomer, *An. Ind. Hyg. Assoc. J.* **32**:153–156.

Ott, M. G., Langner, R. R., and Holder, B. B., 1975, Vinyl chloride exposure in a controlled industrial environment. A long-term mortality experience in 594 employees, *Arch. Environ. Health* 30:333–339.

Ott, M. G., Fishbeck, W. A., Townsend, J. C., and Schneider, E. J., 1976, A health study of employees exposed to vinylidene chloride, *J. Occup. Med.* 18:735–738.

Pagano, G., Esposito, A., Giordano, G., and Hagström, B. E., 1978, Embryotoxic and teratogenic effects of styrene derivatives on sea urchin development, *Scand. J. Work Environ. Health* 4(suppl. 2):136–141.

Pagé, M., Thériault, L., and Delorme, F., 1976, Elevated CEA levels in polyvinyl chloride workers, *Biomedicine* 25:279.

Pantarotto, C., Fanelli, R., Bidoli, F., Morazzoni, P., Salmona, M., and Szczawinska, K., 1978, Arene oxide in styrene metabolism: A new perspective in styrene toxicity? *Scand. J. Work. Environm. Health* 4(suppl. 2):67–77.

Parent, R. A., and Casto, B. C., 1979, Effect of acrylonitrile on primary Syrian golden hamster embryo cells in culture: transformation and DNA fragmentation, *J. Nat. Canc. Inst.* 62:4, 1025–1029.

Parkki, M. G., Marniemi, J., and Vainio, H., 1976, Action of styrene and its metabolites styrene oxide and styrene glycol on activities of xenobiotic biotransformation enzymes in rat liver *in vivo, Toxicol. Appl. Pharmacol.* 38:59–70.

Parkki, M. G., Marniemi, J., Ekfors, T., Louhivuori, A., and Aitio, A., 1979, Hepatotoxic changes of hamsters by styrene, in *Proceedings of the Industrial Toxicology Meeting*, Prague 1977, p. 74.

Paulet, G., and Desnos, J., 1961, Acrylonitrile. Toxicity—mechanism of therapeutic action, *Arch. Int. Pharmacodyn.* 131:54–83.

Patty, F. R., 1963, *Industrial Hygiene and Toxicology*, Interscience Publishers, New York, vol. II, pp. 1319–1321.

Pell, S., 1978, Mortality of workers exposed to chloroprene, *J. Occup. Med.* 20:21–29.

Penttilä, M., Sorsa, M., and Vainio, H., 1980, Inability of styrene to induce nondisjunction in *Drosophila* or a positive micronucleus test in the Chinese hamster, *Tox. Lett.* 6:119–123.

Peter, S., and Ungvary, G., 1980, Lack of mutagenic effects of vinyl chloride monomer in the mammalian spot test, *Mutat. Res.* 77:193–196.

Pessayre, D., Wandscheer, J. C., Descatoire, V., Artigou, J. Y., and Benhamou, J. P., 1979, Formation and inactivation of a chemically reactive metabolite of vinyl chloride, *Toxicol. Appl. Pharmacol.* 49:505–515.

Philippe, R., Lauwerijs, R., Buchet, J. P., and Roels, H., 1971, Evalution de l'exposition des travailleurs au styrène par le dosage de ses métabolites urinaires: Les acides mandelique et phénylglyoxylique. II: Application aux travailleurs fabriquants des polyesters, *Arch. Mal. Prof. Med. Trav. Sec-Soc.* 35(6):631–640.

Picciano, D. J., Flake, R. E., Gay, P. C., and Kilian, D. J., 1977, Vinyl chloride cytogenetics, *J. Occup. Med.* 19:527–530.

Plotnick, H. B., and Weigel, W. W., 1979, Tissue distribution and excretion of $^{14}C$ styrene in male and female rats, *Res. Comm. Chem. Pathol. Pharmacol.* 24(3):515–524.

Plugge, H., and Safe, S., 1977, Vinyl chloride metabolism. A review, *Chemosphere* 6:309–325.

Plugge, H., and Jaeger, R. J., 1979, Acute inhalation toxicity of 2-chloro-1,3-butadiene (chloroprene): Effects on liver and lung, *Toxicol. Appl. Pharmacol.* 50:565–572.

Pollock, J. R. A., and Stevens, R. (eds.), 1965, *Dictionary of Organic Compounds*, 4th ed., Vol. 2, New York, Oxford University Press, p. 681.

Ponomarkov, V., and Tomatis, L., 1978, Effects of long term oral administration of styrene to mice and rats, *Scand. J. Work. Environ. Health* 4(suppl. 2):127–135.

Ponomarkov, V., and Tomatis, L., 1980, Long-term testing of vinylidene chloride and chloroprene for carcinogenicity in rats, *Oncology* 37:136–141.

Popper, H., and Thomas, L. B., 1975, Alterations of liver and spleen among workers exposed to vinyl chloride, *Ann. N. Y. Acad. Sci.* **246:**172–194.

Popper, H., 1979, Hepatic cancers in man: quantitative perspective, *Environm. Res.* **19:**482–494.

Poteryaeva, G. E., 1966, Effect of hexachlorobutadiene on the offspring of albino rats, *Gigiena i, Sanit* **31-33.** Abstracted in *Chem. Abs.* **65:**1281 f.

Prodan, L., Suciu, I., Pislaru, V., Ilea, E., and Pascu, L., 1975, Experimental acute toxicity of vinyl chloride (monochlorethylene), *Ann. N. Y. Acad. Sci.* **246:**154–158.

Purchase, I. F. H., Richardson, C. R., Anderson, D., Paddle, G. M., and Adams, W. G. F., 1978, Chromosomal analyses in vinyl chloride-exposed workers, *Mutat. Res.* **57:**325–334.

Purchase, I. F. H., Richardson, C. R., and Anderson, D., 1975, Chromosomal and dominant lethal effects of vinyl chloride, *Lancet* **ii:**410–411.

Rabello-Gay, H. N., and Ahmed, E. A., 1980, Acrylonitrile: *In vivo* cytogenetic studies in mice and rats, *Mut. Res.* **79:**249–255.

Radike, M. J., Stemmer, K. L., Brown, P. G., Larson, E., and Bingham, E., 1977, Effect of ethanol and vinyl chloride on the induction of liver tumours: preliminary report, *Environ. Health Perspect.* **21:**153–155.

Radwan, Z., and Henschler, D., 1977, Uptake and rate of metabolism of vinyl chloride by the isolated perfused rat liver preparation, *Int. Arch. Occup. Environm. Health* **40:**101–110.

Ragule, N., 1974, Embryotoxic action of styrene, *Gig. i. Sanit.* **11:**85–86.

Ramsey, J. C., and Young, J. D., 1978, Pharmacokinetics of inhaled styrene in rats and humans, *Scand. J. Work Environm. Health* **4(suppl. 2):**84–94.

Ramsey, J. C., Young, J. D., Karbowski, R. J., Chenoweth, M. B., McCarty, L. P., and Braun, W. H., 1980, Pharmakokinetic of styrene in human volunteers, *Toxicol. Appl. Pharmacol.* **53:**54–63.

Rannug, U., Johansson, A., Ramel, C., and Wachtmeister, C. A., 1974, The mutagenicity of vinyl chloride after metabolic activation, *Ambio* **3:**194–197.

Rannug, U., Göthe, R., and Wachtmeister, C. A., 1976, The mutagenicity of chloroethylene oxide, chloroacetaldehyde, 2-chloroethanol, and chloroacetic acid, conceivable metabolites of vinyl chloride, *Chem. Biol. Interact.* **12:**251–263.

Ravier, E., Diter, J. M., and Pialat, J., 1975, A case of hepatic angiosarcoma in a worker exposed to vinyl chloride monomer (Fr.), *Arch. Mal. Prof., Med. Trav. Sec. Soc.* **36:**171–177.

Reichert, D., Werner, H. W., and Hanschler, D., 1978, Role of liver glutathione in 1,1-dichloroethylene metabolism and hepatotoxicity in intact rats and isolated perfused rat liver, *Arch. Toxicol.* **41:**169–178.

von Reinl, W., Weber, H., and Greiser, E., 1977, Epidemiological study on mortality of VC-exposed workers in the Federal Republic of Germany (Ger.), *Medichem* (September): pp. 2–8.

Reitz, R. H., Watanabe, P. G., McKenna, M. J., Quast, J. F., and Gehring, P. J., 1980, Effects of vinylidene chloride on DNA synthesis and DNA repair in the rat and mouse. A comparative study with dimethylnitrosamine, *Toxicol. Appl. Pharmacol.* **52:**357–370.

Reynolds, E. S., Moslen, M. T., Szabo, S., and Jaeger, R. J., 1975a, Vinyl chloride induced deactivation of cytochrome $P_{450}$ and other components of the liver mixed function oxidase system: an *in vivo* study, *Res. Commun. Chem. Pathol. Pharmacol.* **12:**685–694.

Reynolds, E. S., Moslen, M. T., Szabo, S., Jaeger, R. J., and Murphy, S. D., 1975b, Hepatotoxicity of vinyl chloride and 1,1-dichloroethylene, *Am. J. Pathol.* **81:**219–236.

Reynolds, E. S., Jaeger, R. J., and Murphy, S. D., 1975c, Acute liver injury by vinyl chloride: involvement of endoplasmic reticulum in phenobarbital-pretreated rats, *Environ. Health Perspect.* **11:**227–233.

Roche, J., Fournet, J., Hostein, J., Panh, M., and Bonnet–Eymard, J., 1978, Hepatic angiosarcoma due to vinyl chloride. Report of 4 cases (Fr.), *Gastroenterol. Clin. Biol.* **2:**669–678.

Ryan, A. J., James, M. O., BenZvi, Z., Law, F. L. P., and Bend, J. R., 1975, Hepatic and extrahepatic metabolism of $^{14}C$ styrene oxide, *Environ. Health Perspect.* **17:**135-144.

Salmon, A. G., 1976, Cytochrome $P_{450}$ and the metabolism of vinyl chloride, *Cancer Lett.* **2:**109-114.

Salnikova, L. S., and Fomenko, V. N., 1973, Experimental investigation of the influence of chloroprene on embryogenesis, *Gig. Tr. Prof. Zabol.* **8:**23-26.

Sandberg, E. Ch., and Slanina, P., 1980, Distribution of 1-$^{14}C$ acrylonitrile in rat and monkey, *Tox. Lett.* **6:**187-191.

Sandell, J., Parkki, M. G., Marnicmi, J., and Aitio, A., 1978, Effects of inhalation and cutaneous exposure to styrene on drug metabolizing enzymes in the rat, *Res. Comm. Chem. Pathol. Pharmacol.* **19(1):**109-118.

Sanotskii, I. V., 1976, Aspects of the toxicology of chloroprene: Immediate and long-term effects, *Environ. Health Perspect.* **17:**85-93.

Saric, M., Kulcar, Z., Zorica, M., and Gelic, I., 1976, Malignant tumours of the liver and lungs in an area with a PVC industry, *Environ. Health Perspect.* **17:**394-398.

Sassu, G. M., Zilio-Grandi, F., and Conte, A., 1968, Gas chromatographic determinations of impurities in vinyl chloride, *J. Chromatogr.* **34:**394-398.

Savolainen, H., and Vainio, H., 1977, Organ distribution and nervous system binding of styrene and styrene oxide, *Toxicology* **8:**135-141.

Savolainen, H., and Pfäffli, P., 1977, Effects of chronic styrene inhalation on rat brain protein metabolism, *Acta Neuropath.* **40:**237-241.

Savolainen, H., and Pfäffli, P., 1978, Accumulation of styrene monomer and neurochemical effects of long term inhalation exposure in rats, *Scand. J. Work. Environ. Health* **4(suppl. 2):**78-84.

Sax, N. I., 1968, *Dangerous Properties of Industrial Materials*, Third Edition. Van Nostrand Reinhold, New York, p. 576.

Schwetz, B. A., Smith, F. A., Humiston, C. G., Quast, J. F., and Kociba, R. J., 1977, Results of a reproduction study in rats fed diets containing hexachlorobutadiene, *Toxicol. Appl. Pharmacol.* **42:**387-398.

Seppäläinen, A. M., and Härkönen, H., 1976, Neurophysiological findings among workers occupationally exposed to styrene, *Scand. J. Work Environ. Health* **2:**140-146.

Seppäläinen, A. M., 1978, Neurotoxicity of styrene in occupational and experimental exposure, *Scand. J. Work. Environ. and Health* **4(suppl 2):**181-183.

Seutter-Berlage, F., Delbressine, L. P. C., Smeets, F. L. M., and Ketelaars, H. C. J., 1978, Identification of three sulfur containing urinary metabolites of styrene in the rat, *Xenobiotica* **8(7):**413-418.

Shahin, M. J., 1976, The nonmutagenicity and recombinogenicity of vinyl chloride in the absence of metabolic activation, *Mutat. Res.* **40:**269-272.

Shimkin, M. B., Weisburger, J. H., Weisburger, E. K., Gubareff, N., and Sumtzeff, V., 1966, Bioassay of 29 alkylating chemicals by the pulmonary-tumour response in strain A mice, *J. Natl. Cancer Inst.* **36:**915-935.

Short, R. D., Winston, J. M., Minor, J. L., Hong, C. B., Seifter, J., and Lee, C. C., 1977a, Toxicity of vinylidene chloride in mice and rats and its alteration by various treatments, *J. Toxicol. Env. Health* **3:**913-921.

Short, R. D., Minor, J. L., Winston, J. M., and Lee, C. C., 1977b, A dominant lethal study in male rats after repeated exposures to vinyl chloride or vinylidene chloride, *J. Toxicol. Env. Health* **3:**965-968.

Shugaev, B. B., 1969, Concentrations of hydrocarbons in tissues as a measure of toxicity, *Arch. Environ. Health* **18:**878-882.

Siegers, C. P., Younes, M., and Schmitt, G., 1979, Effects of dithiocarb and (+)-cyanidanol-3 on the hepatotoxicity and metabolism of vinylidene chloride in rats, *Toxicology* **15:**55-64.

Simmon, V., 1977, Mutagenic halogenated hydrocarbons. Presented at Meeting of Structural Parameters Associated with Carcinogenesis, Annapolis, Maryland, Aug. 31–Sept. 2.

Smith, P. M., Williams, D. M. J., and Evans, D. M. D., 1976, Hepatic angiosarcoma in a vinyl chloride worker, *Bull. N. Y. Acad. Med.* **52**:447–452.

Sollenberg, J., and Baldesten, A., 1977, Isotachophoretic analysis of mandelic acid, phenylglyoxylic acid, hippuric acid and methylhippuric acid in urine after occupational exposure to styrene, toluene and/or xylene, *J. Chromatogr.* **132**:469–476.

Spencer, H. C., Irish, D. D., Adams, E. M., and Rowe, V. K., 1942, The response of Laboratory animals to monomeric styrene, *J. Ind. Hyg. Toxicol.* **24**:295–301.

Spirtas, R., and Kaminski, R., 1978, Angiosarcoma of the liver in vinyl chloride/polyvinyl chloride workers. 1977 Update of the NIOSH Register, *J. Occup. Med.* **20**:427–429.

Stoltz, D. R., and Withey, R. J., 1977, Mutagenicity testing of styrene and styrene epoxide in *Salmonella typhimurium*, *Bull. Environm. Contam. Toxicol.* **17**:737–742.

Suciu, I., Drejman, I., and Valaskai, M., 1963, Investigation of the disease produced by vinyl chloride, *Med. Interna* **15**:967.

Suzuki, Y., 1978, Pulmonary tumours induced in mice by vinyl chloride monomer, *Environm. Res.* **16**:285–301.

Szabo, S., and Selye, H., 1972, Effect of phenobarbital and steroids on the adrenal apoplexy produced by acrylonitrile in rats, *Endocrinol. Exp.* **6**:141–146.

Szabo, S., Reynolds, E. S., and Kovacs, K., 1976, Animal model of human disease, *American J. Pathol.* **82**:653–656.

Szabo, S., Bailey, K. A., Boor, P. J., and Jaeger, R. J., 1977a, Acrylonitrile and tissue glutathione: differential effect of acute and chronic interactions, *Biochem. Biophys. Res. Comm.* **79**:1, 32–37.

Szabo, S., Jaeger, R. J., Moslen, M. T., and Reynolds, E. S., 1977b, Modification of 1,1-dichloroethylene hepatotoxicity by hypothyroidism, *Toxicol. Appl. Pharmacol.* **42**:367–376.

Szentesi, I., Hornyak, E., Ungvary, G., Czeizel, A., Bognar, Z., and Timar, M., 1976, High rate of chromosomal aberration in PVC workers, *Mutat. Res.* **37**:313–316.

Tabershaw, I. R., and Gaffey, W. R., 1974, Mortality study of workers in the manufacture of vinyl chloride and its polymers, *J. Occup. Med.* **16**:509–518.

Thiess, A. M., and Fleig, I., 1978a, Analysis of chromosomes of workers exposed to acrylonitrile, *Arch. Toxicol.* **41**:149–152.

Thiess, A. M., and Fleig, I., 1978b, Chromosome investigations on workers exposed to styrene/polystyrene, *J. Occup. Med.* **20**:747–749.

Thiess, A. M., and Friedheim, M., 1978, Morbidity among persons employed in styrene production, polymerization and processing plants, *Scand. J. Work. Environ. Health.* **4(suppl. 2)**:203–214.

Thomas, L. B., and Popper, H., 1975, Pathology of angiosarcoma of the liver among vinyl chloride-polyvinyl chloride workers, *Ann. N. Y. Acad. Sci.* **246**:268–277.

Ungvary, G., Hudak, A., Tatrai, E., Lorincz, M., and Fally, G., 1978, Effects of vinyl chloride exposure alone and in combination with trypan blue—applied systematically during all thirds of pregnancy on the foetuses of CFY rats, *Toxicology* **11**:45–54.

U.S. Consumer Product Safety Commission, 1978. Assessment of acrylonitrile contained in consumer products, Final report, contract No. CPSC-C-77-0009, Task No. 1014K. H.I.A./Economic Analysis, Washington, D.C.

U.S. Department of Labor, 1978, Occupational exposure to acrylonitrile (vinyl cyanide). Proposed standard and notice of hearing, *Fed. Regist.* **43**:2586–2621.

U.S. Food and Drug Administration, 1975, Vinyl chloride polymers in contact with food. Notice of proposed rulemaking. *Fed. Regist.* **40**:40,529–40,537.

U.S. Environmental Protection Agency, 1975a, Preliminary assessment of suspected carcinogens in drinking water, Washington, D.C., p. II-3.

U.S. Environmental Protection Agency, 1975b, Preliminary assessment of suspected carcinogens in drinking water, Report to Congress, Washington, D.C., pp. II-7.

U.S. Environmental Protection Agency, 1975c, Scientific and technical assessment report on vinyl chloride and polyvinyl chloride. EPA-600/6-75-004, Springfield, Va., National Technical Information Service, pp. 7-42.

Vainio, H., Pääkkönen, R., Rönnholm, K., Raunio, V., and Pelkonen, O., 1976, A study on the mutagenic activity of styrene and styrene oxide, Scand. J. Work. Environ. Health 3:147-151.

Vainio, H., and Mäkinen, A., 1977, Styrene and acrylonitrile induced depression of hepatic nonsulfhydryl content in various rodent species, Res. Comm. Pathol. Pharmacol. 17(1):115-124.

Vainio, H., Hemminki, K., and Elovaara, E., 1977, Toxicity of styrene and styrene oxide on chick embryos, Toxicology 8:319-325.

Vainio, H., and Elovaara, E., 1979, The interaction of styrene oxide with hepatic cytochrome $P_{450}$ in vitro and effects of styrene oxide inhalation on xenobiotic biotransformation in mouse liver and kidney, Biochem. Pharmacol. 28:2001-2004.

Vainio, H., Järvisalo, J., and Taskinen, E., 1979, Adaptive changes caused by intermittent styrene inhalation on xenobiotic biotransformation, Toxicol. Appl. Pharmacol. 49:7-14.

Van Bladeren, P. J., Delbressine, L. P. C., Hoogeterp, J. J., Beaumont, A. H. G. M., Breiner, D. D., Seutter-Berlage, F., and Van der Gen, A., Formation of mercapturic acids from acrylonitrile, crotononitrile and cinnamonitrile by direct conjugation and via an intermediate oxidation process, . . .in "The Dual Role of Glutathione Conjugation in the Biotransformation of Xenobiotics," P. J. Van Bladeren, Academic dissertation 8th April 1981, Klokke, Netherlands.

Van Duuren, B. L., Nelson, N., Orris, L., Palmes, E. D., and Schmitt, F. L., 1963, Carcinogenicity of epoxides, lactones and peroxy compounds, J. Natl. Cancer Inst. 31:41-55.

Van Duuren, B. L., Langseth, L., Orris, L., Teebor, G., Nelson, N., and Kuschner, M., 1966, Carcinogenicity of epoxides, lactones and peroxy compounds. IV. Tumour response in epithelial and connective tissue in mice and rats, J. Natl. Cancer Inst. 37:825-834.

Van Duuren, 1975, On the mechanism of carcinogenic action of vinyl chloride, Ann. N. Y. Acad. Sci. 246:258-267.

Venitt, S., Bushell, C. T., and Osborne, M., 1977, Mutagenicity of acrylonitrile (cyanoethylene) in Escherichia coli, Mutat. Comm. Res. 45:283-288.

Venitt, S., 1978, Mutagenic studies with acrylonitrile. Reply to author's comments, Mutat. Res. 57(1):113.

Verburgt, F. G., and Vogel, E., 1977, Vinyl chloride mutagenesis in Drosophila melanogaster, Mutat. Res. 48:327-336.

Viola, P. L., Bigotti, A., and Caputo, A., 1971, Oncogenic response of rat skin, lung and bone to vinyl chloride, Cancer Res. 31:516-522.

Viola, P. L., and Caputo, A., 1977, Carcinogenicity studies on vinylidene chloride, Environ. Health Persp. 81:45-47.

Vogel, E., 1979, Mutagenicity of chloroprene, 1-chloro-1,3-trans-butadiene, 1,4-dichlorobutene-2 and 1,4-dichloro-2,3-epoxybutane in Drosophila Melanogaster, Mutat. Res. 67:377-381.

Von Oettingen, W. F., Hueper, W. C., Deichmann-Grubler, W., and Wiley, F. H., 1936, 2-chloro-butadiene (chloroprene): Its toxicity and pathology and the mechanism of its action, J. Ind. Hyg. Toxicol. 18:240-270.

Wagoner, J. K., 1978, Vinyl chloride and pulmonary cancer, J. Environ. Pathol. Toxicol. 1:361-362.

Ward, A. M., Udnoon, S., Watkins, J., Walker, A. E., and Darke, C. S., 1976, Immunological mechanisms in the pathogenesis of vinyl chloride disease, Brit. Med. J. 1:936-938.

Watanabe, P. G., Hefner, R. E., Jr., and Gehring, P. J., 1976, Vinyl chloride-induced depression of hepatic non-protein sulfhydryl content and effects on bromosulfophtalein (BSP) clearance in rats, Toxicology 6:1-8.

Watabe, T., Isobe, M., Yoshikawa, K., and Takabatake, E., 1978a, Studies on metabolism and toxicity of styrene to styrene glycol via styrene oxide by rat liver microsomes, *J. Pharm. Dyn.* **1:**98–104.

Watabe, T., Isobe, M., Sawahata, T., Yoshikawa, K., Yamada, S., and Takabatake, E., 1978b, Metabolism and mutagenicity of styrene, *Scand. J. Work Environ. Health* **4(suppl. 2):**142–155.

Watabe, T., Isobe, M., Yoshikawa, K., and Takabatake, E., 1978c, Studies on metabolism and toxicity of styrene II. Mutagenesis in *Salmonella typhimurium* by metabolic activation of styrene with 3-methylcholanthrene pretreated rat liver, *J. Pharm. Dyn.* **1:**301–309.

Watson, W. A. F., 1972, Studies on a recombination-deficient mutation of *Drosophila*. II. Response to X rays and alkylating agents, *Mutat. Res.* **14:**299–307.

Waxweiler, R. J., Stringer, W., Wagoner, J. K., Jones, J., Falk, H., and Carter, C., 1976, Neoplastic risk among workers exposed to vinyl chloride, *Ann. N.Y. Acad. Sci.* **271:** 40–48.

Williams, D. T., and Miles, W. F., 1975, Gas-liquid chromatographic determination of vinyl chloride in alcoholic beverages, vegetable oils, and vinegars, *J. Assoc. Off. Anal. Chem.* **58:**272–275.

Wilson, R. H., Hough, G. V., and McCormick, W. E., 1948, Medical problems encountered in the manufacture of American-made rubber, *Ind. Med.* **17:**199–207.

Wilson, R. H., and McCormich, W. E., 1954, Toxicity of plastics and rubber. Plastomers and monomers, *Ind. Med. Surg.* **23:**479.

Windholz, M., (ed.) 1976, The Merck Index, 9th ed., Rahway, N.Y., Merck & Co., pp. 986, 1283.

Winell, M., Holmberg, B., and Kromevi, T., 1976, Biological effects of vinyl chloride: An experimental study, *Environ. Health Perspect.* **17:**211–216.

Withey, J. R., 1976, Quantitative analysis of styrene monomer in polystyrene and foods including some preliminary studies of the uptake and pharmacodynamics of the monomer in rats, *Environ. Health Perspect.* **17:**125–133.

Withey, J. R., and Collins, P. G., 1977, Pharmacokinetics and distribution of styrene monomer in rats after intravenous administration, *J. Toxicol. Environ. Health* **3:**1011–1020.

Withey, J. R., and Collins, P. G., 1978, Styrene monomer in foods. A limited Canadian survey, *Bull. Environ. Contam. Toxicol.* **19:**86–94.

Withey, J. R., and Collins, P. G., 1979, The distribution and pharmacokinetics of styrene monomer in rats by the pulmonary route, *J. Environ. Pathol. Toxicol.* **2:**1329–1342.

Wolf, M. A., Rowe, V. K., Collister, D. D., Hollingsworth, R. L., and Oyen, F., 1956, Toxicological studies of certain alkylated benzenes and benzene, *Arch. Ind. Health* **14:**381–398.

Wolff, M. S., 1976, Evidence for existence in human tissues of monomer for plastics and rubber manufacture, *Environ. Health Perspect.* **17:**183–187.

Wolff, M. S., Lorimer, W. V., Lilis, R., and Selikoff, I. J., 1978, Blood styrene and urinary metabolites in styrene polymerisation, *Brit. J. Ind. Med.* **35:**318–329.

Yagen, B., Hernandez, O., Bend, J. R., and Cox, R. H., 1981, Synthesis and relative stereochemistry of the four mercapturic acids derived from styrene oxide and $N$-acetyl cysteine, *Chem. Biol. Interact.* **34:**57–87.

Yllner, S., 1971, Metabolism of chloroacetate-1-$^{14}$C in the mouse, *Acta Pharmacol. Toxicol.* **30:**69–80.

Yoshikawa, K., Isobe, M., Watabe, T., and Takabatake, E., 1980, Studies on metabolism and toxicity of styrene. III. The effects of metabolic inactivation by rat liver S9 on the mutagenicity of phenyloxirane towards *Salmonella typhimurium*, *Mutat. Res.* **78:** 219–226.

Zajdela, F., Croisy, A., Barbin, A., Malaveille, C., Tomatis, L., and Bartsch, H., 1980, Carcinogenicity of chloroethylene oxide, an ultimate reactive metabolite of vinyl chloride and bis (chloromethyl)ether after subcutaneous administration and in initiation-promotion experiments in mice, *Cancer Res.* **40:**352–356.

Zil'Fyan, V. N., Fichidzhyan, B. S., Garibyan, D. K., and Pogosova, A. M., 1977, Experimental study of chloroprene for carcinogenicity, *Vop. Onkol.* **23:**61–65.

Zimmermann, F. K., and Vig. B. K., 1975, Mutagen specificity in the induction of mitotic crossing over in *Saccharomyces cerevisiae, Mol. Gen. Genet.* **139:**255–268.

*Chapter 5*

# Mutagenicity, Carcinogenicity, and Teratogenicity of Halogenated Hydrocarbon Solvents

## M. Mercier, M. Lans, and J. de Gerlache

Seven chlorinated solvents (methylene chloride, chloroform, carbon tetrachloride, trichloroethylene, 1,1,1-trichloroethane, 1,2-dichloroethane, and tetrachloroethane) widely used in industry for metal degreasing, in extraction processes, as refrigerants or aerosol propellants, paint removers, and starting material for the manufacture of fluorocarbons have been reviewed.

The physical and chemical properties, metabolism, mutagenicity, carcinogenicity, and teratogenicity are presented and discussed. Some of these solvents are hepatotoxic after acute or long-term exposure; chloroform and carbon tetrachloride present some nephrotoxic properties and, as methylene chloride, are also reported to be teratogenic and/or embryotoxic. Although negative or only weakly positive in mutagenicity tests, carbon tetrachloride and chloroform are carcinogenic in several species (rats, mice). Evidence of carcinogenicity has also been demonstrated for 1,2-dichloroethane.

The only relevant data available concerning trichloroethane and tetrachloroethane are insufficient to draw a final conclusion concerning their carcinogenicity and teratogenicity; the long-term effects at industrial and environmental concentrations are not well known and need to be studied. Therefore, except for specific industrial situations, the available data are too limited to permit a general conclusion.

**M. Mercier** • International Program for Chemical Safety, Management Unit, W.H.O, Geneva, Switzerland.    **M. Lans and J. de Gerlache** • Laboratoire de Biochemie Toxicologique et Cancerologique, U.C.L., B-1200 Brussels, Belgium.

## 1. INTRODUCTION

Seven halogenated hydrocarbon solvents have been reviewed and commented on with special emphasis on mutagenicity, teratogenicity, and carcinogenicity.

Carbon tetrachloride and chloroform have been used as fumigants and for the manufacture of fluorocarbon; 1,2-dichloroethane is used as a fumigant and in the manufacture of vinyl chloride, 1,1,1-trichfloroethane is used in the manufacture of vinylidene chloride. Tetrachloroethylene, trichloroethylene, and dichloromethane are widely used as degreasing solvents.

Several reviews of these chlorinated solvents are available. Carbon tetrachloride and 1,1,1-trichloroethane have been reviewed by Mercier (1977); chloroform by Berkowitz (1978a), Mercier (1977), and Winslow and Gerstner (1977); dichloromethane by Berkowitz (1978b), and Mercier (1977); tetrachloroethylene by Berkowitz (1978b) and NIOSH (1976); trichloroethylene by Mercier (1977) and Lyman (1978). The seven halogenated hydrocarbon solvents have been reviewed by IARC (1979).

Some of these solvents are hepatotoxic or nephrotoxic. All of these compounds are readily metabolized *in vivo*, and their degradation products are rapidly excreted, mainly in the urine. There is little long-term storage in fat tissues. With the intention of enlarging the sections concerning metabolism, teratogenicity, mutagenicity, and carcinogenicity of the solvents, their formulas, production, uses, properties and occurrence are summarized in Tables I to V.

## 2. CHLOROFORM

### 2.1. Absorption, Distribution, Metabolism, and Excretion

As for other volatile solvents, inhalation is considered the main route of entry of chloroform in man. Rapidly absorbed and distributed in all organs, chloroform is exhaled for the most part unchanged, but a part of it is exhaled as carbon dioxide. The results of experiments undertaken to investigate the excretion of labeled chloroform showed great discrepancy. These were reviewed in detail (Charlesworth, 1976). The discrepancy was partly due to the technique used to recover metabolites, but also to striking differences among species.

The conversion rate into carbon dioxide was only 20% in monkeys, while mice receiving 60 mg/kg orally over a 5-day period converted 80% of the dose into carbon dioxide (Brown *et al.*, 1974a). Experiments with rats demonstrated that, in this species, only 4 to 5% of chloroform administered

**Table I**

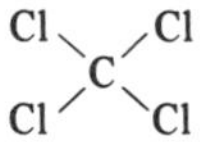

| Cl—C(Cl)(Cl)—Cl | Cl—C(Cl)=CH₂ | Cl—CH(Cl)—Cl |
|---|---|---|

$$\begin{array}{ccc}
\text{Cl}\diagdown\phantom{C}\diagup\text{Cl} & \text{Cl}\diagdown\phantom{C}\text{CH}_2 & \text{Cl}\diagdown\phantom{Cl}\text{CH} \\
\phantom{Cl}\text{C}\phantom{Cl} & \text{Cl}\diagup & \text{Cl—CH} \\
\text{Cl}\diagup\phantom{C}\diagdown\text{Cl} & & \text{Cl}\diagup
\end{array}$$

Carbon tetrachloride 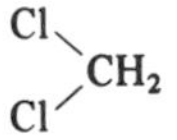 · Dichloromethane 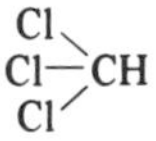 · Chloroform

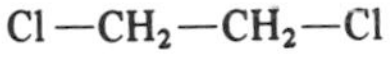

$Cl-CH_2-CH_2-Cl$

Dichloroethane

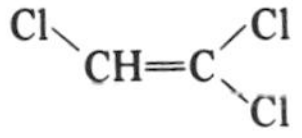

$$\begin{array}{cc}
\text{Cl}\diagdown\phantom{CH}\diagup\text{Cl} \\
\phantom{Cl}\text{CH=C} \\
\phantom{ClCHC}\diagdown\text{Cl}
\end{array}$$

Trichloroethylene

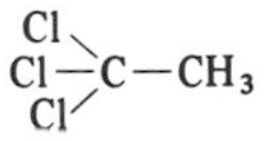

$$\begin{array}{c}
\text{Cl}\diagdown \\
\text{Cl—C—CH}_3 \\
\text{Cl}\diagup
\end{array}$$

1,1,1-Trichloroethane

$$\begin{array}{cc}
\text{Cl}\diagdown\phantom{C=C}\diagup\text{Cl} \\
\phantom{Cl}\text{C=C} \\
\text{Cl}\diagup\phantom{C=C}\diagdown\text{Cl}
\end{array}$$

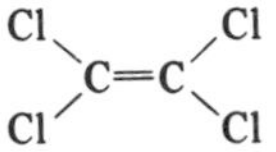

Tetrachloroethylene

intraduodenally was converted into carbon dioxide and 70% excreted unchanged (Paul and Rubinstein, 1963).

The pharmacokinetics of chloroform in humans under anesthesia has been studied (Smith *et al.*, 1973). Two volunteers who received labeled chloroform exhaled about 50% of the dose as $CO_2$ (Charlesworth, 1976). In another experiment, male and female volunteers who received orally 500 mg of chloroform, exhaled from 20 to 66% as chloroform after as long as 40 to 120 minutes.

A difference in the elimination rate between males and females was observed and was explained by the affinity of chloroform for adipose tissue, which predominates in women (Fry *et al.*, 1972).

Differences in tissue concentrations between the sexes are sometimes striking. Taylor *et al.* (1974) showed that, in mice receiving labeled chloroform, radioactivity was found predominantly in the liver and kidneys of males and

**Table II**
**Production[a]**

| Chemical | Annual world production ($10^6$ kg) |
|---|---|
| Carbon tetrachloride | 806 |
| Chloroform | 300 |
| 1,2-Dichloroethane | 5000 |
| Dichloromethane | >270 |
| Tetrachloroethylene | 950 |
| 1,1,1-trichloroethane | ≈600 |
| Trichloroethylene | 500 |

[a]Cited by IARC (1979).

## Table III
### Uses

| | |
|---|---|
| Dichloromethane | Paint remover, solvent in insecticide, formulations, aerosol propellant |
| Chloroform | Chemical synthesis of chlorodifluoro-methane for use as refrigerant propellant (50%) and plastic synthesis (25%). Drugs and cosmetics (23%), grain fumigation, general solvent, extraction processes, and anaesthesic |
| Carbon tetrachloride | Synthesis of chlorofluoromethanes (85%), grain fumigation, fire extinguisher, rodenticide, and industrial solvent |
| 1,2-Dichloroethane | Production of vinyl chloride (80%) and other halogenated hydrocarbons |
| Trichloroethylene | Vapor degreasing of metal parts, analgesic and anaesthesic food technology (decaffeinated coffee) |
| Trichloroethane | Cold cleaning of metals (35%), vapor degreasing (35%) for removal of greases, oils and waxes, chemical intermediate for vinylidene chloride (25%), and aerosols |
| Tetrachloroethylene | Dry-cleaning (80%), degreasing agent, intermediate in synthesis of fluorocarbons |

in the intestine and bladder of females, but no difference in metabolism was observed.

The dehalogenation of compounds including chloroform could proceed, as sulfhydryl radicals are present, by a nonenzymatic pathway (Bray *et al.*, 1952; Butler, 1961). Sulfhydryl groups could be derived from glutathion (Booth *et al.*, 1961).

Dechlorination also occurs in liver microsomes and is dependent on NADPH and oxygen (Van Dyke and Chenoweth, 1965; Van Dijke, 1966). Various factors affecting the drug metabolism system modify chloroform toxicity, thus indicating the role of the metabolic activation system in chloroform toxicity (McLean, 1970).

Moreover, the selective effects of these factors on renal or hepatic toxicity has been described (Kluwe *et al.*, 1978). Strong evidence exists that phosgene could be formed by the mixed-function-oxidase system (Mansuy *et al.*, 1977; Pohl *et al.*, 1979).

## 2.2. Toxicity

The acute toxicity of chloroform is dependent on species, sex, age, strain, and even mode of administration (Kimura, 1971; Thompson, 1974). The oral $LD_{50}$ in male mice ranges from 120 to 490 mg/kg while it is about 1200 mg/kg for rats, and because of the difference in distribution in males and females, organ susceptibility is not the same.

The males of many strains of mice were susceptible to renal tubular necrosis, whereas females showed no renal effects even at lethal doses (Klaassen, 1967; Deringer, 1953). Liver damage, however, was the cause of death in both rats and mice after acute administration of chloroform (Doyle, 1967; Brown, 1974b).

From its use as an anesthetic in humans, chloroform is known to cause hepatic and renal toxicity. Hepatic necrosis has also been reported in man following ingestion of pharmaceutical preparations containing 12.5% chloroform (Colon, 1963).

Chloroform anesthesia is accompanied by a decreased cardiac output and a tendency to hypotension; it appears to be the most cardiotoxic of all anesthetics and its effects are the least reversible (Strobel, 1961). Stimulation of the vagus nerve or direct toxic action may on occasion be fatal to man and may be attributed to cardiac arrest; other toxic signs include coma, and renal and liver damage (Challen et al., 1958; Matsuki et al., 1974).

Numerous studies have shown that chloroform causes fatty infiltration and necrosis of the liver as early as 15 minutes after ingestion, inhalation, or intravenous administration (Jones, 1958, Plaa et al., 1958; Klaassen and Plaa, 1967; Palmer et al., 1979).

Guinea pigs given 3.5 mg/kg daily for 5 months died during the course of the experiment. All showed a decrease in the albumin–globulin ratio of blood proteins, and those that died showed structural lesions of the liver, heart, muscle, and stomach wall on microscopic examination. In the same experiment rats receiving 125 mg/kg of chloroform showed during the 4th and the 5th month an impaired ability to develop new conditioned reflexes and decreased cholinergic activity (Miklashevski et al., 1966).

Of the male and female mice given a toothpaste containing chloroform 6 days a week for 6 weeks, all subjects in the 425 mg/kg group and 8/10 males in the 150 mg/kg group died within the first week. There were no deaths at 60 mg/kg, but moderate retardation in weight gain indicated toxicity at this level of exposure (Roe et al., 1979).

Repeated inhalation for 7 hours daily for 130 days at 125 mg/m$^3$ caused reversible damage to the kidneys and liver of rats (Torkelson et al., 1976); such damage did not occur after only 4 hours of inhalation. At higher concentrations mortality and observable histopathological changes were increased. Reports on human occupational exposure to chloroform are rare (Von

## Table IV
## Properties[a]

| | Boiling point | Density ($D_{20}^{20}$) | Solubility | Volatility | Stability and reactivity | Impurities and technical products |
|---|---|---|---|---|---|---|
| Dichloromethane | 40.1°C | $D_4^{15}$ 1.33 | In water, phenol miscible with chlorinated solvents | 400 mm (24°C) | Nonflammable; stable at room temperature, reacts with aluminium chlorinated in chloroform and tetrachlorure in the presence of a catalyst. | Commercial grade contains phenol hydroquinone, paracresol, resorcinol water, acids, and chloroform |
| Chloroform | 61.2°C | 1.48 | Slightly soluble in water; soluble in ethanol and benzene | 200 mm (25°C) | Slowly decomposed under prolonged sunlight exposure Oxidized by strong oxidizing agents Reactive with halogenated agents, and primary amines and phenols. | Stabilized by 0.5–1% ethanol Several halogenated hydrocarbons and water. |
| Carbon tetrachloride | 76.7°C | $D_4^{25}$ 1.58 | Miscible with ethanol diethylether; chloroform, insoluble in water | 91.3 mm (20°C) | Decomposed in phosgene in presence of limited quantity of water at 250°C when dry; nonreactive with metals; sometimes explosive in contact with aluminium alloys | May contain other hydrocarbons impurities. |

| | | | | | | |
|---|---|---|---|---|---|---|
| 1,2-Dichloroethane | 83.5°C | 1.25 | Slightly soluble in water; soluble in most organic solvents. | 64 mm (20°C) | Stable at room temperature when dry; resistant to oxidation; hydrolyzed to ethylene glycol in presence of water or alkali | Polychlorinated ethanes; mixed with tetrachlorure (3:1) to reduce fire hazard. |
| Tetrachloroethylene | 121°C | 1.62 | Insoluble in water; soluble in ethanol and oil. | 20 mm (26°C) | Decomposes slowly in contact with water, oxidized by strong oxidizing agents | Stabilized by a mixture of amines, epoxydes, and esters. |
| Trichloroethylene | 87°C | $D_4^{20}$ 1.46 | Miscible with water, acetone, chloroform, and oils | 77 mm (25°C) | Nonflammable; oxidative breakdown by atmospheric oxygen | Stabilized by amines; presence of epoxydes, and epichlorhydrin. |
| Trichloroethane | 74°C | $D_2^{25}$ 1.34 | Sparingly soluble in water; soluble in acetore, benzene, and carbon tetrachloride | 103 mm (20°C) | Decomposes at ambient temperature in the presence of water and metals. Forms phosgene with atmospheric oxygen at high temperatures. Forms 1,1-dichloroethylene in the presence of aqueous Ca(OH)$_2$. | Stabilized with n-methylpyrrole dioxine, nitromethane (3.8%), alcohol ketones, and nitriles. |

[a]From IARC Monographs, On the evaluation of the Carcinogenic Risk of Chemicals to Humans, vol. 20 (1979).

**Table V**
**Occurence**[a]

| | Air | Water | Food | Marine organism | Humans | Occupational exposure |
|---|---|---|---|---|---|---|
| Methylene chloride | 5 ppt in rural samples | 5 g/liter found by chlorination of water | In coffee, oleoresins hopes extracts | — | Expired air: 0.12–340 g/h[f] | Chemical plants 0–5,000 ppm Plastic manufactures 3–5 ppm |
| Chloroform | In troposphere by solar photochemical reaction of TCE[b]; max. 0.01–15 ppb[c] | 1.7–91.0 g/liter | Residue of fumigant mixtures; meat dairy products (U.K.) | 56–1040 g/kg in some fish species[d] | Post-mortem: 1–68 g/kg of wet tissue[e] | Hospital, department stores, biological products, internal combustion engines |
| Carbon tetrachloride | Max 20 ppb[i] | 1 ppb[e] | Resulting of fumigation—decline during storage | Up to 200 g/kg in fish | 1–10 ppm wet weight[e] | Blast furnace, steel mills |
| 1,2-Dichloroethane | 1–8% of production (1974) | 0–6 g/liter[h] | — | — | Expired air at 0–0.8 g/kg | Hospital; industrial solvent[g] |

| Compound | | | | | | |
|---|---|---|---|---|---|---|
| Trichloroethylene | As result of tap losses during degreasing operations 2–28 mg/m3 | 0.2 g liter; equilibred with air concentration | Meat products (12–20) butter, oil, and tea (60 ppb) | 0–500 mg/g/dry weight | Post-mortem 1–3 g/kg[c]; Expired air: 0–3.9 g/h | Workshops, degreasing rooms, nurses |
| Trichloroethane | 0.02–2 ppb near production sites, mainly by evaporation | Up to 3.3 g/liter tap water equilibred with air | Up to 10 ppb in everyday foodstuffs (meat, oils, fruits, bread) | 30 ppb | Expired air: 0.03 140 g/liter/kg bw | — |
| Tetrachloroethylene | 1–10 ppm | 0.1 g/liter by chlorination of water | Diary products, meat, oils 1 g/kg | 1–20 g/kg | Post-mortem: 0.5 30 g/kg | Industrial installations 2–300 mg/m3 Expired air: up to 12 g/h |

[a] If no other indications, IARC (1979).
[b] Appleby et al., (1976).
[c] Lillian et al., (1975).
[d] Dickson and Riley, (1976).
[e] McConnel et al., (1975)
[f] Conckle et al., (1975).
[g] NIOSH, (1977).
[h] Symons et al., (1975).
[i] Singh et al., (1975).

Oettingen, 1964). No evidence of liver injury has been found after 3–4 years of exposure. On the other hand, epidemiological studies on workers exposed to chloroform over long periods showed enlarged livers, fatty degeneration, and even toxic hepatitis (Bomski *et al.*, 1967). A report on long-term exposure (1–5 years) to chloroform contained in mouthwashes and toothpastes produced no evidence of liver damage, according to serum-enzyme levels (De Salva *et al.*, 1975).

Kidney damage in animals generally involves degenerative changes in Henle's loop, such as an accumulation of lipoid material.

## 2.3. Mutagenicity and Carcinogenicity

Following administration of chloroform to mice, a dose-dependent relationship was observed between liver necrosis and the subsequent incidence of hepatomas, although many mice died during the experiment (Eschenbrenner and Miller, 1945).

A metabolite could be responsible for the liver necrosis (MacLean, 1970; Sholler, 1970), and covalent binding to liver and kidney proteins occurs (Ilett *et al.*, 1973). This indicates that a carcinogenic metabolite could be formed. That specific factors affect glutathion availablility (Brown, 1974b), and that the mixed-function-oxidase system modifies the toxicity of chloroform reinforces this hypothesis.

However, mutagenicity tests with *Salmonella* TA 1535, TA 1538, and *E. coli* in the presence of microsomal preparations from mouse, rabbit, or rat liver were negative (Uehleke *et al.*, 1976, 1977). Other experiments on cultured cells using the azaguanine test system (Sturrock, 1977) showed no mutagenicity. Similarly, sister chromatic exchange (SCE) was not increased by chloroform (White *et al.*, 1979).

However, several *in vivo* studies have indicated that chloroform is a carcinogenic agent. The National Cancer Institute (1976) conducted a study with groups of 50 male and 50 female mice receiving 2.5% chloroform in corn oil for 78 weeks at initial doses of 100 and 200 mg/kg for males and 200 to 400 mg/kg for females. The incidence of kidney epithelial tumors in males was significantly greater with doses of 90 and 180 mg/kg (N.I.H., 1976).

At high doses, chloroform was considered carcinogenic for rat liver (females being more susceptible), and for the kidneys of male rats but not, in contrast with the liver, of females. This could be because chloroform is not as well metabolized in the liver of male rats, so that more of the chemical reaches the kidneys (Reuber, 1979).

Chloroform is carcinogenic for the thyroid in female rats and, at low doses, for the mammary glands and endocrine organs. It is also carcinogenic in mice, Both males and females develop a high incidence (100% in the high-dose groups) of carcinoma of the liver.

Carcinogenicity studies were also conducted with toothpaste containing chloroform (3.6%) in strains of mice and dogs (7.5 mg/kg/day) during 1.5 years (Roe, 1979). A significant increase in kidney adenomatous tumors appeared in male mice receiving 60 mg/kg/day over 100 weeks, but not in other strains and species.

Chloroform, administrated to mice in their drinking water (15 mg/kg/day) significantly increased metastasis and the number of cells of an Ehrlich ascite (Capel et al., 1979). Guinea pigs given doses of 35 mg/kg chloroform had cirrhosis of the liver after three months (Miklashevski et al., 1966).

Despite its nonreactivity in mutagenic tests, chloroform can thus be considered carcinogenic since its carcinogenicity in more than one mammalian species is sufficiently documented. As Barcelona (1979) has observed, chloroform emissions due to the chlorination of the public water supply or cooling waters exceed those due to its use as a solvent, and urban dwellers receive at least 1.2 times the dose predicted as background levels. The problem of chloroform should, therefore, be considered not only as a polluant in industrial or occupational areas.

## 2.4. Embryotoxicity and Teratogenicity

Chloroform has been found in cord blood in quantities equal to or greater than those in maternal blood (Dowty et al., 1976), reflecting transplacental acquisition. Chloroform was not teratogenic when given to rats and rabbits by gavage at toxic doses (25 and 50 mg/kg, respectively) that were lethal for some animals (Thompson et al., 1974). Fetotoxicity was manifest only as reduced birth weight at the highest dose level in both species.

However, the exposure of mice and rats for up to 1 hr to anesthetic concentrations of chloroform (25–37,000 ppm) during organogenesis proved to be highly embryotoxic (Schwetz et al., 1974).

Moreover, when pregnant Sprague–Dawley rats were exposed to 30, 100, and 300 ppm for 7 hrs/day on days 6 to 15 of gestation, a decreased conception rate, a high incidence of fetal resorption, retarded fetal development, and body measurements or acaudia reflecting high embryotoxicity and some teratogenicity were observed (Schwetz et al., 1974).

More recent work on another species, the mouse, has also indicated that inhaled chloroform interferes with implantation and produces a low incidence of fetal malformation (Murray et al., 1979), depending on the dose administered.

Fetal mortality and decreased fetal weight, rather than teratogenicity, were also reported by Dilley *et al.* (1977) when pregnant rats were exposed to 20 g/m$^3$ of chloroform during days 7–14 of gestation.

## 3. CARBON TETRACHLORIDE

### 3.1. Absorption, Distribution, Metabolism, and Excretion

Carbon tetrachloride is absorbed through the lungs, gastrointestinal tract, and skin. Because of its liposolubility, the highest concentrations are found in fatty tissues; it is also found in the liver and bone marrow.

There is probably limited metabolism. Elimination of unchanged carbon tetrachloride takes place almost entirely through the lungs in animals and man (Fry *et al.*, 1972). The pattern of distribution of ingested carbon tetrachloride differs from that following inhalation (Recknagel and Litteria, 1960). Absorbed carbon tetrachloride is decomposed to a limited extent by homolytic rupture. *In vitro* studies (Butler, 1961) have demonstrated its biotransformation to chloroform and to carbon dioxide.

Claims have been made for the existence of another metabolite, hexachloroethane, identifiable in the tissues and bile of rabbits receiving toxic doses of carbon tetrachloride (Flower *et al.*, 1969). There may also be biotransformation by heterolytic scission to yield toxic phosgene (Cessi *et al.*, 1966).

### 3.2. Toxicity

Lipid peroxidation towards the activity of microsomal enzymes, presumably initiating a free-radical metabolite, seems to be the most important factor in carbon tetrachloride toxicity (Reynolds 1967; Recknagel, 1967; Garner and McLean, 1969; Glende *et al.*, 1976). Since the toxic action of carbon tetrachloride is dependent upon metabolic activation by the mixed-function-oxidase system, it can be modified by the activators and inhibitors of these enzymes (Cignoli and Castro, 1971; Pani *et al.*, 1973, Uehleke *et al.*, 1977).

Newborn rats are as sensitive as adults to these toxic effccts, while their metabolizing system is not yet completely developed (Cagen and Klaassen, 1979). A similar mechanism could be responsible for extrahepatic tissue damage (Von Oettingen, 1964; Chen *et al.*, 1977; Tsirel'Nikow and Tsirel'Nikova, 1976). Free radical products could attack specific cellular constituents, such as sulfhydryl groups or proteins, by alkylation (Tracey and Sherlock, 1968).

The important specific effects seem to be those on liver and kidney functions. Exposure of different animal species, including man, caused centrolubular necrosis of the liver and acute renal tubular necrosis that were aggravated by alcohol consumption (New *et al.*, 1962). In the hepatic cell, the earliest changes were associated with the endoplasmic reticulum (Recknagel, 1967; Rao and Recknagel, 1969). The ribosomes were dislocated from the membranes (Smuckler *et al.*, 1962), leading to a significant depression of protein synthesis. Lipid peroxidation also appeared very soon after carbon tetrachloride administration (Rao and Recknagel, 1969) and was associated with decreased activity in glucose-6-phosphates (Hathway, 1974).

Oral administration to rats produced decreased cholesterol, phospholipid, and triglyceride plasma concentrations (Stern *et al.*, 1965). Lipoprotein levels also decreased (Lombardi and Ugazio, 1965). Carbon tetrachloride also induced cell necrosis, fat accumulation, and steatosis in the liver.

Human accidental poisoning is relatively frequent owing to carbon tetrachloride's widespread domestic use. Poisoning is usually due to inhalation and sensitivity is variable: jaundice, acute renal failure, and higher serum levels of liver enzymes have usually been observed. The other immediate effects are dizziness, headache, vomiting, and diarrhea. Inhalation leads mainly to kidney damage, while ingestion leads mainly to hepatic lesions (Beecher, 1953; New *et al.*, 1962; Dupont *et al.*, 1975).

After 40–150 exposures of rabbits and guinea pigs to carbon tetrachloride, toxic effects were seen with 50 ppm. The adverse effects were increased liver weight, moderate fatty degeneration, and cirrhosis (Adams *et al.*, 1952).

In rats, long-term studies with carbon tetrachloride in the diet showed that levels of 80 to 200 ppm (corresponding to a daily intake of 15 mg/kg) did not modify growth, sexual development, reproductive activity, or general health. Other studies involving long-term exposure to carbon tetrachloride vapor showed a no-effect level at 5 ppm for rats and 10 ppm for rabbits.

Human deaths have been reported after ingestion of 1.5 ml, while other patients survived after ingesting more than 100 ml. Most cases of death resulted from inhaling the vapor of the solvent when used as a dry-cleaning agent.

### 3.3. Mutagenicity and Carcinogenicity

In plate tests with *S. typhimurium* TA 100, TA 1535, and TA 1538, carbon tetrachloride was nonmutagenic both in the presence or absence of a microsomal-activation system (McCann and Ames, 1976; McCann *et al.*, 1975; Uehleke *et al.*, 1977).

It was also negative in *E. coli* (Uehleke *et al.*, 1976). In an *in vitro* chromosome assay using cultured rat-liver cells, no chromosome damage was observed with carbon tetrachloride (Dean and Hodson-Walker, 1979).

However, its irreversible binding to microsomal lipids, protein, and DNA (Butler, 1961; Tracey and Sherlock, 1968; Rocchi *et al.*, 1973; Diaz-Gomez and Castro, 1980) suggests that its biological reactivity could lead to a carcinogenic intermediate. This is confirmed by several experimental data in animals in which the incidence of carcinoma was significantly increased.

Oral administration of carbon tetrachloride led to the formation of hepatomas in many strains of mice (Hartwell, 1951; Shubik and Hartwell, 1957, 1969). Sixteen hepatomas were seen in a group given 30 doses of 1.6 mg/kg over a period of 30 days, and a significant number of tumors was observed in a group receiving 30 doses of 0.1 mg/kg over a period of 100 days, with a correlation between the degree of necrosis and the incidence of hepatoma (Eshenbrenner and Miller, 1945).

Hepatocellular carcinomas and neoplastic nodules were found ($p < 0.05$) in an experiment where groups of 50 male and 50 female rats were treated 5 times weekly with, respectively, 47 and 94 mg/kg of carbon tetrachloride for males and 80–160 mg/kg for females during 78 weeks (National Cancer Institute, 1976; Weisburger, 1977).

After subcutaneous or intramuscular administration of carbon tetrachloride to rats, a low yield of hepatomas was observed (Kawzaki, 1965; Reuber and Glover, 1967, 1970) at does higher than 2 g/kg body weight. Alpert *et al.* (1972) reported that female rats receiving 1.6 g/kg carbon tetrachloride for two years developed mammary adenocarcinomas (8/30). Of 25 male mice receiving a biweekly intrarectal administration of carbon tetrachloride, 13 developed nodular hyperplasia.

The combined administration of carbon tetrachloride with other agents has indicated that a single dose can promote the carcinogenesis initiated by *N*-nitrosobutyluree (Yokoro *et al.*, 1973), nitrosodiethylamine (Pound, 1978), and fast neutrons in mice (Cole and Nowell, 1964; Curtis and Tilley, 1972). Chronic administration of carbon tetrachloride to rats that received a single dose of aflatoxin (Lemonnier *et al.*, 1974) or 3-methyl-dimethyl aminobenzene (Kanematsu, 1976) has led also to an increased number of liver tumors.

Cases of hepatoma appeared in man several years after carbon tetrachloride poisoning had been reported (Tracey and Sherlock, 1968); laundry and dry-cleaning workers exposed to carbon tetrachloride were found to develop an excess of lung, cervical, and skin cancer. A slight excess of leukemia and cancer was also observed (Blair *et al.*, 1979).

Carbon tetrachloride may thus be considered to present a risk to humans since experimental and epidemiological data have shown it to be carcinogenic. It may well also accelerate the development of preneoplastic cells initiated by other environmental carcinogens but, to date, there is no specific information concerning this particular risk for man.

## 3.4. Embryotoxicity and Teratogenicity

A study of the transplacental migration and accumulation in blood of volatile organic constituents suggests a possible selective one-way transfer of carbon tetrachloride to the fetus (Dowty *et al.*, 1976). Marked injury to the tissues of the placenta and, in particular, to the chorionic epithelium of the labyrinth portion, with maximal degenerative changes on days 14 and 16 of pregnancy, has been observed in female rats receiving high doses of carbon tetrachloride (0.3 ml/ 100 g) (Tsirel'Nikov and Tsirel'Nikova, 1977).

Carbon tetrachloride administered to pregnant rats at 300 and 1000 ppm for 7 hrs on days 6 to 15 of gestation caused a certain degree of retarded fetal development, such as delayed ossification of the sternbrae, rather than embryotoxicity (Schwetz *et al.*, 1974). However, the degree of maternal toxicity was great.

Increased fetal mortality was observed in pregnant mice given single doses of 150 mg/ animal during the last stage of pregnancy. The cause of death was fetal liver damage. Moreover, disturbances and necrosis were found in the placenta (Roschlau and Rodenkirchen, 1969). Since evidence of oetotoxicity has been presented in only one relevant experiment, more information is needed on embryotoxicity and teratogenicity after inhalation of carbon tetrachloride at doses related to environmental or industrial conditions, in order to drawn any conclusions.

## 4. TRICHLORETHYLENE (TCE)

### 4.1. Absorption, Distribution, Metabolism, and Excretion

The most important route of absorption is via the lungs, but moderate absorption can occur through the skin and from the gastrointestinal tract (Gibits and Ploche, 1973). Retention, according to some authors, is as high as 70% (Soucek and Vlachova, 1960; Fernandez *et al.*, 1975), but lower according to others: 55% according to Astrand and Ovrum (1976), and 43% according to Monster *et al.*, (1976). Trichlorethylene is eliminated to only a small extent by exhalation (Fernandez *et al.*, 1975; Monster *et al.*, 1976). Uptake of the solvent after 30 min. is about one third of that after 4 hrs of inhalation. On the other hand, TCE seems rarely to be absorbed through the skin in toxic quantities during industrial uses (Sato and Nakajima, 1978).

Most animal studies have involved parenteral administration of TCE. In the rat, rabbit, and dog, TCE appears to concentrate mostly in the brain and least of all in the skeletal muscle, the lungs, and the liver (Von Oettingen, 1955; Clayton and Parkhouse, 1962).

After a single exposure (50 ppm), TCE was detectable in blood for four days. However, repeated exposure did not cause a continuous increase in blood levels, indicating different pharmacokinetic behavior in acute and chronic exposure (Kimmerle and Eben, 1973a,b).

When human subjects were exposed to 200 ppm TCE for up to three hours (Stewart *et al.*, 1970, 1974), the blood showed a maximum level (6 ppm) after two hours, but TCE may be found in blood and expired air more than 60 hours after exposure (Monster and Boersma, 1975). At higher concentrations an arteriovenous difference in the TCE concentration was observed corresponding to uptake in the tissues.

After absorption in man, more than 70% of the TCE was recovered as metabolites (Fernandez *et al.*, 1975; Monster *et al.*, 1976). The metabolites involved oxidation to chloral hydrate by liver microsomal mixed-function-oxidase (Leibman, 1965; Byington and Leibman, 1965). The formation of an intermediate epoxide suggested by Powell (1945) would explain this oxidation. Chloral hydrate would then be reduced to trichloroethanol (89%) and trichloroacetic acid (TCA) (11%), which are excreted in the urine (Sellers *et al.*, 1972). Trichloroethanol is usually conjugated with glucuronic acid before excretion (Müller *et al.*, 1974).

Five male volunteers inhaled 70 ppm for four hours on five consecutive days; 11% was excreted unchanged by the lungs, 43% as trichloroethylene, and 24% as TCA in urine. These amounts were related to lean body mass (Monster *et al.*, 1976).

Excretion of trichloroethanol glucuronide by the kidneys is rapid (half live, 3 hours), whereas that of TCA is slow (half life 50–99 hours) (Muller *et al.*, 1974.)

The kinetics of elimination in expired air exhibit multi-exponential curves, while elimination of the metabolites varies considerably because of the metabolic reaction rates. Additional pathways of elimination must operate since recovery accounts for only 50–75% of the amount inhaled (Muller *et al.*, 1974; Fernandez *et al.*, 1975).

TCE principally affects the central nervous system; it is essentially a narcotic. As in the case after the absorption of other volatile hydrocarbons, headache and nausea (after short exposure), and CNS depression, neurological signs, hepatorenal failure, and decreased cardiac output (after longer exposures) are observed (Waters *et al.*, 1977).

The acute effects involve ventricular fibrillation and hypotension, and most victims die from primary cardiac arrest with secondary respiratory failure (Gaultier *et al.*, 1971; Konietzko *et al.*, 1978).

Deliberate inhalation of moderate concentrations of TCE induces euphoric effects and, when repeated, may lead to addiction. The most frequent lesions found in addicts at autopsy have been hepatonecrosis and nephropathy (Beisland and Wannag, 1970; Clearfield, 1970; Edh *et al.*, 1973).

The published results of investigations on human volunteers are mainly behavioral. A TLC of 50 ppm has been estimated on the basis of the appearance in several studies of toxic symptoms at this concentration (Nomiyana and Nomiyana, 1977).

Chronic effects of TCE on humans were for a long time considered nonexistent or rare, but now the growing opinion is that the chronic toxicity of TCE could be more important than acute toxicity. Transverse lesions of the spinal cord following accidental exposure to anesthetic levels of TCE have been observed, and neuropsychiatric symptoms and vegetative nervous changes have also been described (Grandjean et al., 1973).

Exposure to TCE may alter the heart rate and cause bradycardia attributable to increased vagal tone. However, continuous exposure to 35 ppm for 90 days caused no visible signs of toxicity in rats, dogs, monkeys, guinea pigs, or rabbits (Prendergast et al., 1967; Gehring, 1968; Kylin et al., 1965).

TCE has also been found to have immunosuppresive properties (Zadorozhnyi, 1973), but incomplete description of the experimental conditions makes these results inconclusive.

## 4.2. Mutagenicity and Carcinogenicity

The similarity in chemical structure of TCE to vinylchloride has given rise to speculations about its possible activation and subsequent carcinogenicity.

Powell (1945) postulated the formation of an epoxide intermediate to explain the urinary excretion of trichloroacetic acid. Metabolic end-products of chlorinated ethylenes are predominantly alcohols and carbonic acids, and recent investigations (Bonse et al., 1975; Bonse and Henschler, 1976) have demonstrated that the mechanism of formation of these end-products is an intramolecular rearrangement of the epoxides. The asymmetric chlorine substitution could give rise to the electrophilic character that intensifies the possibility of alkylating reactions of the epoxide, which overpower the deactivating conjugating mechanisms (Bonse and Henschler, 1976; Henschler and Bonse, 1977). In fact, a parallelism between mutagenic activity and asymmetric substitution of chlorinated ethylene can be established (Greim et al., 1975; Henschler and Bonse, 1977).

TCE has been found slightly mutagenic in a modified Ames mutagenicity testing system (Greim et al., 1975; Shahin and Von Borstel, 1977), but the rearrangement of trichloroethylene epoxide to chloral hydrate in mammalian liver cells, which might not necessarily prevail in microorganisms, could modify the carcinogenic power of TCE (Henschler et al., 1977). On the other hand, experiments on the carcinogenicity of TCE were conducted with technical samples of TCE that contained, as stabilizers, considerable amounts of 1,2-epoxybutane and epichlorhydrin, which are highly mutagenic in the Ames test (Henschler *et al.*, 1977). This could explain the high incidence of hepatocarcinoma in both male and female mice observed after high daily oral doses of TCE for 18 months (National Cancer Institute, 1976).

The question of whether TCE itself is carcinogenic remains open. Baden *et al.* (1979) and Waskell (1978) tested TCE under different experimental conditions for mutagenicity and concluded that TCE was a weak or nonmutagen. No effects of TCE on SCE in Chinese hamster ovary cells have been observed by Stevens *et al.* (1977). Bronzetti *et al.* (1978), however, observed joint mutation and gene conversion in their tests on yeast (*Saccharomyces cerevisiae*). More recently, Henschler *et al.* (1980) exposed mice, rats, and hamsters for 18 months, 5 days a week, 6 hrs a day, to 535 and 2675 mg/m$^3$ of pure TCE without any significant increase in tumor formation in any species tested, except malignant lymphoma to which female NMRI mice are particularly sensitive. However, inhalation studies by Page and Arthur (1978) with rats and mice showed a higher incidence of carcinoma in the test animals.

The fact that [14]C-TCE binds irreversibly to liver endoplasmic proteins *in vitro* and *in vivo* (Allemand *et al.*, 1978; Bolt and Banerjee, 1976), and that microsomal inducers increase its hepatotoxicity, confirms its cellular reactivity. When incubated *in vitro* with rat liver microsomes, TCE metabolites were irreversibly bound to protein and to RNA. However, the binding of TCE to RNA was lower than that of vinyl chloride, which is carcinogenic (Laib *et al.*, 1979). Moreover, TCE exposure did not produce preneoplastic hepatocellular enzymatic deficiencies (ATPase) as observed for vinylchloride under the same conditions.

The carcinogenicity of TCE could thus only be explained by study of the different pathways of metabolic deactivation of this compound, especially in man.

From the epidemiological studies available covering ten or more years of exposure, no significant excess of cancer has been demonstrated (Axelson *et al.*, 1978). However, the small number of cancer cases reported cannot rule out risk, especially with regards to rare cancers such as liver cancer.

Blair *et al.* (1979) reported an excess of lung, cervical, and skin cancer, and a slight excess of leukemia and liver cancer in a group of 330 laundry and dry cleaning workers. On the other hand, Tola *et al.*, (1980) found that cancer mortality was lower than expected among 2117 workers exposed to TCE for 13 years.

## 4.3. Embryotoxicity and Teratogenicity

TCE readily crosses the placenta and is found in fetal blood (Laham, 1970) and may be responsible for the respiratory difficulties of the newborn exposed *in utero* (Kalgenova *et al.*, 1961; Korobko, 1972; Phillips, 1971; Lilleaasen, 1972).

During labor, TCE used as an anesthetic reduces uterine motility (Lakomy *et al.*, 1972). Its use as an analgesic has been accompanied by an increase in maternal and fetal mortality (Thierstein *et al.*, 1960).

Pregnant mice and rats were exposed to 300 ppm TCE, 7 hrs daily, on days 6–15 of gestation without significant manifest maternal, embryonal or fetal toxicity (Schwetz *et al.*, 1975).

Another teratogenicity study in rats fed 5% TCE extracted from instant decaffeinated coffee solids (equivalent to 0.5 ppm of TCE) did not show fetal or skeletal abnormalities, nor was there any excessive resorption (Zeitlin, 1966). However, some signs of teratogenicity have been observed in more recent experiments.

Female rats were exposed by inhalation to TCE vapors at a concentration of 1800 ppm (Dorfmuller *et al.*, 1979). Significant elevations in skeletal and soft tissue anomalies, indicative of developmental delay in maturation rather than teratogenesis, were observed in the group exposed during pregnancy, but there were no observable behavioral effects in the offspring at 10, 20, and 100 days of age.

Earlier, Krasovitskaya and Malyarova (1967) reported that newborn rats exposed continuously to 1 ppm of TCE showed retardation in growth. Teratogenic effects have also been observed in the offspring of female rats exposed by inhalation to 1620 mg/ m$^3$, 6 hrs per day, on days 6–15 of gestation (Page and Arthur, 1978).

## 5. 1,2-DICHLOROETHANE

### 5.1. Absorption, Distribution, Metabolism, and Excretion

Following intraperitoneal injection in mice, 10–42% of 1,2-dichloroethane was expired unchanged, with 12–15% expired as $CO_2$. Most of the remainder was excreted in the urine, mainly as chloroacetic acid and S-carboxymethylcysteine (Yllner, 1971).

Rannug *et al.* (1978) implicated GSH and cytosolic GSH-transferase activity in the activation of 1,2-dichloroethane to metabolites mutagenic to *S. typhimurium* TA 1535.

Alternatively, Banerjee and Van Duuren (1979) reported that 1,2-dichloroethane was activated by microsomal mixed-function-oxidases to metabolites irreversibly bound to proteins and DNA.

*In vitro* studies seem to indicate that several 1,2-dichloroethane activation pathways are operative, producing different metabolites responsible for macromolecular binding, mutagenicity, and toxicity.

*In vitro* studies on the activation of 1,2-dichloroethane (Rannug *et al.*,

1978; Rannug and Beije, 1979; Guengerich *et al.*, 1980) have indicated that the microsomal metabolism of the solvent occured via mixed-function oxidation, and that microsomal GSH transferase catalyzed the formation of metabolites irreversibly bound to DNA. 2-chloroacetaldehyde, *S*-(2-chloroacetaldehyde), *S*-(2-chloroethyl)-GSH and 1-chloroso-2-chloroethane are proposed as the major metabolites involved in this irreversible binding to macromolecules and proteins.

Adducts that give rise to mutagenic activity in *Salmonella* result almost exclusively from a reaction catalyzed by cytosolic GSH transferase systems. These *in vitro* studies have shown that chloroacetaldehyde can also be reduced to 2-chloroethanol by alcohol dehydrogenase (Guengerich and Watanabe, 1979), but that this metabolite is not involved in DNA alkylation.

The similarity of the toxic effects of 2-chloroethanol and 1,2-chloroethane (Ambrose, 1950; Millet *et al.*, 1970; Hayes *et al.*, 1973) suggests that poisoning by 1,2-dichloroethane is due, at least in part, to this metabolic product.

## 5.2. Toxicity

In humans, deaths following the ingestion or inhalation of 1,2-dichloro-ethane have been attributed to circulatory and respiratory failure [National Institute for Occupational Safety and Health (NIOSH), 1976].

In man and in rats, acute poisoning caused disseminated hemorrhagic lesions, mainly in the liver, attributed by Martin *et al.*, (1968) to a reduction in the level of blood clotting factors and to thrombocytopenia.

Chronic exposure caused degeneration of the liver, tubular damage, and necrosis of the kidneys in rats (McCollister *et al.*, 1956). Necrosis of the corneal endothelium was seen in dogs after s.c. injection of the solvent (Kuwabara *et al.*, 1968).

In man, repeated exposure to 1,2-dichloroethane in the occupational environment has been associated with anorexia, nausea, abdominal pain, irritation of the mucous membranes, neurological disorders, and dysfunction of liver and kidneys (Byers, 1943; Watrous, 1947; Delplace *et al.*, 1962).

## 5.3. Mutagenicity and Carcinogenicity

1,2-dichloroethane is mutagenic in *S. typhimurium* TA 1530, TA 1535, and TA 100, presumably causing base pair substitution mutations (Brem *et al.*, 1974; McCann *et al.*, 1975; Bignami *et al.*, 1977; Rosenkranz, 1977; Rannug *et al.*, 1978; Rannug and Beije, 1979).

It caused no chromosome breaks in *Allium* root tips or in human lymphocytes, nor did it induce lysogeny in *E. coli* K39 (Kristoffersson, 1974), but it increased the frequency of sex-linked recessive lethals in *Drosophila melanogaster*, larvae or adults (Rapoport, 1960; Shakarnis, 1969, 1970), and single strand breaks in hamster cell DNA (Ehrenberg *et al.*, 1974).

Chloroacetaldehyde, a metabolite of 1,2-dichloroethane, is mutagenic in *S. typhimurium* TA 100 (McCann *et al.*, 1975; IARC, 1979).

1,2-dichloroethane was tested in experiments in mice and in rats by oral administration. Following lifetime gavage (100–200 mg/kg/day) of mice, this solvent produced benign and malignant tumors of the lungs and malignant lymphomas in animals of both sexes, hepatocellular carcinomas in males, the mammary and uterine adenocarcinomas in females (Weisburger, 1977; National Cancer Institute, 1978). In rats, lifetime gavage of 100–150 mg/kg/day produced carcinomas of the forestomach in male animals, benign and malignant mammary tumors in females, and hemangiosarcomas in animals of both sexes (Weisbuger, 1977; National Cancer Institute, 1978).

In contrast, 1,2-dichloroethane did not induce any treatment-related tumors in lifetime inhalation studies (150 ppm daily exposure) on rats and mice (Maltoni, 1980), or after i.p. injections (thrice weekly, 100 mg/kg for 8 weeks) of the solvent in male mice (Theiss *et al.*, 1977).

Carcinogenesis has been observed in rodents following gavage, but no carcinogenic response has been observed in rodents exposed daily over a lifetime to 1,2-dichloroethane by inhalation. This compound is mutagenic in *S. typhimurium* and *Drosophila melanogaster*, can form a reactive chloroethyl sulphide intermediate, but can be metabolized by microsomal and/or cytosolic enzyme systems; the main route of human exposure is by inhalation. Therefore, studies are needed on the potential differences in the pharmacokinetics of 1,2-dichloroethane following different routes of exposure, to determine the potential carcinogenic risk to humans. At this time, however, it is reasonable to regard 1,2-dichloroethane as presenting a carcinogenic risk for humans (IARC).

### 5.4. Teratogenicity and Embryotoxicity

No data on embryotoxicity and teratogenicity were available.

## 6. TETRACHLOROETHYLENE

### 6.1. Absorption, Distribution, Metabolism, and Excretion

Tetrachloroethylene vapors and liquid are readily absorbed through the lungs (Stewart *et al.*, 1961), and to some extent from the gastrointestinal tract (Von Oettingen, 1964). They can be absorbed by the skin in mice (Tsuruta, 1975) and in man (Stewart and Dodd, 1964; Hake and Stewart, 1977).

After dermal absorption of the liquid, the half-life of t. chloroethylene in alveolar air is approximately 8 hr (Steward and Dodd, 1964). Its intestinal absorption is facilitated by fats and oils (Lamson *et al.*, 1929). According to Paulus (1951) very little enters the blood stream after inhalation.

In man, following exposure, about 80–100% of the uptake was excreted unchanged by the lungs (Monster et al., 1979). This confirmed the results obtained with mice (Yllner, 1961) and rats (Daniel, 1963; Pegg et al., 1979). However, its biological half-life is 3–5 days, and the inhaled t. chloroethylene is excreted very slowly (Stewart et al., 1970). The total body half-life was calculated to be 71 hr (Guberah and Fernandez, 1974).

The metabolites identifed in the urine of mice exposed to t. chloroethylene were mainly TCA, oxalic acid and traces of dichloroacetic acid (Yllner, 1961). Rats given inhalation with labelled ($^{14}$C)tetrachloroethylene expired approximatively 70% unchanged; 26% was either expired as $CO_2$ or excreted as nonvolatile metabolites in the urine and feces; 3–4% remained in the body (Pegg et al., 1979).

In man, inhalation of t. chloroethylene is followed by long-lasting excretion of metabolites in the urine (Ikeda and Iamura, 1973). Exposure to t. chloroethylene vapors (0.6 g/m$_3$) in air for 3 hrs produces urinary excretion of TCA, representing about 1–2% of the inhaled dose during 70 hrs (Ogata et al., 1971; Monster et al., 1979). Workers exposed to t. chloroethylene vapors may reach a concentration higher than 10 mg/l trichloroacetic acid in their urine and show some signs of poisoning (Munzer and Heder, 1972).

An oxidative metabolism of t. chloroethylene in the liver (Bonse et al., 1975) is suggested by the fact that hepatotoxicity is enhanced in rats pretreated with phenobarbital or aroclor, and by the urinary excretion of chlorinated metabolites (Moslen et al., 1977). Tri- and dichloroacetic acids were also urinary metabolites in humans exposed to t. chloroethylene vapors (Bolanoswska and Golacta, 1972; Munzer and Hender, 1972). These data suggest the presence of an oxirane intermediate (Bartsch et al., 1979; Shumann et al., 1980).

## 6.2. Toxicity

Repeated exposure to t. chloroethylene vapors produced a variety of pathological changes in the liver, ranging from fatty degeneration to necrosis, in rats, rabbits, guinea pigs (Rowe et al., 1952; Pegg et al., 1979), and dogs (Hall and Shillinger, 1925).

Oral doses of t. chloroethylene have lesser effects on the kidneys. Only a near lethal dose caused swelling of the convoluted tubules and hydropic degeneration in male mice (Plaa and Larson, 1965; Klaassen and Plaa, 1966), and i.p. doses of 1.6–2.3 g/kg t. chloroethylene caused slight calcification of tubules in dogs (Klaassen and Plaa, 1967).

Acute intoxication in man has been reported principally in industry, from degreasing operations. In the fetal cases reported by Baader (1954) and Vallaud et al. (1956), pulmonary edema, and hepatonephritris were determined as the cause of death. Inhalation of various concentrations of t. chloroethylene caused mucous membrane and skin irritations (Von Oettingen, 1964b) and lung edema (Patel *et al.*, 1977) while neurological effects have been described (Tuttle *et al.*, 1977) in dry cleaners.

Chronic exposure to t. chloroethylene vapors caused irritation of the respiratory tract, nausea, headache, sleeplessness, abdominal pain, and constipation (Coler and Von Rossmiller, 1953; Lob, 1957; Von Oettingen, 1964; Stewart *et al.*, 1970b; Chmielewski *et al.*, 1976). Liver cirrhosis, hepatitis, and nephritis are rare (Stewart, 1969), but a case of "obstructive jaundice" in a 6-week old infant was attributed to t. chloroethylene in breast milk (Bagnell and Ellenberger, 1977).

## 6.3. Mutagenicity and Carcinogenicity

Although the data on metabolism suggest the presence of an oxirane intermediate, t. chloroethylene was not detected as a bacterial mutagen in the presence of a liver microsomal fraction (Greim *et al.*, 1975; Bartsch *et al.*, 1979). In this last study, no mutagenicity was observed in *S. typhimurium* TA 100 with concentrations up to $4.10^{-3}$ M in the presence of a liver S9 fraction from phenobarbital-treated mice, with or without cofactors.

In a host-mediated assay in mice using *S. typhimurium* TA 1950, TA 1951, and TA 1952, there was a significant increase in the number of revertants with doses equivalent to the $LD_{50}$ or to half the $LD_{50}$ (Cerná and Kypènova, 1977).

T. chloroethylene did not induce detectable mutations in *E. coli* K 12 m (Greim *et al.*, 1975), nor did it induce chromosomal aberrations in the bone marrow cells of mice receiving either single (half $LD_{50}$) or 5 daily i.p. injections ($1/6 LD_{50}$) of the chemicals (Cerná and Kypènová, 1975).

Tetrachloroethylene was tested for carcinogenicity in mice and rats by gavage and by inhalation. Gavage in mice (450 mg/kg/day in male and 300 mg/kg/day in females for 78 weeks) produced a shorter lifespan in treated animals, due to early toxicity. A high incidence of hepatocellular carcinomas in animals of both sexes was found 90 weeks from the beginning of the experiment (National Cancer Institute, 1977).

After gavage in rats (500 mg/kg/day), no increase in tumor incidence was observed, but toxic nephropathy was observed in those treated animals that died in the early weeks of the experiment (National Cancer Institute, 1977). Nevertheless, because of the poor survival of treated animals, this experiment was inadequate for measuring carcinogenic effects. Inhalation of t. chloroethylene rats (2–4 g/m3) for 12 months did not produce a statistically significant difference in tumor incidence between the treated and control groups (Rampy *et al.*, 1978).

After receiving t. chloroethylene in i.p. injections (400 mg/kg) twice weekly during 24 weeks, the average number of lung tumors per mouse was not greater than that in the controls (Theiss *et al.*, 1977).

Only one experiment showing carcinogenic effects in mice has actually been reported; the others are inadequate because the high toxicity or the long exposure killed the animals.

In conclusion, it seems difficult to demonstrate that t. chloroethylene has a carcinogenic effect.

Indirect data, obtained from tests for mutagenicity, are also ambigous. T. chloroethylene proved negative in cytogenetic tests in mice, nonmutagenic in *E. coli*, and is also the exception in the halo-olefins group; it was not mutagenic in the bacterial tests using microsomal activation, although it is practically certain that in the metabolic process, an oxirane intermediate is produced.

In man, lymphocytic leukemia has been reported, but only in dry-cleaning workers exposed also to carbon tetrachloride and trichlorethylene (Blair, 1978).

### 6.4. Embryotoxicity and Teratogenicity

The only available data concern rats and mice exposed on days 6–15 of gestation to $2 \, \text{g}/\text{m}^3$ t. chloroethylene. No effects were observed on the average number of implantation sites per litter, litter sizes, incidence of fetal resorptions, fetal sex ratios, or fetal body measurements. No treatment-related increase in the incidence of skeletal or visceral malformations was observed (Schwetz *et al.*, 1975).

## 7. DICHLOROMETHANE

### 7.1. Absorption, Distribution Metabolism, and Excretion

Dichloromethane, also known as methylene chloride, is absorbed by the lungs (75% of inhaled vapor), through the skin (Stewart and Dodd, 1964), and taken up into the blood stream (Astrand and Ovrum, 1975). It is rapidly excreted almost unchanged in expired air and in the urine (Riley *et al.*, 1966).

Several *in vitro* and *in vivo* studies have demonstrated that dichloromethane is metabolized to CO (Carlsson and Hultengren, 1975; Fodor *et al.*, 1973; Kubic *et al.*, 1974). It has been reported that human exposure for 1–2 hours to dichloromethane (500–1,000 ppm) results in the formation of carboxyhemoglobin (Stewart and Hake, 1976; Stewart *et al.*, 1972), while in rats, labeled CO and $CO_2$ were found to account for 76% of the administered labeled dichloromethan (Carlsson and Hultengre, 1975; Kubic *et al.*, 1974;

Rodkey and Collison, 1977a and 1977b). However, the affinity of CO for hemoglobin is not modified by dichloromethane (Dill *et al.*, 1978).

The mechanism of this transformation seems to be enzymatic, either by microsomal-heme oxygenase (Coburn, 1973) or by the hepatic microsomal-monooxygenase system (Hogan *et al.*, 1976; Di Vincenzo *et al.*, 1975). A free radical mechanism does not appear to be a satisfactory explanation (Reynolds, 1972; Ugazio *et al.*, 1973).

Phenobarbital, a microsomal enzyme inducer, produced a 300% increase in carbon monoxide formation, while SKF 525-A, a microsomal inhibitor, was found to inhibit carbon monoxide formation (Kubic *et al.*, 1974).

The fate and distribution of dichloromethane has been studied in the rat (Carlsson and Hultengre, 1975; Di Vincenzo, 1972) following inhalation or i.p. administration. The highest specific concentration was found in the liver, kidneys and adrenal glands, although there was no accumulation in fat.

Human exposure to 100–200 ppm showed a half-life of dichloromethane in the blood of approximately 40 min. (Dill *et al.*, 1978).

## 7.2. Toxicity

The acute toxic effects of dichloromethane were seen mainly in the CNS (NIOSH, 1976). The LD$_{50}$ was generally higher than 1000 mg/kg for the animal species tested (Mercier, 1977).

It induced fatty liver (Morris *et al.*, 1979), and hepatotoxic effects were also observed in mice following a single lethal dose (Gehring, 1968). No renal dysfunction was detected.

Following the accidental exposure (2300 ppm) of four men to dichloromethane vapor, one died; in the others, excessive inhalation produced nausea, acute bronchitis, irritation, and anemia. They were found to have low hemoglobin values and red-blood-cell counts, which could, however, be due to previous moderate exposure (Moskowitz and Shapiro, 1949).

The neurological picture of acute dichloromethane poisoning is generally characterized by vestibular and cerebellar brain stem signs with marked disturbances of cortical dynamics and subcortical relationships (Klinkova, 1957, cited by Mercier, 1977).

Exposure to dichloromethane vapor at a level of 1000 ppm for two hours, a breathing-zone concentration readily reached when using a paint-remover in a basement shop, resulted in a carboxy-hemoglobin concentration in excess of that encountered in industry with carbon monoxide exposure (5–10%).

Moreover, the biological half-life of carbon monoxide was greatly prolonged during exposure to dichloromethane. In such cases, the half-life is approximately 2–5 times that observed in subjects excreting CO from the atmosphere (Ratney *et al.*, 1974). It is well known that an increase greater than 5% of the carboxyhemoglobin concentration can adversely affect patients suffering from angina pectoris or cardiovascular diseases (Anderson, 1973; Stewart and Hake, 1976).

Dichloromethane produced an inflammatory response and cell damage when administered by inhalation to rats at 3700 ppm 5 hrs/day, 5 days/week for 4 weeks (Sahu *et al.*, 1980).

## 7.3. Carcinogenic and Mutagenic Effects

Methylene chloride has proved to be mutagenic in *S. typhimurium* strains TA 98 and TA 100. The addition of liver homogenate slightly increased the number of mutations (Jongen, 1978). Dichloromethane, when tested in the vapor phase, was shown to be mutagenic in *S. typhimurium* TA 100 with rat liver homogenate, but did not increase mitotic recombination in *S. cerevisiae* (Andrews, 1976). It induced transformed cells in agar, which formed tumors when injected into immunosuppressed mice (Price, 1976).

Only one carcinogenicity study (Theiss *et al.*, 1977) is reported where groups of mice received up to 800 mg/kg (maximal dose tolerated) thrice weekly, in a total of 16–17 injections. Surviving mice were analysed after 24 weeks for lung tumorigenesis, which was not significantly different from that in control groups.

A two-year inhalation study, in which animals (species unspecified) exposed to methylene chloride levels as high as 3500 ppm showed no evidence of cancer, has been reported (Dow Chemical, 1968) but the incomplete results are insufficient to draw any conclusion.

The mutagenicity of dichloromethane in some strains needs to be confirmed by other tests, and some long-term experiments on the carcinogenicity of this solvent are needed to make an evaluation possible.

The lack of case of epidemiological studies could indicate that there are fewer toxicity problems with this solvent than with the others reviewed in this chapter.

## 7.4. Teratogenicity and Embryotoxicity

In a study in which rats, rabbits, dogs, and guinea pigs of both sexes were exposed to levels of up to 5000 ppm of dichloromethane for periods of up to 6 months, no effects of reproduction parameters were seen (Heppel *et al.*, 1944).

Groups of male and female rats given 125 ppm dichloromethane in drinking water during 91 days were mated. Post-exposure reproduction was normal.

In another study, pregnant rats and mice were exposed to 1250 ppm dichloromethane on days 6–15 of gestation (7 hrs daily). Exposure had no effect on the average number of implantation sites per litter, litter size, fetal resorption, sex ratio, or body measurements in either species, but incidence of lumbar ribs or spurs was significantly lower than that of the controls, whereas the incidence of delayed sterbrae ossification was significantly greater for exposed rats.

In mice, a significant number of litters contained pups with a single extra center of ossification in the sternum, but microscopic examination revealed no abnormalities of organs, tissues or cells as a result of maternal exposure to dichloromethane (Schwetz, 1975).

Similar results were obtained by Hardin and Manson (1980) who found no significant anomalies in the test animals after subchronic exposure at 4500 ppm. However, postnatal evaluation is important since pregnant women, fetuses, and newborn infants are particularly susceptible to the carboxy-hemoglobin levels produced by dichloromethane metabolism (Longo, 1977).

Bornschein et al. (1980) demonstrated that the exposure of rats to dichloromethane (4500 ppm 21 days before, and 17 days during gestation) caused altered rates of behavioral habituation to a new environment. These effects were detectable as early as 10 days of age and were still demonstrable in male rats 15 days old. These results, reported as preliminary by the authors, suggest that dichloromethane could affect the functional development of the progency of exposed dams.

## 8. 1,1,1-TRICHLOROETHANE

### 8.1. Absorption, Distribution, Metabolism, and Excretion

1,1,1-trichloroethane is rapidly absorbed through the lungs and the gastrointestinal tract. It may also be absorbed through intact skin and enter the blood stream. Following absorption, most of the compound is eliminated unchanged via the lungs (Stewart and Dodd, 1964; Stewart, 1968).

Hake et al., (1960) estimated that nearly 98% was eliminated unchanged in the expired air of rats receiving an intraperitoneal injection of the $^{14}$C labelled compound; 0.5% is metabolized as carbon dioxide, and the remainder appeared in the urine as the glucuronide of 2,2,2,-trichloroethanol and TCA. Repeated exposure increased the amount of TCA in the urine but not in proportion to the concentration and duration of exposure to 1,1,1-trichloroethane (Tada et al., 1968).

Subacute inhalation (20 ppm/day) studies in rats by Eben and Kimmerle (1974) demonstrated an increase of trichloroethanol urinary excretion reaching a maximum after 10 weeks.

Since there is no accumulation of 1,1,1-trichloroethane in the tissues, it can be assumed that this solvent causes the induction of hepatic enzyme activities responsible for the increased formation of trichloroethanol.

The metabolic pathway in man seems very similar to that in animals. The solvent may be absorbed through the lungs, gastrointestinal tract, or skin (Fukabori *et al.*, 1977; Stewart, 1968), and is excreted unchanged via the lungs for many hours after exposure (Astrand *et al.*, 1973; Stewart *et al.*, 1961).

A small percentage is metabolized to 2,2,2-trichloroethanol and TCA, and excreted in the urine (Stewart, 1968; Stewart *et al.*, 1969; Seki *et al.*, 1975; Fukabori *et al.*, 1976).

## 8.2. Toxicity

Data on the exposure of human subjects using this solvent (which, in general, are similar to those concerning animals) give a good picture of the acute toxicity of 1,1,1-trichloroethane and cover experimental exposure of human volunteers (Stewart, 1968; Torkelson *et al.*, 1958). Fatalities resulting from the abuse of decongestant aerosols or from inhalation of cleaning solvents were reported (Torkelson *et al.*, 1958; Stewart *et al.*, 1961; Gazzaniga *et al.*, 1969; Salvini *et al.*, 1971; Gamberale and Hultengren, 1973; Hall and Hine, 1966; Travers, 1974). Others authors reported death after accidental ingestion (Stewart and Andrews, 1966), after general anesthesia (Frantz *et al.*, 1959; Dornette and Jones, 1966), or among workers exposed to very high concentrations of 1,1,1,-trichloroethane in solvent tanks (Kleinfeld and Feiner, 1966; Stewart, 1968; Hatfield and Maykoski, 1970; Caplan *et al.*, 1976). Anesthesia lasting up to two hours did not produce hepatoxicity, and 1,1,1-trichloroethane appeared to have a minimal potential for producing liver or kidney damage in man when fatalities occurred; the only significant finding at autopsy was moderate to marked pulmonary edema.

The principal toxic effect of excessive simple exposure to the solvent, either via the gastrointestinal tract or the lungs, is a functional depression of the CNS, leading to death from respiratory arrest or shock. It may also sensitize the heart muscle in a similar manner to chloroform, and sudden death from ventricular fibrillation may occur in those exposed to anesthetic concentrations.

Psychophysiological functions, such as reaction time, perceptual speed, and normal dexterity, were all impaired when subjects were exposed to 1,1,1-trichloroethane in concentrations of 250 ppm for 30 minutes.

Long-term inhalation studies have been performed on rats, rabbits, guinea pigs, and monkeys (Adams *et al.*, 1950; Torkelson *et al.*, 1958; Eben and Kimmerle, 1974), on dogs (Prendergast *et al.*, 1967), and in mice (McEwen *et al.*, 1974; McNutt *et al.*, 1975).

Slight retardation in growth, slight fatty degeneration of the liver (but not necrosis), and increased liver weight were the only ill effects reported, except in the study by McNutt on mice exposed to 1000 ppm for 12 weeks, where necrosis of individual hepatocytes occurred in 40% of the animals.

No long-term results of human exposure to 1,1,1-trichloroethane have been described, but one survey was carried out in Japanese factories where a total of 196 printing press operators were exposed for more than 5 years to the solvent at a concentration that reached 53 ppm (Seki *et al.*, 1975). Respiratory function tests and routine laboratory examinations revealed no abnormalities.

### 8.3. Mutagenicity and Carcinogenicity

The only study available on the mutagenic effect of 1,1,1-trichloroethane (Simmon *et al.*, 1977) demonstrated that this solvent was weakly mutagenic when tested with *S. typhimurium* strain TA 100, with or without a microsomal activation system.

It should be noted that 1,1,1-trichloroethane has been examined for possible carcinogenicity in Osborne–Mendel rats and $B_6C_3F_1$ mice. It was administered orally by gavage to 50 animals of each sex and species 5 days per week for 78 weeks.

The incidence of neoplasms did not differ significantly from that observed in untreated animals (National Cancer Institute, 1977). However, because of the shortened life span among both animal species, the NCI considered the test inadequate to make a positive or negative determination of cancer-causing potential.

In Sprague–Dawley rats exposed to the vapors (1750 ppm) of 1,1,1-trichloroethane in air for 6 hrs per day, 5 days a week, for 12 months, followed by observations up to 30 months, no increased tumor incidence was observed (Rampy *et al.*, 1977).

The available data do not permit an evaluation of the carcinogenicity of 1,1,1-trichloroethane, but it must be remembered that its two analogs, chloroform and 1,1,1-trichloroethane, are carcinogenic.

### 8.4. Embryotoxicity and Teratogenicity

The administration of 1,1,1-trichloroethane to fertilized chicken eggs (25 $\mu$mol/egg) exhibited a clear dose-response relationship in terms of survival of the embryos, whether the eggs were treated on the 3rd or 6th day of development. The malformation frequency was increased 5- to 6-fold (Elovaara *et al.*, 1979).

In rodents, however, 1,1,1-trichloroethane did not produce embryonic or fetal toxicity. Groups of rats and mice were exposed by inhalation for 7 hr daily on days 6–15 of gestation to 4.7 gm/$^3$ in air of 1,1,1-trichloroethane; no effects were observed on the average number of implantation sites per litter, litter size, incidence of fetal resorption, fetal sex ratio, or fetal body measurements. No treatment-related increase in the incidence of skeletal or visceral malformations was observed (Leong *et al.*, 1975; Schwetz *et al.*, 1975).

## 9. CONCLUSIONS

A summary of the information available is presented in Table VI. For most of the solvents reviewed, the data are too limited to permit a general conclusion. Some results, however, present clear evidence of carcinogenicity or embryotoxicity in several animal species.

Carbon tetrachloride produces liver tumors in several animal species following different routes of administration. Moreover, human cases of hepatomas appearing several years after overexposure to this solvent are reported, as well as an excess of lung, cervical, and skin cancers; a slight excess of leukemia and liver cancers are observed (Blair *et al.*, 1979). This last study on dry-cleaning area exposure also concerns exposure to trichloroethylene and tetrachloroethylene. For these solvents, however, there is only limited evidence of carcinogenicity and even of mutagenicity. From the very limited epidemiological studies so far reported, no evidence is known which associates trichloroethylene with an increased risk of cancer.

For methylene chloride, although there is no indication of potential carcinogenicity in animal experiments, the information available is not complete enough to draw conclusions. Methylene chloride has been shown to be mutagenic in bacterial test systems, and produced positive results in cell transformation assays.

Tumors have been produced after long-term exposure of experimental animals to chloroform and 1,2-dichloroethane (hepatic tumors in mice and renal tubular necrosis in male rats), while negative results were observed in several *in vitro* mutagenicity tests sytstems. IARC (1979) considers that there is sufficient evidence that these solvents present a carcinogenic risk to humans.

### Table VI
### Summary of Results

|  | Teratogenicity | Mutagenicity | Carcinogenicity |
|---|---|---|---|
| Dichloromethane | No effect observed | Positive | No sufficient data |
| Chloroform | Embryotoxic | Negative | Positive in several species |
| Carbon tetrachloride | Few evidences of foetotoxicity | Negative | Positive |
| 1,2-Dichloroethane | No data | Positive | Positive by gavage Negative by inhalation |
| Trichlorethylene | Teratogenic | Weak or not | Limited evidence in mouse |
| Tetrachloroethylene | Negative in one experiment | Negative | No sufficient data |
| Trichloroethane | No effect on rodents | Weak in one test | No sufficient data |

Trichloroethylene is the only solvent that presented evidence of teratogenicity. Chloroform and carbon tetrachloride showed embryotoxic properties but no teratogenic effects have been reported. For the other solvents the results available are too limited to allow any conclusion.

The possible role of organochlorinated solvents in the promoting step of carcinogenesis should also be considered. Carbon tetrachloride is the only solvent for which such an effect has been described in several experiments (Yokoro *et al.*, 1973; Pound, 1978; Kanematsu, 1976), but no specific test for this effect has so far been developed. This kind of effect could explain the higher incidence of cancer in animal experiments associated with the negative results observed in most mutagenicity tests for these solvents.

# REFERENCES

Adams, E. M., Spencer, H. C., Rowe, V. K., and Irish, D. D., 1950, Vapor toxicity of 1,1,1-trichloroethane (methylchloroform) determined by experiments on laboratory animals, *Arch. Ind. Hyg.* 1:225–236.

Adams, E. M., Spencer, H. C., Rowe, V. K., McCollister, D. D., and Irish, D. D., 1952, Vapor toxicity of carbon tetrachloride determined by experiments on laboratory animals, *AMA Arch. Ind. Hyg.* 6:50–66.

Allemand, H., Pessayre, D., Descatoire, V., Degott, C., Feldmann, G., and Benhamou, J.-P, 1978, Metabolic activation of trichloroethylene into a chemically reactive metabolite toxic to the liver, *J. Pharmacol. Exp. Ther.* 204:714–723.

Alpert, A. E., Arkhangelsky, A. V., Lunts, A. M., and Panina, N. P., 1972, Experimental hepatopathies and carcinomas of the breast in rats (Russ), *Bjull. Eskp. Biol. Med.* 74:78–81.

Ambrose, A. M., 1950, Toxicological studies of compounds investigated for use as inhibitors of biological processes. II. Toxicity of ethylene chlorohydrin, *Arch. Ind. Hyg. Occup. Med.* 2:591–597.

Anderson, E. W., Andelman, R. J., Strauch, J. M., 1973, Effect of low level of carbon monoxide exposure on onset and duration of angiopectoris, *Ann. Intern. Med.* 79:46–50.

Andrews, A. W., Zawistowski, E. S., and Valentine, C. R., 1976, A comparison of the mutagenic properties of vinylchloride and methylchloride, *Mutat. Res.* 40:273–276.

Appleby, A., Kazazis, J., Lillian, D., and Singh, H. B., 1976, Atmospheric formation of chloroform from trichloroethylene, *J. Environ. Sci. Health* A11:711–715.

Astrand, I, and Ovrum, P., 1976, Exposure to trichloroethylene. I. Uptake and distribution in man, *Scand. J. Work Environ. Health* 4:199–211.

Astrand, I., Kilbom, A., Wahlberg, I., and Ovrum, P., 1973, Methylchloroform exposure. I. Concentration in alveolar air and blood at rest and during exercise, *Work. Environ. Health* 10:69–81.

Astrand, I., Ovrum, P., and Carlsson, A., 1975, Exposure to methylene chloride. I. Its concentration in alveolar air and blood during rest and exercies and its metabolism, *Scand. J. Work, Environ. Health* 1:78–94.

Axelson, O., Andersson, K., Hogstedt, C., Holmberg, B., Molina, G., and de Verdier, A., 1978, A cohort study on trichloroethylene exposure and cancer mortality, *J. Occup. Med.* 20:194–196.

Baader, E. W., 1954, *Gewerbekrankheiten Urban and Schwarzenberg*, Munich.

Baden, J. M., Kelley, M., Mazze, R. I., and Simmon, V. F., 1979, Mutagenicity of inhalation anaesthetics: trichloroethylene, divinylethene, nitransoxide, and cyclopropane, *Br. J. Anaesth.* **51**:417–412.

Bagnell, P. C., and Ellenberger, H. A., 1977, Obstructive jaundice due to a chlorinated hydrocarbon in breast milk, *Can. Med. Assoc. J.* **117**:1047–1048.

Banerjee, S., and Van Duuren, B. L., 1979, Binding of carcinogenic halogenated hydrocarbons to cell macromolecules, *J. Natl. Cancer Inst.* **63**:707–711.

Barcelona, M. J., 1979, Human exposure to chloroform in a costal urban environment, *J. Environ. Sci. Health.* **14**:267–283.

Bartsch. H., Malaveille, C., Barbin, A., and Plancke, G., 1979, Mutagenic and alkylating metabolites of Halo-Ethylenes, Chlorobutadienes and Dichlorobutenes produced by rodent or human liver tissues, *Arch. Toxicol.* **41**:249–277.

Beecher, H. K., 1953, Clinical impression and clinical investigation, *J. Am. Med. Assoc.* **151**:45–47.

Beisland, H. O., and Wannag, S. A., 1970, Trikloretylensniffing akutte lever-og nyreskader, *T. Norsk. Laegenforen.* **90**:285–288.

Berkowitz, J. B., 1978a, *Litterature Review—Problem Definition Studies on Selected Chemicals, Chloroform*, Contract No. DAMD17-77-C-7037, Monthly Progress Report 10, Cambridge, MA, Arthur D. Little, Inc.

Berkowitz, J. B., 1978b, *Litterature Review—Problem Definition Studies on Selected Chemicals,* Appendix B, *Methylene Chloride*, Cambridge, MA, Arthur D. Little, Inc., pp. 58–105.

Bignami, M., Cardamone, G., Comba., P., Ortali, V. A., Morprugo, G., and Carere, A., 1977, Relationship between chemical structure and mutagenic activity in some pesticides: The use of *Salmonella typhimurium* and *Aspergillus nidulans* (Abstract No. 79), *Mutat. Res.* **46**:243–244.

Blair, A., Decoufle, P., and Grauman, D., 1978, Mortality among laundry and dry cleaning workers (Abstract), *Am. J. Epidemiol.* **108**:238.

Blair, A., Decoufle, P., and Grauman, D., 1979, Causes of death among laundry and dry cleaning workers, *Am. J. Publ. Health* **69**:508–511.

Bolanowska, W., Golacka, J. 1972, Inhalation and excretion of tetrachloroethylene in man in experimental conditions, *Med. Pr.* **23**:109–119.

Bomski, H., Sobolewska, A., and Strakowski, A., 1967, Toxic damage of the liver by chloroform in chemical industry workers (Germ.), *Arch. Gewerbepathol. Gewerbehyg.* **24**:127–134.

Bolt, H. M., Butcher A., Wolowski, L., Gil, D. L., and Bolt, W., 1977, Incubation of $^{14}$C-trichloroethylene vapor with rat liver microsomes: uptake of radioactivity and covalent protein binding of metabolites, *Int. Arch. Occup. Environ. Health* **39**:103–111.

Bonse, G., and Henschler, D., 1976, Chemical reactivity, biotransformation, and toxicity of polychlorinated aliphatic compounds, *CRC Crit. Rev. Toxicol* **4**:395–409.

Bonse, G., Urban, T., Reichert, D., and Henschler, D., 1975, Chemical reactivity metabolic oxirane formation and biological reactivity or chlorinated ethylenes in the isolated perfused rat liver preparation, *Biochem. Pharmacol.* **24**:1829–1834.

Booth, J., Boyland, E., Sims, P., 1961, An enzyme from rat liver catalyzing conjugations with glutathione, *Biochem J.* **79**:516–524.

Bornschein, R. L., Hastings, L., and Manson, J. M., 1980, Behavioral toxicity of the offspring of rats exposed to dichloromethane (DCM) prior to and/or during gestation, *Toxicol. Appl. Pharmacol* **52**:29–37.

Bray, H. G., Thorpe, W. V., and Vallance, D. K., 1952, The liberation of chloride ions from organic chloro compounds by tissue extracts, *Biochem. J.* **51**:193–201.

Brem, H., Stein, A. B., and Rosenkranz, H. S., 1974, The mutagenicity and DNA-modifying effect of haloalkanes, *Cancer Res.* **34**:2576–2579.

Bronletti, G., Zeiger, E., and Frezza, D., 1978, Genetic activity of trichloroethylene in yeast, *J. Environ. Pathol. Toxicol.* **1**:411–418.

Brown, B. R., Jr., Sipes, I. G., and Sagalyn, A. M., 1974b, Mechanisms of acute hepatic toxicity: chloroform, halothane, and glutathione, *Anesthesiology* **41**:554–561.

Brown, D. M., Langley, P. F., Smith, D., and Taylor, D. C., 1974a, Metabolism of chloroform. I. The metabolism of ($^{14}$C) chloroform by different species, *Xenobiotica* **4**:151–163.

Butler, T. C., 1961, Reduction of carbon tetrachloride *in vivo* and reduction of carbon tetrachloride and chloroform *in vitro* by tissues and tissues constituents, *J. Pharmacol. Exp. Ther.* **134**:311–319.

Byers, D. H., 1943, Chlorinated solvents in common wartime use, *Ind. Med.* **12**:440–443.

Byington, K. H., and Leibman, K. C., 1965, Metabolism of trichloroethylene by liver microsomes. II. Identification of the reaction product as chloral hydrate, *Mol. Pharmacol.* **1**:247–254.

Caplan, Y. H., Backer, R. C., and Whitaker, J. Q., 1976, 1,1,1,-Trichloroethane: Report of a fatal intoxication, *Clin. Toxicol.* **9**:69–74.

Cagen, S. Z., Klaassen, C. D., 1979, Hepatotoxicity of carbon tetrachloride in developing rats, *Toxicol. Appl. Pharmacol.* **23**:541–552.

Capel, I. D., Dorrel, H. M., Jenner, M., 1979, The effect of chloroform ingestion on the growth of some murine tumors, *Environ. J. Cancer* **15**:1485–1490.

Carlsson, A., and Hultengren, M., 1975, Exposure to methylene chloride. III. Metabolism of $^{14}$C-labelled methylene chloride in rats. *Scand. J. Work, Environ. Health.* **1**:104–108.

Cêrná, M., and Kypènová, H., 1977, Mutagenic activity of chloroethylenes analysed by screening system tests (Abstract No. 36), *Mutat. Res.* **46**:214–215.

Cessi, C., Colombini, C., and Mameli, L., 1966, The reaction of liver proteins with a metabolite of carbon tetrachloride, *Biochem. J.* **101**:46c–47c.

Challen P. J. R., Hickish, D. E., and Bedford, J., 1958, Chronic chloroform intoxication, *Br. J. Ind. Med.* **15**:243–249.

Charlesworth, F. A., 1976, Patterns of chloroform metabolism, *Food Cosmet. Toxicol.* **14**:59–60.

Chen, W. J., Chi, E. Y., and Smuckler, E. A., 1977, Carbon tetrachloride-induced changes in mixed function oxidases and microsomal cytochromes in the rat lung, *Lab. Invest.* **36**:388–394.

Chmielewski, J., Tomaszewski, R., Glombiowski, P. Kowalewski, W., Kwiatkowski, S. R., Szczekocki, W., and Winnicka, A., 1976, Clinical observations of the occupational exposure to tetrachloroethylene, *Biul. Inst. Med. Morskiej.* **27**:197–205.

Cignoli, E. V., and Castro, J. A., 1971, Effect of inhibitors of drug metabolizing enzymes on carbon tetrachloride hepatotoxicity, *Toxicol. Appl. Pharmacol.* **18**:625–637.

Clayton, J. I, and Parkhouse J., 1962, Blood trichloroethylene concentrations during anesthesia under controlled conditions, *Br. J. Anaesth.* **34**:141–148.

Clearfield, H. R., 1970, Hepatorenal toxicity from sniffing spot remover (trichloroethylene), *Am. J. Dig. Dis.* **15**:851–856.

Coburn, R. F., 1973, Endogenous carbon monoxide metabolism, *Ann. Rev. Med.* **24**:241–250.

Cole, L. J., and Nowell, P. C., 1964, Accelerated induction of hepatomas in fast neutron-irradiated mice injected with carbon tetrachloride, *Ann. N.Y. Acad. Sci.* **114**:259–267.

Coler, H. R., and Rossmiller, H. R., 1953, Tetrechloroethylene Exposure in a small industry, *Arch. Ind. Hyg.* **8**:227–232.

Conkle, J. P., Camp, B. J., and Welch, B. E., 1975, Trace composition of human respiratory gas, *Arch. Environ. Health.* **30**:290–295.

Conlon, M. F., 1963, Addiction to chlorodyne, *Br. Med. J.* **2**:1177–1178.

Curtis, H. J., and Tilley, J., 1972, The role of mutations in liver tumor induction in mice, *Radiat. Res.* **50**:539–542.

Daniel, J. W., 1963, The metabolism of $^{36}$Cl-labelled trichloroethylene and tetrachloroethylene in the rat, *Biochem. Pharmacol.* **12**:795–802.

Dean, B. J., and Hodson-Walker G., 1979, An *in vitro* chromosome assay using cultured rat liver alls, *Mut. Res.* **64**:329–337.

Delplace, Y., Cavigneaux, A., and Cabasson, G., 1962, Occupational diseases due to methylene chloride and dichloroethane (Fr.), *Arch. Mal. Prof. Med. Trav. Secur. Soc.* **23**:816–817.

Deringer, M. K., and Dunn, T. B., 1953, Results of exposure of strain C3H mice to chloroform, *Proc. Soc. Exp. Biol. (N. Y.)* **83**:474–478.

De Salva, S., Volpe, A., Leigh, G., and Regan, T., 1975, Long-term safety studies of a chloroform-containing dentrifice and mouth rinse in man, *Food Cosmet. Toxicol.* **13**:529–532.

Diaz-Gomez, M. I., and Castro, J. A., 1980, Covalent binding of carbon tetrachloride metabolites to liver nuclear DNA, proteins, and lipids, *Toxicol. Appl. Pharmacol.* **56**:199–206.

Dickson, A. G., and Riley, J. P., 1976, The distribution of short-chain halogenated aliphatic hydrocarbons in some marine organisms, *Marine Pollut. Bull.* **7**:167–169.

Dill, D. L., Watanabe, P. G., and Norris, J. M., 1978, Effect of methylene chloride on the oxyhemoglobin dissociation curve of rat and human blood, *Toxicol. Appl. Pharmacol.* **46**:125–129.

Dilley, J. V., Chernoff, N., Kay, D., Winslow, N., and Newell, G. W., 1977, Inhalation teratology studies of five chemicals in rats (Abstract No. 154), *Toxicol. Appl. Pharmacol.* **41**:196.

DiVincenzo, G. D., and Hamilton, M. L., 1975, Fate and disposition of ($^{14}$C) methylene chloride in the rat, *Toxicol. Appl. Pharmacol.* **32**:385–393.

DiVincenzo, C. D., Yanno, F. J., Astill, B. D., 1972, Human and canine exposures to methylene chloride vapor. *Am. Indust. Hyg. Assoc. J.* **33**:125–135.

Dorfmuller, M. A., Henne, S. P., York, R. G., Bornschein, R. L., and Manson, J. M., 1979, Evaluation of teratogenicity and behavioral toxicity with inhalation exposure of maternal rats to trichloroethylene, *Toxicology* **14**:153–166.

Dornette, W. H. L., and Jones, J. P., 1960, Clinical experiences with 1,1,1-trichloroethane; a preliminary report of 50 anesthetic administrations, *Anesth. Analg. (Cleveland)* **39**:249–255.

Dow Chemical Co., Unpublished report submitted to W.H.O. 1968.

Dowty, B. J., Laseter, J. L., and Storer, J., 1976, The transplacental migration and accumulation in blood of volatile organic constituents, *Pediat. Res.* **10**:691–701.

Doyle, R. E., Woodard, J. C., Lewis, A. L., and Moreland, A. F., 1967, Mortality in Swiss mice exposed to chloroform, *J. Am. Vet. Med. Assoc.* **151**:930–934.

Dupont, P., Bernis, P. Paduart, and P. Vereerstraeten, P., 1975, A propos de 45 cas d'intoxication au tetrachlorore de carbone. *Acta Clin. Belg* **30**:485–493.

Eben, A., and Kimmerle, G., 1974, Metabolism excretion and toxicology of methylchloroform in acute and subacute exposed rats, *Arch. Toxikil.* **31**:233–242.

Edh, M., Sclerud, A., and Sjöberg, C., 1973, Fatalities in connection with the misuse of organic solvents (in Swedish), *Lakartidningen.* **70**:3949–3961.

Ehrenberg, L., Osterman-Golkar, S., Singh, D., and Lundginst, U., 1974, On the reaction kinetics and mutagenic activity of methylating and $\mu$-halogenoethylating gasoline additives, *Radiat. Bot.* **15**:185–194.

Elovaara, E., Hemminki, K., and Vainio, H., 1979, Effects of methylene chloride, trichloroethane, tetrachloroethyle, and toluene on the development of chick embryos, *Toxicology* **12**:111–119.

Eschenbrenner, A. B., and Miller, E., 1945, Induction of hepatomas in mice by repeated oral administration of chloroform with observations on sex difference, *J. Natl. Cancer Inst.* **5**:251–255.

Fernandez, J. G., Droz, P. O., Humbert, B. E., and Caperos, J. R., 1977, Trichloroethylene exposure. Simulation of uptake, excretion, and metabolism using a mathematical model, *Br. J. Ind. Med.* **34**:43–55.

Fernandez, J. G., Humbert, B. E., and Droz, P. O., 1975, Exposition au trichloroethylene, bilan de l'absorption de l'excrétion et du métabolisme sur des sujécts humains, *Arch. Mal. Prof.* **36**:397–407.

Fodor, G. G., Prasjnar, D., and Schlipköter, H. W., 1973, Endogenous formation of CO from incorporated halogenated hydrocarbons of the methane series (German), *Staub. Reinhalt. Luft.* **33**:258–259.

Fowler, J. S. L., 1969, A new metabolite of tetrachloride carbon, *Br. J. Pharmacol.* **36**:181.

Fry, B. J., Taylor, T., and Hathway, D. E., 1972, Pulmanory elimination of chloroform and its metabolite in man, *Arch. Int. Pharmacodyn* **196**:98–111.

Fukabori, S., Nakaaki, K. Yonemoto, J., and Tada, O., 1976, Cutaneous absorption of methyl chloroform (Japanese), *Rodo Kagaku* **52**:67–80 (*Chem. Abstr.* **85**:1487 y).

Fukabori, S., Nakaaki, K. Yonemoto, J., and Tada, O., 1977, On the cutaneous absorption of 1,1,1-trichloroethane (2), *J. Sci. Lab.* **53**:89–95.

Gamberale, F., and Hultengren, M., 1973, methylchloroform exposure. II. Psychophysiological functions, *Work Environ. Health.* **10**:82–92.

Garner, R. C., and McLean, A. E. M., 1969, Increased susceptibility to carbon tetrachloride poisoning in the rat after pretreatment with oral phenobarbitone, *Biochem. Pharmacol.* **18**:645–650.

Gaultier, M., Efthymion, M. L., Efthymion, Th., and Pebay-Peyroula, F., 1971, Cardiac manifestations of the chronic trichloroethylene poisoning (French), *Ann. Cardiol. Angeiol.* **20**:185–190.

Gazzaniga, G., Binaschi, S., Sportelli, A., and Riva, M., 1969, L'éliminazione nell'aria elveolare dell'uomo dell' 1,1,1-trichloroetano dopo esposizione a 600 ppm per 3 ore, *Bull. Soc. Ital. Biol. Sper.* **45**:97.

Gehring, P. J., 1968, Hepatotoxic potency of various chlorinated hydrocarbon vapors relative to their narcotic and lethal potencies in mice, *Toxicol. Appl. Pharmacol.* **13**:287–298.

Gibitz, H. J., and Plochl, F., 1973, Orale trichlorathylenvergiftung bei einem 4½ jahre alten kind, *Arch. Toxikol.* **31**:13–18.

Glende, E. A., Jr., Hruszkewycz, A. M., and Recknagel, R. O., 1976, Critical role of lipid peroxidation in carbon tetrachloride-induced loss of aminopyrine demthylase, cytochrome P-450 and glucose 6-phosphatase, *Biochem. Pharmacol.* **25**:2163–2170.

Grandjean, E., Münchinger, R., Turrain, V., Haas, P. A., Knoepfel, H. K., and Rosenmund, H., 1955, Investigations into the effects of exposure to trichlorethylene in mechanical engineering, *Br. J. ind. Med.* **12**:131–142.

Greim, H., Bonse. G., Radwan, Z., Reichert, D., and Henschler, D., 1975, Mutagenicity *in vitro* and potential carcinogenicity of chlorinated ethylenes as a function of metabolic oxirane formation, *Biochem. Pharmacol.* **24**:2013–2017.

Guberan, E., and Fernandez, J., 1974, Control of industrial exposure to tetrachloroethylene by measuring alveolar concentrations: theoretical approach using a mathematical model, *Br. J. Ind. Med.* **31**:159–167.

Guengerich, F. P., and Watanabe, P. G., 1979, Metabolism of $^{14}$C and $^{36}$Cl vinyl chloride *in vivo* and *in vitro*, *Biochem. Pharmacol.* **28**:589–596.

Guengerich, F. P., Crawford, W. M., Domoradzki, J. Y., MacDonald, T. L., and Watanabe, P. G., 1980. *In vitro* activation of 1,2-dichloroethane by microsomial and cytosolic enzymes, *Toxicol. Appl. Pharmacol.* **55**:303–317.

Hake, C. L., and Stewart, R. D., 1977, Human exposure to tetrachloroethylene inhalation and skin contact, *Environ. Health Perspect.* **21**:231–238.

Hake, C. L., Waggoner, T. B., Robertson, D. N., and Rowe, V. K., 1960, The metabolism of 1,1,1-trichloroethane by the rat, *Arch. Environ. Health* **1**:101–105.

Hall, F. B., and Hine, C. H., 1966, Trichloroethane intoxication: a report of two cases, *J. Forensic Sci.* **11**:404.

Hall, M. C., and Shillinger, J. E., 1925, Tetrachloroethylene: a new anthelmintic for worms in dogs, *North Am. Vet.* **9**:41–52.

Hartwell, J. L., 1951, Survey of compounds which have been tested for carcinogenic activity, Washington, D.C., Government Printing Office, *Public Health Service Publication* No. 149.

Hatfield, T. R., and Maykoski, R. T., 1970, A fatal methyl chloroform (trichloroethane) poisoning, *Arch. Environ. Health* **20**:279-284.

Hathway, D. E., 1974, Chemical, biochemical, and toxicological differences between carbon tetrachloride and chloroform. A critical review of recent investigations of these compounds in mammals, *Arzneim Forsch* **24**:173-176.

Hayes, F. D., Short, R. D., and Gibson, J. E., 1973, Differential toxicity of monochloroacetate, monofluoroacetate, and monoiodoacetate in rats, *Toxicol. Appl. Pharmacol.* **26**:93-102.

Henschler, D., and Bonse, G., 1977, Metabolic activation of chlorinated ehtylenes: dependance of mutagenic effect on electrophilic reactivity of the metabolically formed epoxides, *Arch. Toxikol.* **39**:7-12.

Henschler, D., Eder, E., Neudecker, T., and Metzler, M., 1977, Carcinogenicity of trichloroethylene: Fact or artifact? *Arch. Toxikol.* **37**:233-236.

Henschler, D., Romen, W., Elsässer, H. M., Reichert, D., Eder, E., and Radwan, 1980, Carcinogenicity study of trichloroethylene by long-term inhalation in three animal species, *Arch. Toxikol.* **43**:237-248.

Heppel, L. A., Neal, T. L., Perrin, M. L., Orr, M. L., Porterfield, V. J., 1944, Toxicology of dichloromethane (methylene chloride): Studies on effects of daily inhalations, *Industry. Hyg. Toxicol.* **26**:8-16.

Hogan, G. K., Smith, R. G., and Cornish, H. H., 1976, Studies on the microsomal conversion of dichloromethane to carbon monoxide (Abstract No. 49), *Toxicol. Appl. Pharmacol.* **37**:112.

IARC, 1979, *IARC Monographs on the Evaluation of the Carcinogenic Risk of Chemicals to Humans, 19, Some Monomers, Plastics and Synthetic Elastomers, and Acrolein*, Lyon, p. 396.

IARC, 1979, Monographs, *20, Some Halogenated Hydrocarbons*, Lyon, p. 396.

Ikeda, M., and Imamura, T., 1973, Biological half-life of trichloroethylene and tetrachloroethylene in human subjects, *Int.-Arch. Arbeitsmed.* **31**:209-224.

Ilett, K. F., Reid, W. D., Sipes, I. G., and Krishna, G., 1973, Chloroform toxicity in mice: correlation of renal and hepatic necrosis with covalent binding of metabolites to tissue macromolecules, *Exp. Mol. Path.* **19**:215-229.

Jones, W. M., Margolis, G., and Stephen, C. R., 1958, Hepatotoxicity of inhalation anesthetic drugs, *Anaesthesiology* **19**:715-723.

Jongen, W. M. F., Alink, G. M., and Koeman, J. H., 1978, Mutagenic effect of dichloromethane on *Salmonella typhimurium*, *Mutat. Res.* **56**:245-248.

Kalgenova, R. I., Tsigankova S. T., and Chernobai, V. P., 1969, Pokajateligazoobmena i kislotno-shchelochnogo ravnoversiia u ploda priobezb olivanii v roddakh trikhloretilenom s kislorodom i s vojdukhom, *Vopr. Okhr. Materin.* **14**:81-85.

Kanematsu, T., 1976, Promoting effect of carbon tetrachloride on azodye hepatocarcinogenesis in rats, *Fukuoka Igaku Zasshi* **67**:134-145.

Kawasaki, H., 1965, Development of tumor in the course of spontaneous restoration of carbon tetrachloride induced cirrhosis of the liver in rats, *Kurume Med J.* **12**:37-42.

Kimmerle, G., and Eben, A., 1973a, Metabolism, excretion, and toxicology of trichloroethylene after inhalation. I. Experimental exposure in rats, *Arch. Toxikol.* **30**:115-126.

Kimmerle, G., and Eben, A., 1973b, Metabolism, excretion, and toxicology of trichloroethylene after inhalation. 2. Experimental human exposure, *Arch. Toxikol.* **30**:127-138.

Kimura, E. T., Ebert, D. M., and Dodge, P. W., 1971, Acute toxicity and limits of solvent residue for sixteen organic solvents, *Toxicol. Appl. Pharmacol.* **19**:699-704.

Klaassen, C. D., and Plaa, G. L., 1966, Relative effects of various chlorinated hydrocarbons on liver and kidney function in mice, *Toxicol. Appl. Pharmacol.* **9**:139-151.

Klaassen, C. D., and Plaa, G. L., 1967, Relative effects of various chlorinated hydrocarbons on liver and kidney function in dogs, *Toxicol. Appl. Pharmacol.* **10**:119-131.

Kleinfeld, M. and Feiner, B. Health hazards associated with work in confined spaces, *J. Occup. Med.* **8**:358-1966.

Klimkova-Deutschkowa, E., cited by Mercier, M. (1977).

Kluwe, W. M., McCormack, K. M., and Hook, J. B., 1978, Selective modification of the renal and hepatic toxicities of chloroform by induction of drug-metabolizing enzyme systems in kidney and liver, *J. Pharmacol. Exp. Ther.* **207**:566–573.

Konietzko, H., Haberlandt, W., Heilbronner, H., Reill, G., and Weichardt, H., 1978, Cytogenetische untersuchungen an trichloroäthylenarbeiten.

Korobko, S. F., 1972, Techeni rodov ipokazateli kislotnoshchelochnogo sostoianiia ploda pri obezbolivanii trikloretilenom s zakis' iu azota, *Vopr. Okhr. Materin. Det.* **17**:56–58.

Krantz, J. C., Jr., Park, C. S., and Ling, J. S. L., 1959, Anesthesia. LX: The anesthetic properties of 1,1,1-trichloroethane, *Anesthesiology* **20**:635.

Krasovitskaya, M. L., and Malyarova, L. K., 1968, O khronicheskom deistvii malykh kontsentratsii etilena i trikhloretilena na organism novorzhdennvkh zhivotnykh. *Gig. Sanit.* **33**:7–10.

Kristoffcrsson, U., 1974, Genetic effects of some gasoline additives (Abstract), *Hereditas* **78**:319.

Kubic, V. L., Anders, M. W., Engel, R. R., Barlow, C. H., and Caughey, W. S., 1974, Metabolism of dihalomethanes to carbon monoxide. I. *In vivo* studies, *Drug Metab. Disp.* **2**:53–57.

Kuwabara, T., Quevedo, A. R., and Cogan, D. C., 1968, An experimental study of dichloroethane poisoning, *Arch. Ophthal.* **79**:321–330.

Kylin, B., Sümegi, I., and Yllner, S., 1965, Hepatoxicity of inhaled trichloroethylene and tetrachloroethylene. Long-term exposure, *Acta Pharmacol. Toxicol.* **22**:379–385.

Laham, S., 1970, Studies on placental transfer. Trichlorethylene, *Ind. Med. Surg.* **39**:46–49.

Laib, R. J., Stöckle, G., Bolt, H. M., and Kunz, W., 1979, Vinylchloride and trichloroethylene: comparison of alkylating effects of metabolites and induction of preneoplastic enzyme dificiencies in rat liver, *J. Cancer Res. Clin. Oncol.* **94**:139–147.

Lakomy, T., Papierowski, Z., and Kylszejko, Cz., 1972, Resultats cliniques de l'influence du trichloroethylene par la contractilité de l'utérus gravide pendant l'accouchement comparés aux résultats des examens "in vitro," *Gynecol. Obstet.* **64**:665–672.

Lamson, P. D., Robbins, B. H., and Ward, C. B., 1929, The pharmacology and toxicology of tetrachloroethylene, *Am. J. Hyg.* **9**:430–444.

Leibman, K. C., 1965, Metabolism of trichloroethylene in liver microsomes. I. Characteristics of the reaction, *Mol. Pharmacol.* **1**:239–246.

Lemonnier, F. J., Scotto, J. M., and Thuong-Trieu, C., 1974, Disturbances in tryptophan metabolism after a single dose of aflatoxin $B_1$ and chronic intoxication with carbon tetrachloride, *J. Natl cancer Inst.* **53**:745–749.

Leong, B. K. J., Schwetz, B. A., and Gehring, P. J., 1975, Embryo and fetotoxicity of inhaled trichloroethylene, perchloroethylene, methyl chloroform, and methylene chloride in mice and rats, *Abstract of Papers, Society of Toxicology*, 14th Annual Meeting, March, 29 pp.

Lilleaasen, P., 1972, Narkose og anestesi som arsak til loodselsaslyksi, *Tidsskr. Nor. Laegeforen.* **92**:1938–1942.

Lillian, D., Singh, H. B., Appleby, A., Lobban, L., Arnts, R., Gumpert, R., Hague, R., Toomey, J., Kazazis, J., Antell, M., Hansen, D., and Scott, B., 1975, Atmospheric fates of halogenated compounds, *Environ. Sci. Technol.* **9**:1042–1048.

Lob, M., 1957, Les dangers du perchlorethylene, *Arch. Gewerbepathol. Gewerbehyg.* **16**:45–47.

Lombardi, B., Ugazio, G., 1965, Serum lipoproteins in rats with carbon tetrachloride induced fatty liver, *J. Lipid Res.* **6**:498–505.

Longo, L. D., 1977, The biological effects of carbon monoxide on the pregnant woman, fetus, and newborn infant, *Am. J. Obstet. Gynecol.* **129**:69–103.

Lyman, W. J., 1978, Report on trichloroethylene, in Berkowitz, J.B., *Literature Review—Problem Definition Studies on Selected Chemicals*, Cambridge, MA., Arthur D. Little, Inc. pp. 19–69.

McCann, J., and Ames, B. N., 1976, Detection of carcinogens as mutagens in the *Salmonella/*microsome test: assay of 300 chemicals: discussion, *Proc. Natl. Acad. Sci. (Wash.)* **73**:950–954.

McCann, J., Choi, E., Yamasaki, E., and Ames, B. N., 1975b, Detection of carcinogens as mutagens in the *Salmonella*/microsoms test: assay of 300 chemicals, *Proc. Natl. Acad. Sci.* (*Wash.*) **72:**5135-5139.

McCann, J., Simmon, V., Streitzieser, D., and Ames, B. N., 1975a, Mutagenicity of chloro-acetaldehyde a possible metabolic product of 1,2-(dichloroethane ethylene dichloride), chloroethanol (ethylene chlorohydrin), vinyl chloride, and cyclophosphamide, *Proc. Natl. Acad. Sci.* (*Wash.*) **72:**3190-3193.

McCollister, D. D., Hollingsworth, R. L., Oyen, F., and Rowe, V. K., 1956, Comparative inhalation toxicity of fumigant mixtures. Individual and joint effects of ethylene dichloride, carbon tetrachloride and ethylene dibromide, *Arch. Ind. Health.* **13:**1-7.

McConnell, G., Ferguson, D. M., and Pearson, C. R., 1975, Chlorinated hydrocarbons and the environment, **Endeavor 34:**13-18.

MacEwen, J. D., Kinkead, E. R., and Haun, C. C., 1974, A study of the biological effect of continuous inhalation exposure of 1,1,1-trichloroethane (methyl chloroform) on animals, *NASA Contract Rep.* 134323.

McLean, A. E. M., 1970, The effect of protein deficiency and microsomal enzyme induction by DDT and phenobarbitone on the acute toxicity of chloroform and a pyrrolizidine alkaloid, retrorsine, *Br. J. Exp. Path.* **51:**317-321.

McNutt, N. S., Amster, R. L., McConnell, E. E., and Morris, F., 1975, Hepatic lesions in mice after continuous inhalation exposure to 1,1,1-trichloroethane, *Lab. Invest.* **32:**642-654.

Maltoni, C., 1980, Studies on long term effects on rats and mice of ethylene dichloride, administered by inhalation. Final Report, Centro Tumeri and Instituto di Oncologna, Bologna, Italy (in press).

Mansuy, D., Beaune, P., Cresteil, T., Lange, M., and Leroux, J-P., 1977, Evidence for phosgene formation during liver micromal oxidation of chloroform, *Biochem. Biophys. Res. Comm.* **79:**513-517.

Martin, G., and Figert, D. M., 1974, Gas-solid chromatographic determination of volatile denaturants in ethanol solution, *J. Assoc. Off. Anal. Chem.* **57:**148-152.

Martin, G., Knorpp, K., Huth, K., Heinrich, F., and Mittermayer, D., 1968, Clinical features, pathogenesis, and management of dichloroethane poisoning (Germ.), *Dtsch. med. Wschr.* **93:**2002 (Translation in *Germ. Med. Mth.*, 1969, **14:**62-67.

Matsuki, A., and Zsigmond, E. K., 1974, The first fatal case of chloroform anaesthesia in the United States, *Anesth. Analog.* (*Cleveland*), **53:**152-154.

Mercier, M., 1977, Criteria (Exposure/Effect Relationships) for Organochlorine Solvents, Doc. V/F/177-4, Luxembourg, Commission of the European Communities.

Miklashevski, V. E., Tubarinoja, U. N., Rakhamanina, N. L., and Yagovleva, G. P., 1966, Toxicity of chloroform administered orally, *Gig. Sanit.* **31:**320-325.

Miller, V., Dobbs, R. J., and Jacobs, S. I., 1970, Ethylene chlorohydrin intoxication with fatality, *Arch. Dis. Child.* **45:**589-590.

Monster, A. C., Boersma, G., and Duba, W. C., 1976, Pharmacokinetics of trichloroethylene in volunteers, influence of workload and exposure concentration, *Int. Arch. Occup. Environ. Health* **38:**87-102.

Monster, A. C., Bocrsma, G., and Steenweg, H., 1979, Kinetics of tetrachloroethylene in volunteers; influence of exposure concentration and work load, *Int. Arch. Occup. Environ. Health* **42:**3-4, 303-309.

Morris, J. B., Smith, F., German, R., 1979, Studies on methylene chloride-induced fatty liver, *Exp. Mol. Pathol.* **30:**386-393.

Moskowitz, Ch., Shapiro, E., 1949, Accidental exposure to dichloromethane vapor, *Am. Ind. Hyg. Ass. J.* **13:**116-118.

Moslen, M. T., Reynolds, E. S., and Szabo, S., 1977, Enhancement of the metabolism and hepatoxicity of trichloroethylene and perchloroethylene, *Biochem. Pharmacol.* **26:**369-375.

Müller, G., Spassovski, M., and Henschler, D., 1974, Metabolism of trichloroethylene in man. II. Pharmacokinetics of metabolites, *Arch. Toxikol* **32:**283-295.

Münzer, M., and Heder, K., 1972, Results of industrial-medical and technical examination of chemical purification operations (Germ.), *Zentralbl. Arbeitsmed. Arbeitsschutz* **22**:133–138.

Murray, F. J., Schwetz, B. A., Mc Bride, J. G., and Staples, R. E., 1979, Toxicity of inhaled chloroform in pregnant mice and their offspring, *Toxicol. Appl. Pharmacol.* **50**:515–522.

National Cancer Institute, 1976, *Report on Carcinogenesis Bioassay of Chloroform*, Bethesda, Maryland, Carcinogenesis Program, Division of Cancer Cause and Prevention.

National Cancer Institute, 1977a, *Bioassay of 1,1,1-Trichloroethane for Possible Carcinogenicity* (*Technical report Series No. 3.*), DHEW Publication No. (NIH) 77803, Washington D.C., U.S. Department of Health, Education, and Welfare.

National Cancer Institure, 1977b, *Bioassay of Tetrachloroethylene for Possible Carcinogenicity* (*Technical Report Series No. 13*) DHEW Publication No. (NIH)77-813, Washington D.C., U.S. Department of Health, Education, and Welfare.

National Cancer Institute, 1978, Bioassay of *1,2-Dichloroethane for Possible Carcinogenicity* (*Technical Report Series No. 55*), DHEW Publication No. (NIH) 78-1361, Washington, D.C., U.S. Department of Health, Education, and Welfare.

National Institute for Occupational Safety and Health, 1976a, *Criteria for a recommended Standard. Occupational Exposure to Methylene Chloride*, HEW Publication No. (NIOSH) 76-138, Washington D.C., U.S. Government Printing Office.

National Institute for Occupational Safety and Health, 1976b, *Criteria for a Recommended Standard. Occupational Exposure to Ethylene Dichloride (1,2-Dichloroethane)*, DHEW Publication No. (NIOSH) 76-139, Washington D.C., U.S. Government Printing Office.

National Institute for Occupational Safety and Health, 1976c, *Criteria for a Recommended Standard. Occupational Exposure to Tetrachloroethylene (Perchloroethylene)*, DHEW Publication No. (NIOSH) 76-185, Washington D.C., U.S. Department of Health, Education, and Welfare.

National Institute for Occupational Safety and Health, 1976d, Criteria document: recommendations for a carbon tetrachloride standard, *Occup. Saf. Health Rep.* **5**:1247–1253.

National Institute for Occupational Safety and Health, 1977, *National Occupational Hazard Survey*, Vol. III, *Survey Analyses and Supplemental Tables*, Cincinnati, OH, U.S. Department of Health, Education, and Welfare, pp 2864–2866.

New, P. S., Lubash, G. D., Scherr, L., and Rubin, A. L., 1962, Acute renal failure associated with carbon tetrachloride intoxication, *J. Am. Med. Assoc.* **181**:903–906.

Nomiyama, K., and Nomiyama, H., 1971, Metabolism of trichloroethylene in humans. Sex difference in urinary excretion of trichloroacetic acid and trichloroethanol, *Int. Arch. Arbeitsmed.* **28**:37–48.

Nomiyama, K, and Nomiyama, H., 1977, Dose-response relationship for trichloroethylene in man, *Int. Arch. Occup. Environ. Health.* **39**:237–248.

Ogata, M., Takatsuka, Y., and Tomokuni, K., 1971, Excretion of organic chlorine compounds in the urine of persons exposed to vapors of trichloroethylene and tetrachloroethylen, *Br. J. Ind. Med.* **28**:386–391.

Page, N. P., and Arthur, J. L., 1978, *Special Occupational Hazard Review of Trichloroethylene*, DHEW (NIOSH) Publication No. 78-130, Rockville MD, U.S. Department of Health, Education, and Welfare.

Palmer, A. K., Street, A. E., Roe, F. J. C., Worden, A. N., and Van Abbé, N. J., 1979, Safety evaluation of toothpaste containing chloroform. II. Long term studies in rats, *J. Environ. Pathol. Toxicol.* **2**:821–833.

Pani, P., Torrielli, M. V., Gabriel, L., and Gravela, E., 1973, Further observation on the effects of 3-methylcholanthrene and phenobarbital on carbon tetrachloride hepatotoxicity, *Exp. Mol. Pathol.* **19**:15–22.

Patel, R., Janakiraman, N., and Towne, W. D., 1977, Pulmonary oedema due to tetrachloroethylene, *Environ. Health Persp.* **21**:247–249.

Paul, B. B., and Rubinstein, D., 1963, Metabolism of carbon tetrachloride and chloroform by the rat, *J. Pharmacol. Exp. Ther.* **141**:141–148.

Paulus, W., 1951, Zur frage der vortanschung eines blutalkohols durch einatmen von tri-und tetrachloräthylen, *Dent. Z. Ges. Gerichl. Med.* **40:**593–602.

Pegg, D. G., Zempel, J. A., Braunn, W. H., and Gehring, P. J., 1979, Disposition of $^{14}$C tetrachloroethylene following oral and inhalation exposure in rats, *Toxicol. Appl. Pharmacol.* **51:**465–474.

Phillips, T. J., and MacDonald, R. R., 1971, Comparative effort of Pethidine, trichloroethylene, and Entonox on fetal and neonatal acid-base and $pO_2$, *Br. Med. J.* **3:**558–560.

Plaa, G. L., Evans, E. A., and Hine, C. H., 1958, Relative hepatotoxicity of seven halogenated hydrocarbons, *J. Pharmacol. Ex. Ther.* **123:**224–229.

Plaa, G. L., and Larson, R. E., 1965, Relative nephrotoxic properties of chlorinated methane, ethane and ethylene derivatives in mice, *Toxicol. Appl. Pharmacol.* **7:**37–44.

Pohl, L. R., Bhooshan, B., and Krishna, G., 1979, Mechanism of the metabolic activation of chloroform, *Toxicol. Appl. Pharmacol.*, cited by Lenz, 1979.

Pound, A. W., 1978, Influence of carbon tetrachloride on induction of tumours of the liver and kidneys in mice by nitrosamines, *Br. J. Cancer.* **37:**67–75.

Powell, J. F., 1945, Trichloroethylene: absorption, elimination, and metabolism, *Br. J. Ind. Med.* **2:**142–145.

Prendergast, J. A., Jones, R. A., Jenkins, L. J., Jr., and Siegel, J., 1976, Effects on experimental animals of long-term inhalation of trichloroethylene, carbon tetrachloride, 1,1,1-trichloroethane, dichlorodifluormethane, and 1,1-dichfloroethylene, *Toxicol. Appl.-Pharmacol.* **10:**270–289.

Price, P., Personal communication in reference (Andrews, 1976).

Rampy, L. W., Quast, J. F., Leong, B. D. J., and Gehring, P. J., 1978, Results of long-term inhalation toxicity studies on rats of 1,1,1-trichloroethane and perchloroethylene formulations, in *Proceedings of the First International Congress on Toxicology* (edited by G. L. Plaa and W. A. M. Duncan) Academic Press, New York.

Rannug, I., and Beije, B., 1979, The mutagenic effect of 1,2-dichloroethane on *Salmonella typhimurium.* II. Activation by the isolated perfused rat liver, *Chem. Biol. Interact.* **24:**265–285.

Rannug, U., Sundvall, A., and Ramel, C., 1978, The mutagenic effect of 1,2-dichloroethane on *Salmonella typhimurium.* I. Activation through conjugation with glutathion *in vitro*, *Chem. Biol. Interact.* **20:**1–16.

Rao, K. S., and Recknagel, R. O., 1969, Early incorporation of carbon-labeled carbon tetrachloride into rat liver particulate lipids and proteins, *Exp. Mol. Pathol.* **10:**219–228.

Rapoport, I. A., 1960, The reaction of genic proteins with 1,2-dichloroethane (Russ.), *Dokl. Akad. Nauk SSR* **134:**1214–1217 (Translation in *Dokl. Biol. Sci.*, 1960, **134:**745–747.)

Ratney, R. S., Wegman, D. H., and Elkins, H. B., 1974, *In vivo* conversion of methylene chloride to carbon monoxide, Massachusetts Div. Occup. Hyg. Boston, Mass. 02116- Arch. Environ. Health. 28/4 (223–226).

Recknager, R. C., 1967, Carbon tetrachloride hepatotoxicity, *Pharmacol. Rev.* **19:**145–208.

Recknagel, R. O., and Litteria, M., 1960, Biochemical changes: tetrachloride fatty liver: concentration of carbontetrachloride in liver and blood, *Am. J. Path.* **36:**521–531.

Reuber, M. D., 1979, Carcinogenicity of chloroform, *Environ. Health Perspect* **31:**171–182.

Reuber, M. D., and Glover, E. L., 1967, Hyperplastic and early neoplastic lesions of the liver in Buffalo strain rats of various ages given subcutaneous carbon tetrachloride, *J. Natl. Cancer Inst.* **38:**891–899.

Reuber, M. D., and Glover, E. L., 1970, Cirrhosis and carcinoma of the liver in male rats given subcutaneous carbon tetrachloride, *J. Natl. Cancer Inst.* **44:**419–427.

Reynolds, E. S., 1967, Liver parenchymal cell injury. IV. Pattern of incorporation of carbon and chlorine from carbon tetrachloride into chemical constituents of liver *in vivo*, *J. Pharmacol. Exp. Ther.* **155:**117–126.

Reynolds, E. S., 1972, Comparison of early injury to liver endoplasmic reticulum by halomethane, hexachloroethane, benzene, toluene, bromobenzene, ethionine, thioacetamide, and dimethylnitrosamine. *Biochem. Pharmacol.* **21**:2555-2561.

Riley, E. C., Fasset, D. W., and Sutton, W. L., 1966, Methylene chloride vapor in expired air of human subjects, *Ann. Ind. Hyg. Assoc.* **27**:341-348.

Rocchi, P., Prodi, G., Grilli, S., and Ferreri, A. M., 1973, *In vivo* and *in vitro* binding of carbon tetrachloride with nucleic acids and proteins in rat and mouse liver, *Int. J. Cancer.* **11**:419-425.

Rodkey, F. L., Collison, H. A., 1977a, Biological oxidation of $^{14}C$ Methylene chloride to carbon monoxide and carbon dioxide by the rat, *Toxicol. Appl. Pharmacol.* **40**:33-38.

Rodkey, F. L., Collison, H. A., 1977b, Effect of dihalogenated methanes on the *in vivo* production of carbon monoxide and methane by rats, *Toxicol. Appl. Pharmacol* **40**: 39-47.

Roe, F. J. C., Palmer, A. K., Worden, A. N., and Van Abbe, N. J., 1979, Safety evaluation of toothpaste containing chloroform. I. Long term studies in mice, *J. Environ. Pathol. Toxicol.* **2**:799-819.

Roschlau, G., and Rodenkirchen, H., 1969, Histological examination of the diaplacental action of carbon tetrachloride and allyl alcohol in mice embryos (Germ.), *Exp. Path.* **3**:255-263.

Rosenkranz, M. S., 1977, Mutagenicity of halogenated alkanes and their derivatives, *Env. Health Perspect.* **21**:79-84.

Rowe, V. K., McCollister, D. D., Spencer, H. C., Adams, E. M., and Irish, D. D., 1952, Vapor toxicity of tetrachloroethylene for laboratory animals and human subjects, *AMA Arch. Ind. Hyg. occup. Med.* **5**:566-579.

Sahu, S., Lowther, D., and Ulsamer, A., 1980, Biochemical studies on pulmonary response to inhalation of methylene chloride, *Toxicology Letters.* **7**:41-45.

Salvini, M., Binaschi, S., and Riva, M., 1971, Evaluation of the psychophysiological functions in humans exposed to the threshold limit value of 1,1,1-trichloroethane, *Br J. Ind. Med.* **28**:286-291.

Sato, A., and Nakajima, T., 1978, Difference following skin or inhalation exposure in the absorption and excretion kinetics of trichloroethylene and toluene, *Br. J. Ind. Med.* **35**:43-49.

Scholler, K. L., 1970, Modification of the effects of chloroform on the rat liver, *Br. J. Anaesth.* **42**:603-605.

Schumann, A. M., Quast, J. F., and Watanabe, P. G., 1980, The pharmacokinetics and macromolecular interactions of perchloroethylene in mice and rats as related to oncogenicity, *Toxicol Appl. Pharmacol.* **55**:207-219.

Schwetz, B. A., Leong, B. K. J., and Gehring, P. J., 1974, Embryo- and fetotoxicity of inhaled tetrachloride, 1,1-dichloroethane and methyl ethyl ketone in rats, *Toxicol. Appl. Pharmacol.* **28**:452-464.

Schwetz, B. A., Leong, B. K. J., and Gehring, P. J., 1975, The effect of maternally inhaled trichloroethylene, perchloroethylene, methyl chloroform, and methylene chloride on embryonal and fetal development in mice and rats, *Toxicol. Appl. Pharmacol.* **32**:84-96.

Seki, Y., Urashima, Y., Aikawa, H., Ichikawa, Y., Hiratsuka, F., Yoshioka, Y., Shimbo, S., and Ikeda, M., 1975, Trichloro-compounds in the urine of humans exposed to methyl chloroform at subthreshold levels, *Int. Arch. Arbeitsmed.* **34**:39-49.

Sellers, E. M., Lang, M., Koch-Wesser, J., Le Blanc, E., and Kalant, H., 1972, Interaction of chloral hydrate and ethanol in man. I. Metabolism, *Clin. Pharmacol. Ther.* **13**:37-49.

Shahin, M. M., and Von Bortsel, R. C., 1977, Mutagenic and lethal effects of -benzene hexachloride, dibutyl phthalate and trichloroethylene in *Saccharomyces cerevisia. Mutat. Res.* **48**:173-180.

Shakarnis, V. F., 1969, 1,2-Dichloroethane induced chromosome nondisjunction and recessive sex-linked lethal mutation in *Drosophila melanogaster* (Russian), *Genetika* **5**:89-95.

Shakarnis, V. F., 1970, Effect of 1,2-dichloroethane on chromosome nondisjunction and recessive sex-linked lethals in a radio-resistant strain of *Drosophila melanogaster* (Russian), *Vestn. Leningr. Univ., Biol.* **25:**153–156.

Shubik, P., Hartwell, J. L., 1957, Survey of compounds which have been tested for carcinogenic activity, Washington, D.C., Government Printing Office, Public Health Service Publication No. 149. Supplement 1.

Shubik, P., Hartwell, J. L., 1969, Survey of compounds which have been tested for carcinogenic activity, Washington, D.C., Government Printing Office, Public Health Service Publication No. 149, Supplement 2.

Simmon, V. F., Kauhanen, K., and Tardiff, R. G., 1977, Mutagenic activity of chemicals identified in drinking water, in *Progress in Genetic Toxicology,* (edited by Scott, D., Bridges, B. A., and Sobels, F. H.) Amsterdam, Elsevier/North Holland, pp. 249–258.

Singh, B. H., Lillian, D., Appleby, A., and Lobban, L., 1975, Atmospheric formation of carbon tetrachloride from tetrachloroethylene, *Environ. Lett.* **10:**253–256.

Smith, A. A., Volpitto, P. P., Gramling, Z. W., Devore, M. B., and Glassman, A. B., 1973, Chloroform halothane and regional anesthesia: a comparative study, *Anesth. Analg.* (*Cleveland*) **52:**1–11.

Smuckler, E. A., Iseri, O. A., Benditt, E. P., 1962, An intracellular defect in protein synthesis induced by carbon tetrachloride, *J. Exp. Med.* **116:**55–71.

Soucek, B., and Vlachova, D., 1960, Excretion of trichloroethylene metabolites in human urine, *Br. J. Ind. Med.* **17:**60–64.

Stern, P. H., Furukawa, T., Brody, T. M., 1965, Rat liver and plasma lipids after carbon tetrachloride administration, *J. Lipid Res.* **6:**278–286.

Stevens, W. C., White, A. E., Takahisa, S., Eger, E. I., II, and Wolff, S., 1977, Sisterchromatid exchanges induced by inhalated anesthetics, in *American Society of Anesthesiologists Abstracts of Scientific Papers*, pp. 495–497.

Stewart, R. D., 1968, The toxicology of 1,1,1-trichloroethane, *Ann. Occup. Hyg.* **11:**71–79.

Stewart, R. D., 1969, Acute tetrachloroethylene intoxication, *J. Am. Med. Assoc.* **208:**1490–1492.

Stewart, R. D., and Andrews, J. T., 1966, Acute intoxication with methyl chloroform, *J. Am. Med. Assoc.* **195:**904–908.

Stewart, R. D., and Dodd, H. C., 1964, Absorption of carbon tetrachloride trichloroethylene, tetrachloroethylene, methylene chloride, and 1,1,1-trichloroethane through the human skin, *Am. Ind. Hyg. Assoc. J.* **25:**439–446.

Stewart, R. D., and Hake, C. L., 1976, Paint-remover hazard, *J. Am. Med. Assoc.* **235:**398–401.

Stewart, R. D., Baretta, E. D., Dodd, H. C., and Torkelson, T. R., 1970b, Experimental human exposure to tetrachloroethylene, *Arch. Environ. Health* **20:**224–229.

Stewart, R. D., Dodd, H. C., Gay, H. H., and Erley, D. S., 1970a, Experimental human exposure to trichloroethylene, *Arch. Environ. Health* **20:**64–71.

Stewart, R. D., Fisher, T. N., Hosko, M. J., Peterson, J. E., Baretta, E. D., and Dodd, H. C., 1972, Carboxyhemoglobin elevation after exposure to dichloromethane, *Science* **176:**295–296.

Stewart, R. D., Gay, H. H., Erley, D. S., Hake, C. L., and Schaffer, A. W., 1961a, Human exposure to 1,1,1-trichloroethane vapor, relationship of expired air and blood concentrations to exposure and toxicity, *Am. Ind. Hyg. Assoc. J.* **22:**252–262.

Stewart, R. D., Gay, H. H., Erley, D. S., Hake, C. L., and Schafer, A. W., 1961b, Human exposure to tetrachloroethylene vapor. Relationship of expired air and blood concentrations to exposure and toxicity, *Arch. Environ. Health* **2:**516–522.

Stewart, R. D., Gayd, H. H., Schaffer, A. W., Erley, D. S., and Rowe, V. K., 1969, Experimental human exposure to methyl chloroform vapor, *Arch. Environ. Health* **19:**467.

Stewart, R. D., Hake, C. L., and Peterson, J. E., 1974, "Degreaser's flush." Dermal response to trichloroethylene and ethanol, *Arch. Environ. Health* **29:**1–5.

Strobel, G. E., and Wollman, H., 1969, Pharmacology of anesthetic agents, *Fed. Proc.*, **28**:1386–1403.

Sturrock, J., 1977, Lack of mutagenic effect of halothane or chloroform on cultured cells using the azaguanine test system, *Br. J. Anaesth.* **49**:207–210.

Symons, J. M., Bellar, T. A., Carswell, J. K., Demarco, J., Kropp, K. L., Robeck, G. G., Seeger, D. R., Slocum, C. J., Smith, B. L., and Stevens, A. A., 1975, National organics reconnaissance survey for halogenated organics, *J. Am. Water Works Assoc.* **67**:634–647.

Tada, O., Nakaaki, K., and Fukabori, S., 1968, On the methods of determinations of chlorinated hydrocarbons in the air and their metabolisms in the urine, *Rodo Kagaku* **44**:500–504.

Taylor, D. C., Brown, D. M., Keeble, R., and Langley, P. F., 1974, Metabolism of chloroform. II. A sex difference in the metabolism of $^{14}$C chloroform in mice, *Xenobiotica* **4**:165–174.

Theiss, J. C., Stoner, G. D., Shimkin, M. B., and Weisburger, E. K., 1977, Test for carcinogenicity of organic contaminants of United States drinking waters by pulmonary tumor response in strain A mice, *Cancer Res.* **37**:2717–2720.

Thierstein, S. T., Hanigan, J. J., Paul, M. D., and Stuck, P. L., 1960, Trichloroethylene anesthesian obstetrics: report of 10,000 cases, with fatal mortality and electrocardiographic data, *Obstet. Gynecol.* **15**:560–565.

Thompson, D. J., Warner, S. D., and Robinson, V. B., 1974, Teratology studies on orally adminstered chloroform in the rat and rabbit, *Toxicol. Appl. Pharmacol.* **29**:348–357.

Tola, S., Vilhunen, R., Järvinen, E., and Korkala, M. L., 1980, A cohort study on workers exposed to trichloroethylene, *J. Occ. Med.* **22**:117–124.

Torkelson, T. R., Oyen, F., McCollister, D. D., and Rowe, V. K., 1958, Toxicity of 1,1,1-trichloroethane as determined on laboratory animals and human subjects, *Am. Ind. Hyg. Assoc. J.* **19**:353–362.

Torkelston, T. R., Oyen, F., and Rowe, V. K., 1976, The toxicity of chloroform as determined by single and repeated exposure of laboratory animals, *Am. Ind. Hyg. Assoc. J.* **37**:697–705.

Tracey, J. P., and Sherlock, P., 1968, Hepatoma following carbon tetrachloride poisoning, *N. Y. State J. Med.* **68**:2202–2204.

Travers, H., 1974, Death from 1,1,1-trichloroethane abuse: case report, *Mil. Med.* **139**:889.

Tsirel'nikov, N. I., and Tsirel'nikova, T. G., 1976, Morphohistochemical study of the rat placenta after exposure to carbon tetrachloride at different stages of pregnancy, *Byull. Eksp. Biol. Med.* **82**:1007–1009.

Tsirel'nikov, N. I., and Tsirel'nikova, T. G., 1977, Morphohistochemical study of the rat placenta after exposure to carbon tetrachloride at different stages of pregnancy, *U.S.S—Bull. Exp. Biol. Med.* **82/8**:1262–1265.

Tsuruta, H., 1975, Percutaneous absorption of organic solvents. I. Comparative study of the *in vivo* percutaneous absorption of chlorinated solvents in mice, *Ind. Health* **13**:227–236.

Tuttle, T. C., Wood, G. D., and Grether, C. B., Johnson, B. L., and Xintaras, C., 1977, *A Behavioral and Neurological Evaluation of Dry-Cleaners Exposed to Perchloroethyle*, DHEW (NIOSH) Publication No. 77-124, Cincinnati, OH, National Institute for Occupational Safety and Health.

Uehleke, H., Tabarelli-Poplawski, S., Bonse, G., and Henschler, D., 1982, Spectral evidence for 2,2,3-trichlor-oxirane formation during microsomal trichloroethylene oxidation, *Arch. Toxikol.* **37**:95–105.

Uehleke, H., and Poplawski–Tabarelli, S., 1977, Irreversible binding of $^{14}$C labelled trichloroethylene to mice liver constituents *in vivo* and *in vitro*, *Arch. Toxikol.* **37**:289–294.

Uehleke, H., Greim, H. Krämer, M., and Werner, T., 1976, Covalent binding of haloalkanes to liver constituents, but absence of mutagenicity on bacteria in a metabolizing test system (Abstract No. 25), *Mutat. Res.* **38**:114.

Uehleke, H., Werner, T., Greim, H., and Krämer, M., 1977, Metabolic activation of haloalkanes and tests *in vitro* for mutagenicity. *Xenobiotica* **7**:393–400.

Ugazio, G., Burdino, E., Danni, I., and Milillo, P. A., 1973, Hepatotoxicity and lethality of halogenoalkanes, *Biochem—Soc. Trans.* **1**:968–972.

Vallaud, A., Raymond, V., and Salmon, P., 1957, Les solvents chlorés et l'Hygiène industrielle, *Inst. Natl. Securité (Paris)* (cited by Lob.)

Van Duuren, B. L., and Banerjee, S., 1976, Covalent interaction of metabolites of the carcinogen trichloroethylene in rat hepatic microsomes, *Cancer Res.* **36**:2419–2422.

Van Dijke, R. A., 1966, Metabolism of volatile anesthetics. 3. Induction of microsomal dechlorinating and ethercleaving enzymes, *J. Pharmacol. Exp. Ther.* **154**:364–369.

Van Dijcke, R. A., 1965, Metabolism of volatile anesthetics, *In vitro* metabolism of methoxyflurane and holothane in rat liver slices and cell functions, *Biochem. Pharmacol.* **14**:603–609.

Van Dyke, R. A., and Wineman, C. G., 1971, Enzymatic dechlorination. Dechlorination of chloroethanes and propanes *in vitro*, *Biochem. Pharmacol.* **20**:463–470.

Von Oettingen, W. F., 1964, *The Halogenated Hydrocarbons of Industrial and Toxicological Importance*, New York, Elsevier, pp. 77–81, 95–101.

Von Oettigen, W. F., 1964b, *The Halogenated Hydrocarbons of Industrial and Toxicological Importance*, Amsterdam, Elsevier, pp. 107–170.

Von Oettingen, W. F., 1964c, *The Halogenated Hydrocarbons of Industrial and Toxicology Importance*, Amsterdam, Elsevier, pp. 271–283.

Waskell, L., 1978, A study of the mutagenicity of anesthetics and their metabolites, *Mutat. Res.* **57**:41–45.

Waters, E. M., Gerstner, H. B., and Huff, J. E., 1977, Trichloroethylene. 1. An overview, *J. Toxicol. Environ. Health* **2**:671–707.

Watrous, R. M., 1974, Health hazards of the pharmaceutical industry, *Br. J. Ind. Med.* **4**:111–125.

Weisburger, E. K., 1977, Carcinogenicity studies on halogenated hydrocarbons, *Environ. Health Perspect.* **21**:7–16.

White, A. E., Takehisa, S. Eger, E. I., Wolff, S., and Stevens, W. C., 1979, Sister chromatid exchanges by inhaled anaesthetics, *Anesthesiology* **50**:426–430.

Winslow, S. G., and Gerstner, H. B., 1977, *Health Aspects of Chloroform—A Review and An Abstracted Literature Collection 1907 to 1977*, ORNL/TIRC 77/4, Oak Ridge, Tennessee, Oak Ridge National Laboratory.

Yllner, S., 1961, Urinary metabolites of $^{14}$C-tetrachloroethylene in mice, *Nature (London)* **191**:820–822.

Yllner, S., 1971, Metabolism of 1,2-dichloroethane-$^{14}$C in the mouse, *Acta Pharmacol. Toxicol.* **30**:257–265.

Yokoro, K., Takizawa, S., Kawamura, Y., Nakano, M., and Kawase, A., 1973, Multicarcinogenicity of N-nitrosobutylurea in mice and rats as demonstrated by host conditioning, *Gann* **64**:193–196.

Zadorozhnyi, B. V., 1973, Changes in animals due to long-term inhalation exposure to trichloroethylene in low concentrations, *Gig. Truda Prof. Zabol.* **5**:55–57.

Zeitlin, B. R., 1966, Embryotoxic effects of trichloroethylene. Report submitted to W.H.O. by The General Food Corporation.

# Conclusions

## A. Lafontaine

Industrial development, technological progress, and chemical innovation have deeply modified our existence. A better quality of life has been achieved through higher therapeutic capabilities, increased food production, and more comfort in our domestic environment.

This technological advancement, however, has brought with it a number of new environmental problems. The steadily increasing number of chemicals being used extensively (about one thousand every year) call for a systematic evaluation of the potential risks for man, his resources, and his environment. Though the acute and subacute toxicity of those substances is generally known, many of their other biological activities have not been sufficiently investigated with respect to their mutagenic, teratogenic, and carcinogenic effects. Too often these problems have been ignored in the past, and we are now confronted with the long-term effects on man and his progeny, and on animal and plant resources which had not been envisaged or were not predictable.

Some chemicals or their by-products that have been used for years all over the world have now been proved teratogenic to the embryo, mutagenic to the species, or carcinogenic to the individual. Correlations between those three effects have been demonstrated, and it has been necessary to make use of similarities between the three mechanisms of aggression at the cellular level in order to develop easily applicable tests which confirm epidemiological observations and have a predictive value for new substances.

In any case, the influence of cancer, teratogenesis, and all other effects on the genetic patrimony of the germ cells or of the somatic cells must be considered. Currently, we must conceive of a judicious combination of the available means of investigation, which include gathering epidemiological

**A. Lafontaine** • Director of the Institute for Hygiene and Epidemiology, Brussels, Belgium.

data, determining mutagenic, teratogenic, and carcinogenic effects on animals, and assessing the results of short-term mutagenic tests. An appropriate combination of these methods must be able to predict and evaluate the risk for man or mankind.

We are convinced that using existing technology, it should be possible to attain the following objectives:

1. To identify and classify the mutagenic, teratogenic, and carcinogenic substances to which man is exposed by different routes and pathways.
2. To test new chemicals before use, commercialization, or dispersion in the environment.
3. To reduce the exposure of workers and of the public to a minimum.
4. To continue research for better tests to evaluate chemicals already in use and their by-products, and to predict the risks related to new chemicals.

Although many of these objectives are currently not being met, industrialists, governmental authorities, and researchers should be impressed with the dangers of following a *laissez-faire* policy regarding chemical mutagenis in the environment.

The problem of mutagens in the environment has been recognized for more than two centuries. In 1775, Sir Percival Pott attributed scrotum cancer observed among chimney sweeps to the action of soot. Research in the field of environmental mutagens has progressed very slowly, but during recent decades, the number of observations and epidemiological studies has been increasing. These studies made it possible to emphasize the growing frequency of certain types of cancer among those who manipulate or are exposed to certain chemical substances. In addition, experiments have been carried out on several animal species, using substances suspected to have a carcinogenic effect on man.

According to Boyland (1967), 90% of human cancers are chemically induced. This opinion was supported one year later by the IARC which stated: "Thanks to the epidemiologists' conclusions, it is now possible to estimate that 60 to 90% of human cancers are linked with environmental factors."

Five possible effects of environmental agents which may have genetic consequences can be summarized as follows:

1. Breakage of DNA chains, which can lead to cellular death, chromosomal aberrations, recombinations, gene conversions, and mutations.
2. Modification of DNA bases, which can have the same genetic consequences as breakage of DNA chains, but which have quantitatively different effects according to the nature of the alterogen. For example, the ratio of mutation to cellular death will be proportionally

higher for an alterogen affecting bases than for an alterogen affecting DNA strands.

3. Damage caused to centromeres, centrioles, DNA strands, or tubules which can result in the nondisjunction of chromosomes and consequently in polyploidy.
4. Inhibitory effects on cellular multiplication, which impair cellular repair mechanisms.
5. Alteration of repair enzymes and DNA polymerases, which may increase or decrease the damage resulting from spontaneous lesions.

The role of industrial substances as mutagenic, teratogenic, and carcinogenic agents has been extensively debated. In a report of the NIOSH, Bridport predicts that in the U.S.A., the proportion of cancers of occupational origin will grow from 1 to 5% at the present time to a frequency of 25 to 38%. Even if this prediction is not entirely correct, it does draw attention to the necessity of developing research in this field, as well as preventive measures to control the risk of exposure.

While laboratory screening procedures may never become totally reliable and should be supplemented whenever possible with epidemiological data, they are nevertheless useful because they can indicate where preventative and remedial actions are warranted. For this reason, various efforts have been made to develop experimental methods aimed at identification of commercial chemicals which may be potential carcinogens. The best method still remains the classical one, and consists of injecting different doses of a product into laboratory animals over a defined period. In order for the test to be valid, the level of exposure must be of the same degree of magnitude as that to which man can be exposed.

Such investigations are expensive and require a long period of testing. Moreover, it has been impossible to make systematic studies because the technical means up to now have been inadequate. The statistical interpretation of the results can also fail due to methodological restrictions. This problem serves to emphasize the importance of efforts made to detect mutagenic and carcinogenic substances more quickly by multiplying the experiments. Among the various rapid tests, it seems unlikely that rapid induction tests aimed at reducing the latency period can be employed because of difficulties with transplantations, use of new-born animals, etc. We will have to take other rapid predictive tests more into consideration.

This book is largely dedicated to those tests which do not necessarily rely on the development of tumors, but rely rather on induction of predictive modifications in the cell of a potential mutagenic, teratogenic, or carcinogenic nature.

Mutagenesis is only one of a number of harmful environmental effects which are currently being evaluated. Others, such as toxicity, are also being evaluated, and the methods of assessment and monitoring are frequently similar. Efficiency in testing procedures could be increased by appropriate coordination of effort and the joint use of risk data including the files of personal health and family reproductive histories.

The thalidomide incident has alerted people to the possible teratogenic effects of drugs and other chemical constituents of our changing environment. Carcinogenic agents encountered in our environment at work, at home, and elsewhere, and even occasionally unwittingly associated with medical diagnostic and therapeutic measures, are a continuing cause of concern. Geneticists and epidemiologists will, in the future, be as concerned about possible adverse effects of selective pressures, influenced by circumstances prevailing in advanced societies, as they now are about mutagenesis.

Records of clinically encountered congenital anomalies, cancers and teratogenic effects will, in the future, be that sort of data resource that epidemiologists should use to evaluate the predictable or unpredictable risks of chemicals in the environment and their specific or combined actions.

The important categories of tests which are discussed in this volume can be summarized as follows:

1. The search for chromosome and chromatid anomalies *in vivo* in treated animals.
2. The induction of chromosome and chromatid anomalies in the cells cultivated *in vitro*.
3. Investigation of the ability of substances or their metabolites to chemically modify DNA bases.
4. The induction of the DNA synthesis (repair) following the administration of a substance *in vitro* or *in vivo* in cell cultures.
5. The study of some biological reactions observed during the stage of initiation and development of tumors.

Thanks to rapid tests of mutagenesis, it is now possible to detect substances liable to alter DNA, and as a consequence, induce mutations. Many studies have shown the close, but not absolute correlation existing between mutagenic and carcinogenic capacity.

Among the various test systems, we have given special consideration to the following:

(a) Tests employing dominant lethal mutations, a genetic state which kills the individual carrying it at the heterozygotic state.
(b) Tests *in vivo* using bacterial indicators injected in the peritoneal cavity of treated animals, and tests which employ insects (*drosophila*).

(c) Tests *in vitro* on viral, bacterial, fungal, and plant-indicators which include, in principle, a system of enzymatic activation. Among these tests, the best known is the Ames test, which is based on the induction of mutants among the strains of *Salmonella typhimurium*.

(d) Tests *in vitro* on mammalian cells in which the resistance of cells against some drugs is investigated.

These tests are not totally reliable, and can yield false positive or false negative results. It is therefore advisable to carry out a battery of tests covering the various types of expression of the carcinogenetic activity.

These tests are only useful in detecting primary carcinogens, that is, those which are capable of changing the DNA structure directly or indirectly after metabolic activation. The tests are not capable of detecting those substances which are not necessarily carcinogenic themselves, but which, when given to cells exhibiting pre-existing DNA damage from other agents, are able to induce those cells to become transformed. However, in spite of the limitations of these tests, we believe that they can form the essential basis on which to orient decisions. They are, in addition, useful in evaluating commercial substances as well as assessing the effects of possible contaminants.

We can assume that a negative result from a battery of tests must indicate a favorable presumption regarding the carcinogenicity of a substance, as well as a favorable provisional decision for limited applications. These tests must be followed up by long-term tests if the product is meant for extensive use.

If a test gives a positive result, the substance must be considered suspect and it is necessary to wait for the results of long-term tests on two mammalian species before making a decision.

OSHA has listed four conditions, any one of which, if satisfied, is sufficient for a substance to be regarded as carcinogenic or potentially carcinogenic in man:

1. The substance has already been proven carcinogenic to man;
2. The substance has been demonstrated to be carcinogenic to two mammalian species;
3. The substance is carcinogenic in one single mammalian species, but positive results have been obtained in two different experiments;
4. The substance is carcinogenic in one single mammalian species, but it gives positive results in one rapid test. This volume is primarily concerned with this last condition.

The first chapter of the book is devoted to the problems of maintaining genetic stability and the mechanisms which maintain or alter it at the cellular level. This chapter also deals with the biochemistry of the damage caused to DNA, the biochemistry of mutagenesis and teratogenesis, and the relationships between mutations, repair, and carcinogenesis, as well as the relationships between chromosome aberrations and carcinogenesis.

The other four chapters are devoted to the mutagenicity, carcinogenicity, and teratogenicity of four groups of substances: heavy metals, insecticides, monomers of plastics, and chlorinated hydrocarbutized solvents. Among the different kinds of metals, the effects of lead, cadmium and arsenic have been analysed. Among the pesticides, the effects of carbonates and their phosphorylated derivatives have been examined.

Vinyl chloride, styrene, butadiene, acrylonitrile, vinylidene chloride, and chlorobutanedienes are monomers that deserve further attention and warrant the exercise of due caution. Finally, among the chlorinated hydrocarbons, the seven substances which have been studied are: methylene chloride, chloroform, carbon tetrachloride, 1,2-dichloroethane, trichloroethylene, tetrachloethylene, and 1,1,1-trichloroethane. In each case, the uses and the quantities commercially produced have been considered as well as the metabolic data.

We also hope that the data contained in this edition will be helpful in explaining epidemiological data concerning man and his environment. Mutagenic factors from a variety of origins and in various combinations may be present and interact with each other and also with metabolic products in humans, animals, and plants, which may enhance or control the action of mutagens.

Epidemiological monitoring of human beings, combined with the monitoring of biological indicators in the human environment, are the necessary complement of experimental testing, just as long-term assays with experimental animals are the necessary complement of predictive tests applied to industrial pollutants.

Short-term tests have undoubtedly contributed to the greatest progress in environmental mutagenesis. They have earned a dominant place in genetic toxicology and will keep this place in the years ahead, thanks to appropriate modifications of the techniques which take DNA repair pathways into account. However, compilations of epidemiological data need to be prepared in order to supplement the information contained in this book. This task will eventually help us to reach the stage where we may be able to assess realistically mutagenic, teratogenic, and carcinogenic risks for man.

# Index